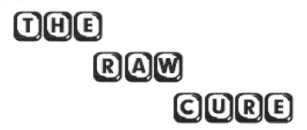

THE RAW CURE

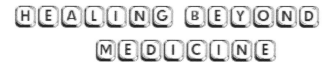

HEALING BEYOND MEDICINE

How self-empowerment, a raw vegan diet, and change of lifestyle can free us from sickness and disease.

JESSE J. JACOBY ©2012

SOULSPIRE PUBLISHING

FORT BRAGG, CA

Soulspire Publishing
Fort Bragg, CA, 95437

ISBN: 978-0-9885920-0-1
Library of Congress Control Number: 2012921011
Dewey CIP: 641.563   **OCLC:** 213839254

Cover art, font, and layout are all original art by Jalen Jacoby.
The book has been edited by Kylene Gott.

Wholesalers to book trade: Nelson's Books and Ingram
Available through Amazon.com, BarnesAndNoble.com

DISCLAIMER

I am not a medical doctor. I chose not to go that route. I believe synthetic medicine is one of the most unnecessary poisons created. It is not possible to cure anything with the use of drugs, medicine, or medical treatment. These options will only treat symptoms of disease. The creation of, and dependence on, synthetic medicine and the money-making machine that it is, has caused disease and the sickness industry to grow uncontrolled. The rate of deaths due to the negative effects of these drugs is skyrocketing. The Food and Drug Administration (FDA) reported 82,724 total deaths in the year 2010 from adverse effects of prescription drugs alone. Additionally, the *Journal of the American Medical Association* has documented a staggering 700,000 emergency room visits annually from adverse drug events.

In the United States, any natural cure for cancer has not been accepted. Cancer patients are instead forced to undergo chemotherapy. Medical doctors who steer their clients away from chemotherapy and warn about the dangers associated with chemo are often stripped of their medical license. A perfect example would be Dr. Tullio Simoncini, an Italian-born physician who cures cancer using an alternative method. Dr. Simoncini had his medical license revoked because other physicians, drug companies, and academic societies that could not eradicate cancer using harmful radiation and chemotherapy were suffering enormous cuts in their profits as a result of his protocol for curing cancer. This is pretty scary when you consider that the Centers for Disease Control and Prevention reported 568,668 deaths from cancer in the year 2009. Many of the processes to alleviate disease are not being revealed to us. With that being said, I must inform you that very little of what I mention in the following pages has been approved or supported by the American Medical Association or the FDA. Nothing I have included as *remedies* or *cures* for any type of disease is meant to replace a prescription from a medical doctor. I am simply relaying alternatives to poisoning your body with poor food choices, synthetic drugs, and dangerous procedures. I have formulated these alternatives from my experience as a raw nutritionist, my research of medical studies, and studying the natural healing processes of the body.

My intention with this book is to educate you on how you can bypass prescription drugs, reach an optimal level of health through a natural, plant-based diet, and refrain from contributing money to the medical industry. I am not claiming to have a cure for any disease, I am suggesting that a change in diet and a change in lifestyle could strengthen the natural defense mechanisms in your body to the point where your body will heal itself. Therefore, the author is not liable for any decisions you make after reading this book. If you feel like you are sick to the point where you must see a doctor, by all means go see one. I suggest however that you see a Naturopathic Doctor who can guide you through an all natural healing process.

TABLE OF CONTENTS

DEDICATION

This book is dedicated to my brother Darin who was a victim of the negligence, human experimentation, and ignorance of the psychotropic drug industry, pharmaceutical industry, and the court system from the age of twelve until his death at the age of twenty-two.

Darin was administered psychotropic drugs in junior high school and was eventually court-ordered into taking them. Because of this heinous government intrusion, he was left to battle with pharmaceutical poisoning from childhood until his death eleven years later. He always felt better without the drugs, but when he refused to take them, he was either hospitalized or they would put him in a straight-jacket and force feed him drugs to sedate him as part of their wicked experimentations.

As an angel of truth, Darin was the most peaceful spirit I have ever known. He was courageous all the way until his moment of death where he held his arms wide open and took on the power of a passenger train going at full speed. For someone to be in that much pain and that much suffering to end his life in that way says a lot about his reality. In the end, he was defeated. He did all he could to fight his way out, but unfortunately the crooked laws in this society protect the medical and pharmaceutical industries to preserve their profits and allow for these tragic events to occur.

In tribute to Darin's life, I have dedicated my life to finding ways to end the greed inspired plots of the medical elite and change the ways of the world. All over the world, millions of people are being misdiagnosed and dying from the negative effects of medicine.

I saw the light and I was not "dumbed-down" or brain-washed by the doctors. At the same time they prescribed him these drugs, they also tried convincing me that I needed them. I refused, and devoted my existence to helping in any way I can to shut down this cycle of abuse and make sure nobody else has to suffer the way my brother suffered - or my family has suffered from his misfortunes.

Thank you Darin for sharing your strength, your courage, and your love with me and the rest of the world.

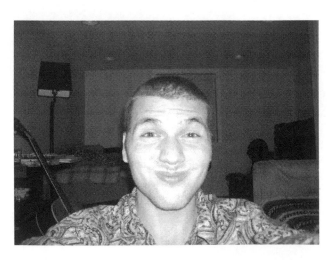

James Darin Jacoby

(1984-2007)

ACKNOWLEDGEMENTS

My life has been a rollercoaster of ups and downs. On my journey, I have encountered some truly amazing people. I have been blessed with good health, a brilliant mind, a longing and desire to seek the truth, great athletic ability, a deep connection with nature, and a joy for living. For this I have to thank my higher power who guides me each day and instructs me through every lesson of life.

I was given the gift of a loving family and raised with encouragement. This helped me to build confidence, and for all of this I have to start by thanking my parents.

My Father, who labored each day in the hot sun and through cold winters while my mother was finishing her degree, made sure we had food to eat, and provided a roof over our heads. After a long day of work, he would still come home and prepare fresh meals for us so we could eat food from nature to build strong bodies and minds. He never imposed any of his ways or beliefs on us, but he found ways to express his discontent for things we did, which he did not agree with. Something that many people do not understand is that you cannot tell a child not to do something if you are doing it yourself. He was never an alcohol drinker. When I had my days of drinking at a young age, he always told me that it was terrible stuff and he would point out the people who were drinkers and let me see for myself where they would end up in life. From seeing this, and from his leading by example, I credit him for my abstinence from alcohol and my disapproval I have of alcohol. Thank you, Dad, for instilling these values in me and for always being there for me. My dad also introduced me to the natural healing world by teaching me that processed foods contain toxic chemicals. Because of his influence, I was eating organic even while attending high school.

My Mother spent each day with us throughout childhood and taught us the ways of living. She nurtured us, she read to us, and she even volunteered to be the class mom so she could be involved in our schooling as much as possible. She demonstrated love in the most appreciative way. Because of her I am the person I am today. She was never a cigarette smoker and she was disgusted by cigarettes. When I was ten or eleven years old, she caught me with cigarettes, and to discipline me, she made me write her an essay on the dangers of smoking. Maybe this is what led me to my love for learning, accumulating knowledge, and researching. I never smoked again. Thank you, Mom, for never giving up on me and for always being fair. I have to thank her as well for supporting me through college and for always welcoming me back home whenever I decided I wanted to go a different route in life. She guided me through the college years and always found ways to make any endeavor or opportunity that presented itself to me, possible.

I would also like to thank the rest of my family. My brother Jalen, who is a brilliant young man, is near the top of his class, and very artistic and talented. He designed the cover for this book. My sister, who has always been one of my favorite people in life, and who believes in me always. To all of my other relatives; thank you for your support throughout the years.

I have to thank all of my teachers, mentors, and friends who have guided me and supported me over the years. Especially Kylene Gott, Tamara Jazwinski, Dave Shutters, Frank Ardito, and JC Santana. Thank you Kylene for editing this book as well and for helping me shape it into what it is.

Thank you to all of the pioneers of natural healing and all of my teachers in the raw food world. I have to start by thanking John McCabe who is a wonderful person and went out of his way to motivate me to finish this book and sent me a copy of his book, *Igniting Your Life*, at just the right time to kick-start my motivation. If you need a good book to motivate you, his is the one you want. Thank you John, for not only going out of your way to help me, but for helping the thousands of others you have reached out to. Without his motivation, this book would not be what it is.

I'd like to acknowledge the works of my idols in the natural healing and raw food world. They are: Dr. Michael Greger, Philip Wollen, Dr. Neal Barnard, Dr. Max Gerson, Dr. John McDougall, Dr. Robert Morse, Charlotte Gerson, Karyn Calabrese, Dr. Ross Horne, Dr. Gabriel Cousens, Dr. Ann Wigmore, Dr. Hereward Carrington, Dr. John Tilden, Arnold Ehret, Dr. Linus Pauling, Dr. Aris Latham, Dr. Norman Walker, Dr. Bernard Jensen, Dr. Herbert Shelton, Rhio, Natasha Kyssa, Cherie Soria, Kristina Carrillo-Bucaram, Mimi Kirk, Dr. Douglas Graham, Sapoty Brook, Dr. Matthias Rath, Steve Meyerowitz, Dr. Udo Erasmus, Dr. Fereydoon Batmanghelidj, John Robbins, Dr. Brian Clement, Dr. Andrew Saul, Dr. Paul Bragg, Patricia Bragg, Dr. Russell Blaylock, Dr. T. Colin Campbell, Dr. Caldwell Esselstyn, Patrick Holford, Dara Dubinet, FreeLee, The DurianRider, and I am sure there are many more. It is because of all of these people that my path to natural healing was made possible.

I have to acknowledge all of the animal activists who dedicate their lives to helping end the Animal Holocaust that is taking place. I would like to honor the folks who put together the film, *Earthlings*, and I urge everyone to view this film to witness the truth about the way animals are being treated. I'd especially like to acknowledge Gary Yourofsky, an educator and activist, who is doing wonderful things to enlighten all of us to the devastating truth behind what happens to the animals that are being raised in horrible factory farms and slaughtered for meat.

Thank you to every person who breaks the links on the chain by eliminating all animal products from their diet. By going vegan, you help save Earth. Thank you Philip Wollen for everything you do, and for creating the Kindness Trust. Thank you John Robbins for the EarthSave foundation and for your book, *The Food Revolution*, which has really helped raise awareness to the dire need for us all to shift the way we are eating and be at peace with the animals.

Thank you to all of the organic farmers in the world. You are heroes to our civilization.

Finally, I want to thank all of those negative people who have come and gone from my life, for they have shown me exactly who I do not want to, and never will be.

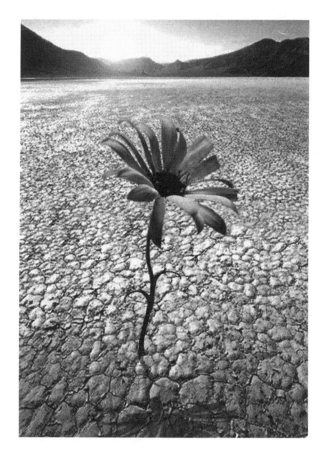

When properly nourished, flowers blossom. Without nutrients, they wither and die. To reach the sunlight, they dance, move, and sway.

GOOD HEALTH IS THE NEW COOL

In society, we have been through all of the different "cools." It has been cool to smoke, cool to drink, cool to eat fast food, cool to drink milk. In school, the coolest kids seemed to have the most processed junk foods packed in their lunches. In college, the "cool" guys went out and partied their lives away — and many of them failed out because of this. Over time, all of these entities we labeled as "cool" turned out to be the exact opposite. They all led to sickness, premature aging, debilitation, and unnatural deaths.

We have not yet advertised good health as being cool. Today, good health is the new cool. To be healthy is the only way to be cool. This is the attitude we all should do our best to abide by:

WE ARE COOL BECAUSE WE ARE HEALTHY!

INTRODUCTION

"Let there be magic in all that you do, it is part of the promise that life made to you." – Mike Dooley

I have spent years of my life diligently researching the work of the best hygienists, natural healers, medical doctors, and raw nutritionists who have ever lived. I cannot count the number of sleepless nights I've encountered while exploring medical studies, reading books, taking notes, writing out my ideas, and embedding the knowledge into my mind. I have dissected nearly two-hundred books in the field of study, and through all of this, I think it is safe to claim that I have discovered my passion. From my work with several hundred consultation clients, who I educated on optimal nutrition, and witnessed heal from degenerative disease, I have become an expert. Although I went through college and spent those years of my life filling my head with everything I needed to learn for my degree, I realized that none of what they taught me is applicable to what I learned on my own through experience and abiding by nature's laws.

As a certified raw nutritionist, nutritionist, lifestyle and weight management consultant, personal trainer, and holistic health coach, I can safely say that I learned far more through my own studying than I did in any educational institution. The world of raw nutrition and raw foods fascinates me more than anything. I never imagined I could open a new book every day and feel surrounded with positive energy, positive people, and creative new ideas, even while being alone. My path to natural healing has granted me this privilege.

On my journey to absorb as much knowledge as possible and reach my optimal level of health, I have enjoyed many of the greatest experiences of my life. Many of these I have been able to generate on my own. Using my mind, imagination, and instinct, I have identified ways to defy science and the dependence on medicine, while abiding by nature's processes, to reach an optimal level of health.

The quest to reach my current level of health consists of many trials and errors. I have experimented on myself by eating an array of foods, mixing up combinations, and also by observing how I feel when adding a little heat to the food I eat. Through all of these encounters, I feel I have discovered the very best way to eat. In this book I share many of my discoveries.

As I continue to eat the foods from Earth and experience the greatest joys possible, I learn the truth about our society and civilization. I have discovered the truth about disease, sickness, and the reasons we are developing heart disease, cancer, diabetes, obesity, and other degenerative diseases. I found that, whenever we purchase processed items from stores, we are eating chemicals rather than foods. I realized that the pharmaceutical industry controls much of our economy and that the reason many of us are sick is because they govern the food industry, medical industry, and parts of the government itself. The fact that the *Food and Drug Administration* clarifies on their website that *they do not review or approve any drug advertisements before they are released, nor do they ban ads for drugs that have serious risks*, should tell us enough in itself.

All over television there are pharmaceutical ads glamorizing the use of prescription drugs. In major cities you find a prevalence of drug stores. *In an August 2007 New England Journal of Medicine article, it was documented that the total spending for all drug-related marketing is at $29.9 billion annually, with around $4.1 billion of that being spent on direct-to-consumer advertising.* When you divide this number, the total comes out to more than $11 million a day. These misleading advertisements, along with all of the profits being made, contribute to us getting sicker by the minute.

My ultimate goal in life is to find a way for a new revolution of people to come together and shift our economy and level of consciousness by developing our own industry similar to the pharmaceutical industry. We will do everything they did to attain the power they have, however we will profit from the well being and good fortunes of our people by spreading good health in the form of education, knowledge, raw foods, organic farming and gardening, and peace between all living creatures. By uniting as a civilization, standing up for our rights, and speaking out against the Animal Holocaust, prescription drugs, chemical additives, fast foods, genetically modified crops, and the laws that keep us sick, we can erase the pharmaceutical, meat, food, dairy, and egg industries' plot to destroy Earth while they lay back, collecting trillions of dollars in profits from our misfortunes, sickness, and premature death.

To help me achieve this goal, and to help you be a part of this revolution, I want to show you how simple it is to adapt a healthy lifestyle. I want you to understand that diseases and conditions such as cancer, emphysema, heart disease, diabetes, atherosclerosis, high cholesterol, and all of the others that we are plagued with as a society are not necessary and largely can be reversed or, at least, greatly reduced. No person should ever have to rely on toxic chemical drugs for much of anything – outside of emergency procedures. Not only is it unrealistic to believe eating pills will protect you from your death, it is not a valid belief. Pills and drugs often make things worse, have serious side effects, and lead you closer to debilitation and death.

In this book, I will properly inform you of what food is. I will educate you on what you are currently eating juxtaposed with what you should be eating. I will guide you through the cycle of disease; how it begins, how to eliminate it, and how to "disease-proof" your body so you will lower your risk of

14

ever being sick again. I will introduce you to a new community of people who are compassionate, loving, and dedicated to making the world a better place. I will awaken you to the truth behind the medical, pharmaceutical, dairy, egg, meat, and mass-marketed food industries. I will present you with evidence that the consumption of animal products is directly linked to a majority of the diseases and conditions that many are suffering from. I will teach you that being sick is not a medical issue and that many of the medical doctors, who are relying on toxic drugs to go along with risky and invasive surgeries, have no idea how to make you better or cure you of what is causing your body to degenerate. This does not mean all doctors cannot help you. If you go to a doctor for any reason, consider doctors like Caldwell Esselstyn and T. Colin Campbell, who are featured in the extraordinary, eye-opening documentary *Forks over Knives.* Put your trust in doctors such as John McDougall, Neal Barnard, Michael Greger, Richard Oppenlander, Jeff Novick, Doug Lisle, Thomas Lodi, Gabriel Cousens, or Robert Morse.

I want to raise awareness to the fact that our current way of living, and the structure of our economy is damaging the health of our children and future generations. The food that is served to our children is often deleterious to their health, and the majority of food products being advertised to target children are leading to the behavioral problems, learning disorders, weight issues, and degenerative diseases – including cancer and diabetes – that are afflicting them. To assure that we end this battle to avoid being sick, and to reach an optimal level of health, we must first educate our youth about the importance of eating real food, and the dangers associated with eating animal products.

These are my views on life. I hope you enjoy and learn from them. After reading this book you should see the world from a different perspective. You will no longer want to eat other living creatures. You will no longer desire food containing synthetic chemicals. You will be more in tune with nature. Life will feel brand new. You will look better, feel better, and live more efficiently.

Please enjoy the journey, prepare to improve your life from every angle, and remember, our children, and a healthy environment, are our future.

There are two types of people in this world:

There are those who win, and those who spend their lives not understanding the concept of winning. Some of us see the big picture and we go places in life, while others lay around in the small frame watching others do great things, wondering why they could never get where those others fought to be.

To win in life, you do not always need to be victorious over opponents, or win the race to acquire the most stuff. Winning is about finding that very thing you are passionate about, winning is about finding your life's purpose, eating the best foods nature has to offer, having compassion for all living creatures, being important in the life of a child, spreading knowledge to as many people as you can, and spreading love everywhere you go.

Some people fail to look further than what is already in front of their eyes, while some choose to dig deep and uncover the truth no matter how costly or how difficult it may be to conquer. I choose to win, and in doing so, I make the world a better place.

ENJOYING LIFE

"Good health is about being able to fully enjoy the time we do have. It is about being as functional as possible throughout our entire lives and avoiding crippling, painful, and lengthy battles with disease. The enjoyment of life is greatly compromised if we cannot see, if we cannot think, if our kidneys do not work, and if our bones are fragile or broken." – Dr. T. Colin Campbell, *The China Study*

After reading this quotation, I think of all of the people who try to pressure others into poisoning their bodies with meat, processed foods, refined foods, cigarettes, alcohol, and drugs saying, "Come on, you only live once."

When I read this quotation, I think of all of the people who act like I am crazy when they realize I do not eat mixtures of chemicals that they refer to as food, but instead, I eat real, wholesome, raw foods. They often say, "come on, you might as well enjoy life while you are living."

Enjoy life? And then I look at the shape of their bodies. I look at the discoloring of their skin and the blemishes on their faces. I look at their prematurely aged features and their clear signs of poor health. I see glimpses of what were once beautiful lives that have faded, as I watch them take another drink of alcohol, I see them smoke another cigarette, I witness them find pleasure from the dead flesh of some poor animal, and stuff their faces with fast food poison.

If I had to guess, I would imagine they do not enjoy their low levels of energy, they do not enjoy constipation or irritable bowel syndrome; they do not enjoy living life without any vibrancy, without any joy, without any passion. I assume they do not enjoy waking up every morning with hangovers from the depletion of their B vitamins after drinking alcohol. They surely cannot enjoy coughing themselves to sleep at night and waking up coughing every morning because of cigarette smoking. I imagine they feel there is something lacking, unknowing that it is because of the vitamins, minerals, and antioxidants that are lacking in their foods. I assume they do not like cancer or heart disease. They are simply living to die. This is not what I would consider enjoying life.

So to throw an accusation at me or anyone else following a raw food diet claiming we do not "enjoy life" because we instead choose to indulge in the best food on Earth, possess the best health, and neglect the poisons which contribute to *"The Dumbing Down of Society"* is absurd. I choose to live freely, away from poisons of the mind, poisons of the soul, and poisons of the spirit. I live to learn, spread knowledge, love, create passion, and to share my positive energy with all of nature. This is what it is like to truly "enjoy life."

<u>The 14 Healthiest Things You Could Ever Do</u>

1.) Never start smoking
2.) Quit smoking if you already do
3.) Refrain from using prescription drugs
4.) Refrain from drinking alcohol
5.) Avoid eating fast foods, processed foods, and fried foods
6.) Avoid eating meat, dairy, eggs, whey, and other animal products
7.) Refrain from using opiates or cocaine
8.) Exercise daily (running, yoga, qigong, circuit training, biking, ball games)
9.) Administer colonics or enemas as needed
10.) Drink good water
11.) Eat organic, raw foods
12.) Grow at least some of your own food and support local organic farmers
13.) Abide by a regular sleep pattern
14.) Keep your home air fresh with living house plants in each room

<u>The 14 Habits That Are Killing You</u>

1.) Eating meat (beef, chicken, pork, fish, etc)
2.) Medicine and pharmaceutical drugs
3.) Smoking cigarettes
4.) Consuming dairy products (milk, cheese, ice cream, whey, yogurt, butter, etc)
5.) Drinking alcohol
6.) Using opiates and/or cocaine
7.) Wearing suntan lotion or sunscreen
8.) Eating processed and/or fast foods
9.) Eating foods that contain processed sugars, and/or bleached and gluten grain flours
10.) Coffee and sugary coffee drinks
11.) Chewing gum
12.) Consuming fried, sauteed, and cooked oils
13.) MSG, artificial sweeteners, and other excitotoxins
14.) Microwaves, ovens, grills, broiling, and cooking your food

THE RAW CURE IN A 'NUTSHELL'

The most amazing thing about *The Raw Cure* philosophy is that we can prevent and reverse many diseases by simply eliminating a few things from our diet and incorporating "real" food into our everyday lives.

No matter what degenerative condition you may have, you can reverse or greatly reduce this condition by removing the following things from your life:

1.) **Meat and all animal flesh**
2.) **Dairy and all dairy products**
3.) **Eggs**
4.) **All Processed foods**
5.) **All fast foods**
6.) **All sodas and processed drinks**
7.) **Cigarettes and nicotine**
8.) **Alcohol**
9.) **Fried oils**
10.) **All clarified sugars and artificial sweeteners**
11.) **All flours**
12.) **Gluten grains**
13.) **All chemical, pharmaceutical drugs**
14.) **Beauty products containing parabens and sulfates**

By removing these items from your diet and incorporating real, organic raw foods, you will vastly reduce your chances of experiencing degenerative diseases and seasonal illnesses, and you will live a much more vibrant, healthful life. You will begin the process of removing the overload of toxins that have been stored in your body for years. In doing so, you will experience a boost in energy, a positive outlook on life, a healthy physique, more mental clarity, and a level of satisfaction you may have never felt before.

You may ask, is it really this simple? The answer is yes, the chemicals that are being added to processed foods and are lurking in meat, dairy, eggs, cigarettes, chemical drugs, beauty products, and alcohol, and the variety of common unhealthful foods are solely responsible for the majority of illnesses in this world. Eliminating these chemicals and deadening foods, and altering our current lifestyle could be the best form of healthcare.

By simply adding the following into your lives as replacements for the items I suggested you remove, you may guarantee yourself a much more enjoyable future:

1.) **Raw, organic fruits, vegetables, superfoods, nuts, and seeds**
2.) **Clean water**
3.) **Internal cleansing**
4.) **A positive attitude always**
5.) **Sunlight**
6.) **Nature**
7.) **Exercise**
8.) **Laughter**
9.) **Love**
10.) **Education and practicing talents**
11.) **Positive people**

You will soon discover that synthetic, over-the-counter, and prescription medications most often complicate things. They largely make things worse. Many of the degenerative diseases today are directly linked to bad dietary choices and nutritional deficiencies. It is important to note that radiation, air pollution, tainted water, bad relationships, and even lack of love also contribute to disease.

Most medical doctors have no clue what optimal nutrition is, as they are not taught true nutrition in medical school. Instead, they are taught chemistry and surgery. A study published in a September 2010 issue of *Academic Medicine*, titled, *Nutrition Education in U.S. Medical Schools*, revealed that *only twenty-five percent of all medical schools studied offered a dedicated course on nutrition. The students received around 19.6 hours of nutritional education throughout their entire medical school program.* The conclusion of their study was that the amount of nutrition education that medical students receive continues to be inadequate.

If you are sick, it can almost always be associated with a nutritional deficiency that comes from eating unhealthful foods, or from toxin overload stemming from the lifestyle choices you make. Because most medical doctors do not include nutrition in their practices, to assist your body through a full recovery, you should either see a raw organic nutritionist or simply change your diet. In addition, avoid seeing a dietitian who follows the absurd and useless USDA food pyramid, and seek someone who studies nature's medicine, which is plant-based nutrition.

If you do see a nutritionist or dietitian and she tells you it is okay to eat meat or drink milk, thank her for the advice, and do not allow any of the misinformation to absorb into your head. Instead, search for someone else. They are living in the past and believing in antiquated, disproved nutritional theories. They are still living in a world full of medicine, sickness, and disease that lacks compassion and truth, but that depends on misinformation, non-foods, drugs, and surgery. You must find someone who understands food and abides by nature's laws. The good news is that there are thousands of us out there who can help you. The most convenient helper, though, is a better educated you, fueled by real nutrition, which can only be found in a plant-based diet rich in raw, organic fruits and vegetables.

"It is not so cool to think of yourself as 'green' or sustainable because you recycle or you change to energy-efficient light bulbs when you still eat animal products that have a much more profoundly negative impact on our environment." – Dr. Richard Oppenlander, Comfortably Unaware

What ails you or brings you down likely has a nutritional aspect that you have not yet recognized or have neglected. This book is the invitation to open your eyes. We greatly benefit by eating the foods that grow from Earth in their raw and natural state. Without real food we can only live for a few years until we become sick, and in most cases develop a degenerative disease and die.

Once we discover the truth, we do a little research, and we change our ways, it all starts to make sense. We have to dedicate more time to our health and well-being than we devote to worrying about our "social" status.

Now, let us begin. First, we will discuss the importance of food.

The First Lesson:

WHY FOOD IS IMPORTANT

The more people I meet, and the more people I observe, the more it dawns on me that most of us will eat anything we are told is food without knowing what it really is. What if I told them they were eating disease? Would they still eat that slice of meaty, cheesy pizza? Would they still stuff their faces with fast food, french fries, burgers, bleached gluten grains, and chemical-laden "soft" drinks? Would they still eat hot dogs if they knew that, in addition to causing pancreatic cancer, the chance of developing leukemia and colon cancer also skyrockets by a large percentage from eating them?

The sad truth is that many people are already aware that the reason why we have so much disease in the world is because people are contining to eat poisonous food. They simply do not know any other way to eat. The way the economy is structured makes it easiest to eat whatever is most convenient, cheap, fast... and, unhealthful.

It does not help that the most popular forms of entertainment, including TV shows, films, sporting events, carnivals, and amusement parks are saturated with poor food choices, and are financially supported by the companies that create these foods and chemical drugs. The advertisements you see all over these events and on TV shows for fast food and pharmaceutical drugs are paying for the entertainment to take place. Seeing these poor quality foods makes it seem as if the food is okay to eat. Good, healthy foods are not to be seen on advertisements at these events.

The food that is most nourishing is not readily available to most people, especially those living in poor neighborhoods. So instead of vibrant health, they are filled with vile foods and depend on toxic drugs in attempts to make them healthful. They are filled with chemical poisons in the form of processed foods, synthetic food additives, and farming chemical residues, and are handed over to the fate of the medical industry. Their food choices become the beginning of their end.

Chapter 1: *WHAT IS FOOD AND WHY IS IT IMPORTANT?*

"Food is that material which can be incorporated into and become a part of the cells and fluids of the body. Non useful materials, such as chemical additives and drugs, are all poisonous. To be a true food, the substance must not contain useless or harmful ingredients." – Dr. Herbert Shelton, *Food Combining Made Easy*

Many people do not eat real food. In fact, many have no idea what they put into their bodies each time they eat. What the average American considers to be food is often a mixture of some sort of over-processed material with a variety of extracts and chemicals. This is not the material that we want becoming a part of the cells and fluids of the body. We want the nutrients from foods that are only present in their natural state. When these combinations of extracts and chemicals become a part of our cells and bodily fluids, we weaken as individuals. We lose our passion, we lose our vitality, our IQ's lower, and we lose our desire to express our true selves. We miss out on many of the joys of life. This is the reason why we prematurely age and start to feel like we are "getting old." We are simply not eating real food. Food is not the processed, packaged garbage that the average person fills his belly with.

Real food is grown in nature. It consists of fresh, sun ripened fruits and vegetables. Some fungi, greens, and sprouts are considered food. Food consists of various organic nuts and seeds, and even a variety of algae and seaweeds. Meat is not a good source of food for the human body. The milk from other animals is also not to be considered food for humans. Eggs are far from an ideal food. I will explain why animal products are not healthful foods in chapter two.

When we deprive ourselves of real food and instead fill up on processed, chemical-laden concoctions, we starve ourselves of nutrients and vitality. We chase our youth away and we invite premature aging. If we have children, we almost guarantee they will not have healthy parents as they age and they will likely lose one or both parents early from a degenerative condition. By consuming unhealthy foods, we throw away our happiness and bring misery upon ourselves. By eating poorly and not taking care of ourselves, we degrade our families and invite illness, frustration, and hatred into our souls. This is why we would greatly benefit by improving our nutrition, cleaning up our diets, and especially, educating ourselves on what we feed to our children.

Low level nutrition and toxic food choices are why *one of every two Americans develops cancer, heart disease, or diabetes and many develop obesity, arthritis, and osteoporosis.* Poor food choices and the lack of true nutrition are why we become stressed and frustrated, lack belief in ourselves and others, and why some resort to crime. We find ourselves depressed, marriages fall apart, and the ecosystem of the world crumbles. We have become a "chemical civilization" that has altered our culture and disconnected us from our true intellect, talents, and nature.

"Either it is appropriable material for tissue building (a food) or it is not. If not, then it is a foreign substance – a poison – and as such can only damage and cannot possibly ever benefit the organism." – Dr. Hereward Carrington

According to Carrington, to qualify as being a real food source, our body must be able to use the food for tissue building and energy consumption. Additionally, Dr. Shelton states that a substance must not contain useless or harmful ingredients to be a true food. With this being considered, I can justly state that fast food restaurants serve items that are not really food. Gas stations and convenient store chains sell products that are so overloaded with chemicals and unhealthy oils, sugars, and salts that they cannot be considered food. Burgers, buns, fries, apple pies, and tacos from various fast food chains; subs from many commercialized sandwich shops; soft drinks; candy bars; pizzas; frozen packaged products that go in microwaveable sleeves, TV dinners, packaged products like toaster pastries, cookies with filling, doughnuts; breads; meats, dairy, eggs; and sugars; none of these are food for humans. They are chemical fillers and diseased pieces of dead flesh, or chemically loaded secretions from other animals, that are strategically marketed to consumers as being nutritious, natural, and healthy, for the sole purpose of increasing profits, while those eating them gradually become sicker and heftier. These food products do not build tissues, instead they are damaging to the human organism.

Many grocery stores sell conventional produce that is degraded. By conventional, I am referring to produce that was not grown organically. Much of it has been genetically modified and is lacking in its natural nutrient spectrum. The bread sold in stores is simply refined flours mixed with refined sugars, yeast, and some chemicals. The beef sold is from animals that were stolen at birth from their mothers' and pumped with chemical feed until they were fattened and then slaughtered.

Understand that the nutrients meat provided at one point in history came from animals consuming grasses and natural foods that they had eaten in nature. These animals no longer eat their natural diet, so they do not receive their natural array of nutrients, and the result is that their meat is not nourishing for humans, nor is it food. The meat that is sold in supermarkets all over the world is therefore lacking in the nutrient profile of wild-raised meat. To obtain the nutrients we need, we must go directly to the source where the animals go for their nutrients in the wild. That source is the fruits, vegetables, and other edible plants that nature provides for all living creatures. Much of the meat served in restaurants where it is heated at high temperatures contains more cancer-causing compounds such as heterocyclic amines, sodium nitrite, sodium nitrate, trans-fats, and polycyclic aromatic hydrocarbons, than it does nutrients. Each of these contributes to cancer and disease. In fact, some fast food meat, dairy, and egg products are considered among the most toxic of all foods.

"The answer to the American health crisis is the food that each of us chooses to put in our mouths each day. It's as simple as that." – Dr. T. Colin Campbell, *The China Study*

The milk and dairy products sold in common markets have been pasteurized, which destroys nutrients and creates health-depleting chemicals, and therefore they cannot be considered food either. They often contain grotesque amounts of pus, blood, antibiotics, and growth hormones, and this is causing disease.

Finally, all of the canned and packaged products on shelves and in the frozen aisles of grocers are rich in preservatives, additives, and even petroleum extracts. They also cannot be correctly labeled as "food."

What this means is the only way we can eat real food is by educating ourselves on how to prepare food, growing our own crops, finding good organic restaurants, shopping at organic grocers, and supporting local organic farmers at farmer's markets. John McCabe wrote an excellent book titled, *The Sunfood Traveler*, which provides readers with all of the best spots to find real food in each community. This is a book you may want to carry with you whenever you are traveling.

Remember, for true nutrition, food can only be correctly called food if it contains nutrients that can be assimilated throughout the body and utilized properly. Even processed foods that are "fortified" with vitamins and minerals cannot be honestly labeled as food. They lack enzymes and biophotons, and the vitamins they contain may be useless synthetic substances.

In order for minerals to be efficient for use in our bodies, they must first be absorbed from the Earth by the plants. The plants then convert these minerals into assimilable form so when we eat them, we are able to properly assimilate these nutrients. Nothing that is synthetic is organic. It does not matter how hard she tries, no chemist can duplicate nature. It simply cannot be done.

A bee pollen granule is the perfect example of how nature cannot be duplicated. Even after each identifiable piece of material found within is matched and the granules look identical to those provided by nature; when these synthetically made granules are fed to the bees, they die off within a couple of weeks. The reason for this is that the vitality and the *life force energy* coming from the fresh, living bee pollen granules made from nature cannot be duplicated. You cannot duplicate life; you cannot duplicate nature in a lab.

Pasteurized cow's milk is another example of the problems associated with an altered food. When you feed baby calves pasteurized milk, such as the milk we are offered to purchase in stores around the world, they often become sick and it can even be fatal. The reason for this is simple: pasteurization damages enzymes, alters the chemistry of, and destroys the vitality and *life force energy* in the milk. When humans drink this stuff, they become fat; their arteries begin to accumulate calcifications of plaque, and their health degenerates. The chemical drugs we then take allow for us to continue consuming this garbage, and as a result, we prematurely age, and our average lifespan is cut shorter every year from unnatural causes. We are seeing an increase in deaths from these unnatural causes because we are providing our bodies with unnatural substances rather than natural foods.

"The ways in which humans use plants, foods, and drugs cause the values of individuals and, ultimately, whole societies to shift. Eating some foods makes us happy, eating others, sleepy, and still others alert. We are jovial, restless, aroused, or depressed depending on what we have eaten." – Terrence McKenna, *Food of the Gods*

Each part of your body, from the cells to the organs, from your level of energy to your current mood, is composed of and/or impacted by material that is derived from food. We are dependent on food from birth in order to make hormones, synthesize vitamins, and create enzymes. Food gives us fuel. Food provides us with the nutrients we need to grow. Food helps us maintain each cell in our body. When cells die off, our body relies on the energy from foods to rid itself of cellular waste. When we generate new cells, it is the nutrients from foods that determine whether these cells will be strong or weak. Our entire process of life revolves around food.

When you discover how vital real food is, and the light turns on inside of your mind, and you realize that for all of these years you have not been providing your body with this real food that is of utter importance to your well-being, this is when you begin to awaken. You discover why your body has been gradually deteriorating over the years. You understand why your relatives and your elders have developed disease and are suffering, or have already passed away. You realize that you have been deceived all of your life. You start to get curious and you start asking questions. Why had I not previously realized this? How come nobody told me about this many years ago? Why are these corporations allowed to get away with this? Why are there advertisements for the most toxic foods being continually presented to us through every form of media? What is wrong with this world?

It is okay to ask these questions. I have asked them myself. I have also found answers for many of them. The most important part of all of this is that there is still time to change. You still have time to introduce real food into your life. The best way to start is by getting rid of all of the old stuff you used to call food and not allowing it back into your life. No more fast food restaurants. No more late night stops at the convenience store. No more late night pizza deliveries. No more microwaveable dinners. Say goodbye to it all and get rid of the microwave, toaster oven, and fryer forever. This will start a new chapter in your life.

Now that you have an understanding of what food really is and why it is important, we can discuss the importance of eating organic, real foods.

EATING ORGANIC: A WISE DECISION

The sales of organic foods and beverages increased annually from around one billion dollars in 1990 to over twenty-one billion in 2008. As people become aware of the health benefits that come along with eating organic foods, the trend continues to grow.

The difference between eating organic foods and choosing to eat conventional can be compared to how you choose to pay your credit card bill. The more you spend towards paying it off, the less interest you will pay over time. If you pay the minimum, you will keep getting by while the interest adds up. When you pay it off in larger payments, you also build more credit and more creditors will want to offer you lines of credit. This is how your body and its level of health relate to spending more on organic and less on conventional foods. If you spend more on organic produce, you will avoid the chemicals used on conventional produce that have been identified as carcinogenic, and that can interfere with nerve, and other tissues. You begin to build your credit with good health.

When you eat conventional, chemically grown foods, and spend as little as possible on food so you can afford to go out drinking, dining, or buying fancy things that you do not need, you may get by for a little while; however, the poor food choices catch up with you. By consuming conventional foods, you are more likely to ingest chemicals that can alter your immune and nerve systems, and can degrade your cell function. Where many of these chemically grown foods are contained is as ingredients in packaged foods that also contain other substances, such as food additives, preservatives, and low-quality oils that also can alter cellular functions. This means that you are more likely to become frustrated, sick, and tired, and also more likely to seek help from medications, doctors, and surgery. In the long run, you lose and you end up spending a lot more. Keep this in consideration the next time you have the choice to spend a bit extra on more nutritious organic, or continue to choose low-quality foods.

Anyone who claims there is no difference between conventional produce and organic also declares their ignorance. Aside from the pesticides, which really are a big deal, conventional crops are grown in nutrient-deficient soils. Without these nutrients, the plants grow to be deficient. One may ask, "Well, how does the plant still grow?" It is a question from someone who does not clearly understand. The answer is that the plants still grow the same way some children grow when they are deprived of nutrients while in the womb or soon after birth. Their growth retards, they are weak, they are frail, their immune system is compromised, and they are more likely to experience a variety of health issues. In some cases, they are born with birth defects. This happens to our plants and our crops just as it so sadly happens to our children when their diet is inadequate. Our children are diseased just as our conventional crops are diseased.

In September 2012, the *Annals of Internal Medicine* published the results of a study conducted at *Stanford University* in an article titled, *Are Organic Foods Safer or Healthier than Conventional Alternatives.* In this flawed study, researchers looked at data from 240 separate studies published in medical journal databases over the years to determine whether or not organic food is healthier than conventional. Stanford researchers concluded that, *"The published literature lacks strong evidence that organic foods are significantly more nutritious than conventional foods. Consumption of organic foods may reduce exposure to pesticide residues and antibiotic-resistant bacteria."* If reducing exposure to pesticides and antibiotic-resistant bacteria is not enough to persuade you to continue eating organic, consider that only seventeen of the 240 studies used to gather information for this particular study actually looked at the health outcomes of people eating organic and conventionally grown foods. Of the seventeen that did so, only three of them compared health outcomes. These three studies compared only allergy-related outcomes and *symptomatic campylobacter infection.* Not a single study included in this report did research on health outcomes such as cancer, childhood illness and developmental issues, immune disorders, or any of the thousands of other serious health conditions identified by the medical industry.

In addition to the many flaws and loopholes attached to this *Stanford University* study, what I find interesting is that *Stanford University* is partnered with the agricultural empire *Cargill,* and their study is suggesting that organic food is no better than its big-agriculture competition. On *Cargill's* website they include a page detailing their partnership with *Stanford University. Stanford* also lists *Cargill* as a donor in their 2011 Annual Report. Is this is a conflict of interest? I would say yes, without a doubt.

Many studies have been done proving that conventional crops produce far less phytochemicals than organic crops do. Phytochemicals are compounds produced by plants that are of great benefit to the body. Dr. Brian Clement, in his book *Life Force,* mentions a study from the 2002 *European Journal of Nutrition* which proved that *organic vegetables contain nearly six times as much salicylic acid as non-organic vegetables. The salicylic acid is disrupted by the pesticides used in non-organic farming.* Studies have been done both at *Rutgers* and *Tufts University* which have proven organic crops have up to eighty-eight percent more minerals than do conventional. According to the *Organic Consumers Association, organic food contains qualitatively higher levels of essential minerals such as calcium, magnesium, iron, and chromium, which are severely depleted in chemical foods grown on pesticide and nitrate fertilizer-abused soil. UK and US government statistics indicate that levels of trace minerals in (non-organic) fruit and vegetables fell by up to seventy-six percent between 1940 and 1991.*

Eating produce deficient in basic nutrients is like going shopping and forgetting your wallet, or any form of payment at home. Yes, you get the pleasures of shopping for new items, but when you get to the register, you realize nothing of use has come from your shopping experience. When you eat nutrient-deficient food, you fool your body into believing it is getting the nutrients, but once you assimilate the contents throughout the body, you realize all you have done is waste energy. Some people argue that there is no difference in the nutrient content of non-organic fruits and vegetables. This is not true. These are the people who are also likely to not understand the difference between macronutrients and micronutrients.

Minerals, vitamins, and phytochemicals are nutrients, they happen to be among our most important nutrients. They are referred to as micronutrients. If you compare the macronutrient content of organic to conventional produce it remains the same. This is only comparing proteins, carbohydrates, and fats though, not vitamins and minerals. What is most important is the micronutrient content. Organic fruit contains much higher amounts of these irreplaceable micronutrients than the opposing conventional produce. *A comprehensive review of ninety-seven published studies comparing the nutritional quality of organic and conventional foods revealed that organic plant-based foods contain higher levels of eight of the eleven vital micronutrients that were studied. This includes significantly greater concentrations of polyphenols and antioxidants. In this comprehensive review, the team of scientists concluded that organically grown, plant-based foods are twenty-five percent more nutrient dense, on average, and deliver more essential nutrients per serving or calorie consumed.* This review was published in the March 2008 edition of the *State of Science Review* by the *Organic Center* and is titled: *New Evidence Confirms the Nutritional Superiority of Plant-Based Organic Foods.*

Please purchase organic food. You are not only boosting your immunity by eating it, you are also helping to build our top soil back up to an adequate level. Without topsoil, little plant life is possible. Topsoil is the outermost layer of soil. Because it has the highest concentration of organic matter and microorganisms, the roots of plants obtain their nutrients from this layer. The conventional monocropping methods common today are destroying this vital layer of Earth. Conventional monocropping can be defined as growing an excess of one particular type of crop when it is not needed. The Earth and the soil need a variety of crops for nourishment. Planting a variety of organic crops, as organic farmers are more likely to do, helps rebuild the topsoil.

By eating organic, you are helping to save the environment. You are supporting the organic farmers who work hard day-after-day to be sure they are providing us with our optimal nutrients. We must thank these courageous farmers. They are the ones that are keeping our planet alive. They bring us hope. They keep the hopes of sharing unity with all of nature lingering around.

A great way to get involved with the organic movement is to join an organic co-op. In Houston, TX there is an amazing organic coop called *Rawfully Organic*. This coop is the largest organic coop in the country. The organizer is Kristina Carrillo-Bucaram. She is beautiful, charismatic, charming, and incredibly inspiring. You can find out more by accessing *fullyraw.com* or *rawfullyorganic.com*. If we could do what she is doing in Houston all over the country, and in every city all over the world, we could also cut our healthcare costs, improve the environment, and reduce the extinction of species.

In most areas across the country there are *Community Supported Agriculture* (CSA) groups offering organic crop-shares where you pay a certain amount of money every couple of weeks and you get organic produce delivered to you, or have the option of picking it up locally. Check out *coopdirectory.org* to find one nearest you.

You can either pay the organic farmers a little extra for their hard work and dedication towards providing real food for us, or you can pay the hospitals a few years later a lot more to misdiagnose you, and give you erroneous treatments for your ailments that are a result of eating foods stripped of their nutrients and loaded with toxic chemicals that destroy nature. The choice is yours. The *Pesticide Action Network* reported that *organic farmers in the U.S. produced more than $20 billion worth of pesticide-free food in 2007, and at a twenty percent annual growth rate, organics are the fastest growing agricultural sector.* Together we can keep this trend going. We do not need pesticides or GMO's to grow our own food or to feed the world.

My word of advice to anyone trying to argue for the production of conventional crops is this: Even if you truly believe that somehow conventional crops are equally nutritious, this does not give you any reason to go against supporting organic farming. There are very sick people out there who need organic food, they need to be taught about the dangers of consuming meat, dairy, and eggs, and they need our help. When you try to publicly speak out for a cause which you know nothing about, you confuse these poor people and they curl back up and give in to the medical trap. In a way, you are nurturing their health ailments. By reverting to organic food, the way food was naturally created to be, we help the environment. Whether you choose to believe it or not, we save each other. Rather than playing the devil's advocate, being vocal about your lack of understanding and lack of education, or expressing your lack of compassion for our environment, I urge you to do some research. Do not simply type in Google searches looking for argument's favoring the other side. Visit the websites of the *Organic Consumers Association* (organicconsumers.org) and The *Organic-Center* (organic-center.org). Read actual books, such as *Comfortably Unaware* by Dr. Richard Oppenlander, *The Food Revolution* by John Robbins, *Sunfood Diet Infusion* by John McCabe, and *Organic Manifesto* by Maria Rodale. Discover the truth about food. Taste the difference. Feel the difference in energy as you indulge in the delights of organic produce.

WHAT IS GMO & WHY SHOULD WE AVOID IT?

"The future of our world depends on how we steward our land, soil, water, and seeds, and pass them on to future generations." – Dr. Vandana Shiva

Another dilemma one faces when eating conventional food is the support of the GMO industry. The concept of genetically modifying crops was explored as a way to simplify the growing process. Before long, it began to destroy the quality of food. Genetically modified foods (GMO) are made by artificially transferring genes between organisms. The cell membrane of the organism is penetrated by the DNA from the other species. In 1983, an antibiotic resistant tobacco plant became the first genetically modified crop. The first GMO food created was a tomato. The tomato was modified to ripen before it would soften, as a way to preserve it for sales in supermarkets.

Because of huge companies like Monsanto, most of the common food crop seeds these days have been genetically modified, and produce crops that fail to provide the natural medicines which the real, organic, unaltered versions of the same crops do. When a seed or crop is genetically altered, the result is a plant that has an unnatural assortment of genetic material and cellular activity. Monsanto is the largest producer of GMO seeds and crops. They are also merged with Pfizer (the richest pharmaceutical company in the world) and together they could take over our food supply if we do not act soon. This would result in the produce we buy from grocers and farmers contributing to our sickness, and would lead to us relying on their synthetic medicines for "relief." These crops are also sprayed with loads of pesticides that trigger allergies and disease in humans and wildlife, and end up in the soil, air, streams, rivers, lakes, marshes, and oceans.

The pesticides alter the presence of enzymes and biophotons in the food. Enzymes and biophotons provide our life force energy. In Sunfood Diet Infusion, John McCabe describes biophotons as *the tiny specs of light which are stored in the cells of the plant and carry different levels of vibrational energy fields*. Enzymes control the metabolic processes in the body. Without foods rich in enzymes and biophotons, we prematurely age, develop disease, and have digestive issues. The vitamins are also altered by a slew of farming chemicals and pesticides.

Additional GMO companies are *Bayer CropScience* (Germany), *DOW Chemical* (US), *DuPont* (US), and *Aventis* (France). If you want to avoid genetically modified foods, it is important to refrain from consuming food products containing ingredients that are owned by any of the GMO companies. Some of the food companies using genetically engineered ingredients are those that sell food items such as processed meats and cheeses; crackers, chips and other similar savory items; cookies; pancake, cake, and muffin mixes; cereals; chocolate products; canned soups; condiments such as mayonnaise, mustard and ketchup, frozen TV dinners; microwaveable packaged meals; commercialized veggie and fruit juices that are in cans, bottles, or juice-boxes; pasta sauces; sodas, and the list goes on. Many of these food items are made with genetically modified organisms and are examples of foods that should always be avoided. Each person who consumes these corporate junk foods has been deceived. He has been deceived by the marketing strategies of the richest corporations in the world. He has been fooled by the corporations that constitute the GMO industry, dairy industry, factory-farming industry, commercialized food industry, and most of all, the pharmaceutical industry. All of these industries are run and managed by the biggest swindling criminals alive.

It is common sense that organic food is more nutritious than conventional, genetically modified food look-a-likes. We, as consumers, are fooled into buying the big, artificially enhanced crops that look appealing thinking we are eating more healthfully. In reality, the foods may be lacking in nutrients and contain toxins. By eating them we may develop a nutritional deficiency, and the chemical residues and GMO alterations may be triggering, or contributing to the development of various diseases.

The next time you shop, look at the difference between the conventional and organic crops. The conventional crops often do not appear to be real. They are modified to look perfect. They look plastic. The reason for this is that they really are unnatural. Don't be superficial when it comes to purchasing the food that becomes your source of energy, buy organic.

An example of how GMO foods can be damaging to our health is that there is an altered mineral balance in GMO fruits. Because of this, the sugars from the fruit may become more absorbable into our blood, causing spikes in our blood sugar levels. This makes the pancreas work extra hard and eventually triggers Type II Diabetes. On the flipside, eating a vegan diet rich in raw, organic fruits that are high in nutrients can be a huge help in reversing diabetes.

In a September 2012 edition of the *Le Nouvel Observateur*, the results of a two year French study exposing the dangers of GMO's were published. The study was conducted using two-hundred rats that were fed *Round-up* tolerant, genetically modified corn from *Monsanto* to evaluate long-term health effects.

Over the course of two years, the rats developed massive breast tumors, suffered excessive kidney and liver damage, and other serious health problems. The major onslaughts of these diseases started to emerge around the thirteenth month.

In July 2012, the *Cornucopia Institute* published an article titled, *Obesity, Corn, and GMO's*. In the article they include the results of a ten-year experimental feeding study carried out by scientists at the *Norwegian Veterinary College* in Norway. The study included rats, mice, pigs, and salmon, and found that genetically engineered (GMO) feed led to obesity in the animals. In addition to becoming obese, these poor animals suffered significant changes to the digestive system and major organs, including the liver, kidneys, pancreas, and genitals. It was also discovered that female rats that ate genetically-engineered *Round-up* tolerant corn died early and more rapidly, two to three times more than those not fed GMO corn.

I suggest that you read any of Dr. Vandana Shiva's books to learn more about the concept of GMO foods and how they are destroying the environment. Dr. Shiva founded the *Research Foundation for Science, Technology and Ecology*, and this led to the creation of *Navdanya* in 1991. *Navdanya* is a national movement established to protect the diversity and integrity of living resources. Most importantly, native seed, the promotion of organic farming, and fair trade. Dr. Shiva speaks out against GMO companies and is doing everything she can to protect Earth from the dangers of the GMO technology. She chairs for the Commission on the Future of Food, and is also the councilor of the World Future Council. Look for her books, ***Making Peace with the Earth, Manifestos on the Future of Food and Seed; Soil Not Oil; Stolen Harvest; Earth Democracy; and Staying Alive***. You can also learn more about GMO foods by watching the documentaries, *The World According to Monsanto* and *The Future of Food*. Visit the website of the ***Organic Consumer's Association***. They have a page dedicated to educating us on the dangers of genetically altered seeds (organicconsumers.org/monsanto). You can also request to join the Facebook group called Millions against Monsanto.

I always support, encourage, and strongly recommend growing at least some of your own food while purchasing and eating only crops that are organic. Not only is this helping to support the organic farmers who work extremely hard to assure us a future free from disease, but it is also supporting our future, our children's futures, our longevity, and the health of wildlife.

Now that you are more aware of why you should be eating and purchasing organic, let's talk about enzymes and why we should not cook our food.

ZAP IT

While growing up, I was constantly listening to my grandmother in the kitchen as she would prepare meals using the microwave. She liked to use the phrase, "zap it." I believe she may have been a little "zap crazy." She would put everything in the microwave without knowing she was damaging many of the nutrients in the food and partially defeating the purpose of eating it. Today, sadly, she is paying for it with poor health.

Most people who buy conventional foods also use a microwave to *cook* these foods. Using a microwave changes the molecular structure of food and greatly decreases its nutritional value. Microwaves alter nutrients and create cancer causing chemicals such as acrylamides and glycotoxins.

On *YouTube* there are many videos that show the effect of radiation and how it is emitted from microwaves. In a video I recently viewed, a guy turned on a microwave, measured the radiation, and backed away from it, going into the next room. The radiation could still be measured. He closed the door, and it was reduced, but was still measurable. This demonstrates how harmful microwaves can be in terms of exposing us, and our food, to radiation.

Hans Hertel, a Swiss food scientist, when discussing the impact of microwaves on nutrients, stated that, *"There are no atoms, molecules, or cells of any organic system able to withstand such a violent, destructive power for any extended period of time, not even in the low energy range of mill watts. This is how microwave cooking heat is generated – friction from this violence in water molecules. Structures of molecules are torn apart, molecules are forcefully deformed (called structural isomerism), and thus become impaired in quality."* He initiated tests on microwaved food to determine its effect on human physiology and the blood and concluded that microwaves lead to food degeneration, which causes changes in the blood. Some of these changes include increased cholesterol levels, decreased hemoglobin and red blood cell levels, and an increase in leukocytes.

In his book, *Heal Yourself 101*, Markus Rothkranz makes an interesting statement about microwaves. He states that, *"Microwaving water and then watering seeds with that water will result in the seed not growing."* Although some people claim to have been able to successfully grow seeds using microwaved water, I have not heard one claim that microwaving the water and the seed together will result in any growth. Think about this now, if a microwave will alter a seed so it will no longer germinate or sprout, imagine what the microwave is doing to the structure of the food you eat after being "zapped." It deadens the food, and it deadens you.

A study published in the November 2003 *Journal of the Science of Food and Agriculture*, indicated for us that *microwaving broccoli with a little bit of water results in a loss of up to ninety-seven percent of its antioxidant content.*

When they steamed broccoli there was only a loss of eleven percent. When eaten raw, broccoli contains all of its antioxidant content.

When microwaves were first introduced to Russia, the Russians conducted extensive testing to determine the biological effects of microwaves. They found that nearly all foods tested formed carcinogenic compounds after being microwaved. Milk and grains formed carcinogenic compounds through the conversion of amino acids. Plant alkaloids were converted into carcinogens. Meat formed heterocyclic amines, which are chemicals formed when muscle meat from beef, pork, chicken, or fish is heated at high temperatures. These chemicals cause changes in DNA, leading to an increased risk of developing many cancers. Processed meats containing nitrates become even more toxic when heated. The heterocyclic amines form when the amino acids, sugars, and creatine in the meat react at high temperatures. These results were enough for the Soviet Union to ban microwaves. As the food industry created more and more processed foods and the westernized diet gained popularity, the ban was eventually lifted.

What can we do to avoid the dangers associated with the microwave? We can simply recycle our microwaves. Give them to the guys who collect scrap steel. Get up right now and remove that nutrient-destroying device from your life. There is no reason for a microwave to be in your kitchen; it is a waste of space, a waste of energy, a destroyer of nutrients, and its use will degrade your health and shorten your life span.

ENZYMES

"What is the great secret that has been eluding the investigations of scientists and lives of laypersons for centuries? Enzymes. You are only alive because thousands of enzymes make it possible. Every breath you take, thought you think, or sentence you read, is a result of thousands of complex enzyme systems and their functions operating simultaneously." – Ann Wigmore, The Hippocrates Diet

In addition to using a microwave, using the stove, oven, fryer, or any other heating appliance can also degrade the nutrients in your food, and degrade your health. Cooking causes chemical changes to occur and shifts the molecular structure of foods. When you heat foods to high temperatures, you destroy the enzymes and the biophoton life force energy contained within.

Enzymes are biological molecules that catalyze, or increase the rates of, chemical reactions. They are long, linear chains of amino acids, as are proteins, and each amino acid sequence produces its own specific structure, containing unique properties. In the body, enzymes control every metabolic process. They also aid in the digestion of foods. Enzymes help to control whether you will age prematurely or age regularly, they play a role in whether you are sick or healthy, and they ultimately keep you alive.

In his book *Enzyme Nutrition*, Dr. Edward Howell points out one of the many roles of enzymes being the *conversion of nutrients into new muscle, flesh, bone, nerves, and glands.* He also mentions how they *assist the kidneys, lungs, liver, skin, and colon with their eliminative duties.* Without enzymes our bodies would not work efficiently. Many of us do not know what enzymes are. By way of low-grade food choices, we are speeding up the process of aging related to a lack of restorative enzymes.

"Life could not exist without enzymes." – Dr. Edward Howell

There are tens of thousands of enzymes in the body. However, there are three main enzyme types. The three main categories of enzymes are: metabolic enzymes, digestive enzymes, and dietary enzymes. Metabolic enzymes activate each of the metabolic processes in the body, such as metabolism, anabolism, and cellular respiration. Each of these processes provides energy for sustaining life and growth. For example, metabolism occurs through a series of enzymatic reactions which convert one substance into another for the storage or release of energy. Digestive enzymes digest the foods that contain no enzymes, being processed and cooked foods. Dietary enzymes are the enzymes found in raw plant matter and these are important for preserving our health and maintaining our youth. These are the enzymes that digest foods for us because they are already present within the foods when we eat them.

For each of the macronutrients we ingest in our food (proteins, carbohydrates, and fats), we have a specific enzyme group to digest them and break them down into amino acids, simple sugars, and fatty acids. The enzymes that digest proteins are protease enzymes. The enzymes that digest carbohydrates are amylase enzymes, and the enzymes that break down fats are lipase enzymes.

We are said to store limited amounts of digestive and metabolic enzymes, which we were given at birth. Therefore, we must obtain adequate amounts of enzymes by eating raw, edible plants in order to avoid using up enzyme reserves. Processed and fast foods are either lacking in, or do not contain enzymes. Aside from a few raw fruits or vegetables, many of the foods served in restaurants do not contain enzymes. When food is cooked, the enzymes become denatured. Heat disrupts the structure of the amino acid sequence. This also results in the formation of heterocyclic amines. When we eat the cooked food, we are forced to use up the enzymes in our reserves. This explains the aging process and how enzymes can impact aging.

In addition to a lack of enzymes; irregular sleep patterns, lack of exercise, and stress also play major roles in the aging process. The quicker you use up enzyme reserves and the more sedentary you become, the quicker you will age. I repeat myself here for a reason. It is highly important that you provide your body with enzymes from raw fruits and raw vegetables.

"Cooking destroys life. I do not say that these articles should never be cooked, but only that there is loss in cooking them, especially if we can eat them perfectly fresh and alive. The life and soul of fruits are lost in cooking." – Dr. Martin Luther Holbrook

In 1930 a Swiss physician by the name of Paul Kouchakoff discovered a process which he referred to as Leucocytosis. This occurs when the enzymes in food are destroyed by the cooking process. After we eat the "dead" food, the white blood cells are falsely triggered to attack the cooked food as if it were a foreign organism invading the body. These white blood cells are triggered because food that contains unnatural substances formed by cooking is exactly that, a foreign organism. When a substance contains unnatural substances that interfere with cellular function, it becomes a poison to the body. When we falsely trigger these white blood cells, we weaken our immune system. This explains how enzymes play a major role in health. As we eat cooked food, we force our pancreas to do extra work secreting digestive and metabolic enzymes. Our pancreas then enlarges, leading to the fluctuation of blood sugar. These issues may worsen into hypoglycemia and diabetes. A lack of sufficient enzymes in the food we eat can be linked to many of the common degenerative diseases in the body.

To avoid this burden on your pancreas, to preserve your enzymes, and to bypass the leucocytosis process, it is important to eat at least sixty percent of your diet "raw," in the form of unheated fruits and vegetables, so you are always ingesting enzymes. This means that if you choose to eat cooked food, you should have fresh veggies with each cooked meal, and be sure to eat a larger portion of the raw food than cooked. Not only will your body be much better off, you will feel better and have more energy after you eat.

WHY GO RAW?

"The act of cooking – and the resultant loss of nutrients, enzymes and oxygen – impairs our digestion and elimination, which are the two most controlling factors of nutrient absorption that regulate our metabolism." – Dr. Brian Clement, LifeForce

Making the transition to a raw vegan diet could possibly be the best decision you ever make for yourself. Not only will you likely add years to your life and preserve your youth, but you will also begin the process of "bullet-proofing" your body so that no sickness, food-induced diseases, or ailments will ever again interfere with your schedule. Most raw foods such as sprouts, fruits, and fresh veggie juices are easily digestible and this means they require little energy from the body for digestion compared to unhealthful foods. As a result, when eating this way, we are able to utilize our energy to fuel our minds and repair damaged cells and tissues so we are more mentally alert and rejuvenated.

Many people immediately reject the idea of following a raw vegan diet and they make uninformed comments such as, "vegan food tastes terrible," or "I like to taste my food." They say this and then go off eating chemically induced combinations of mutilated "foods" lacking natural flavors, but with taste-stimulating synthetic chemical poisons added. Unfortunately for them they have never tried real raw cuisine. If they had tried it they would not likely make these comments. They would have discovered the best food in the world and passed the great news along to their friends and family. When I hear people make these remarks, my first impression is that they are closed-minded. In the new paradigm of the world and in the "healthy is cool" phase of living, we cannot be closed-minded. We have to open our minds and allow new opportunities to find their way to us.

Following a low-fat raw vegan diet rich in fruits and vegetables will transform your body into being the way nature intended for it to be. Every day you will be more likely to wake feeling positive, with more energy. Your creative side will have a presence again. As many of us have already discovered, you will soon notice that sickness is not inevitable, but rather a choice.

"People who eat only raw, plant based foods have an unmistakable shine, like a pregnant woman in her second trimester or someone newly in love. They have a radiant, positive energy. It's easy to spot a raw foodist in a crowd of people living on the Standard American Diet. Just look for unusually clear skin, glossy hair, and shining eyes." – Sarma Melngailis, Raw Food Real World

Food is our fuel. When we use the wrong food for fuel, we generate negative energy and emit this from within. This results in uncharacteristic behavior, anger, and hostility. Anxiety is a common result of making the wrong food choices, especially if those foods contain dairy, gluten grains, fried oils, and synthetic and processed sweeteners.

Because I see the worst concoctions of chemicals possible being eaten and referred to as food, I feel the need to educate my readers on what they are truly eating. You will be surprised to discover that most of what you have been filling your belly with for the majority of your life is harmful to your health and has been weakening your immune system, compromising your organs, and prematurely aging you, while leaving chemical and other residues in your organs.

Finally you will know the truth about what you are eating from a source that is not being paid off by the pharmaceutical, dairy, egg, or meat industries. Some of it is disturbing to discover but once you make the change and eliminate these foods from your life, you will be thankful for your discovery of reinvigorated health and vibrant energy.

Chapter 2: WHAT ARE WE EATING?

"Men dig their graves with their own teeth, and die more by those instruments than by all weapons of their enemies." – Pythagoras

If it is not food that we are eating, then what exactly is it?

"We add salt, sugar, butter, and spices. We remove the germ and husk from the wheat to use the flour for baking. We polish the rice, we refine the sugar. We remove the skin, seeds, and cores of apples and pears. We peel the potatoes and scrape the carrots. The meat, fish, eggs, and cheese supply us with an enormous surplus of animal protein. We make beverages out of coffee, cocoa beans, and tea, which contain stimulating poisons. We use the grapes for wine and brandy (intoxicating poisons) which stimulate the grey cortex of the brain, and later paralyze it. We preserve foods with chemicals such as benzoic acid, sodium benzoate, nitrates, and boric acid in order that it may keep well." – Dr. Kirstine Nolfi, cancer survivor

The food crisis in our country is something the majority of society remains unaware of. By shopping at Wal-Mart, and other commercial grocers that sell processed and refined food products marketed as being nutritious, these consumers reveal their lack of awareness. They have placed their trust in the companies who make the fake food, and government organizations that regulate the food industry, and both of these organizations are controlled by the pharmaceutical industry.

There are not many politicians out there following a vegan diet, and most likely not any, who eat raw or understand the way food works. They also make money from kickbacks that come from the pharmaceutical industry, the GMO industry, and the food chemical industry, by assuring them they will vote for their laws to preserve their profits, while the same companies contribute to the destruction of the environment and wildlife. We cannot expect these political morons to want this type of change when they are blind to the fact that they are poisoning themselves, and their children, daily with the food choices they make. Perhaps this is part of the reason why congress has not stepped up and forced many changes within the food industry. Or maybe the kickbacks they are receiving from huge corporations and industry trade groups are more important to them than their health or the health of their families. I think it may be a little of both.

"What does a fish know about the water in which he swims all of his life?" – Albert Einstein

The sad truth is that many of us were raised eating the same food we now eat and have grown accustomed to filling ourselves with poison rather than nourishing ourselves with real foods, so we know no other way. This is the reason why the "genetic myth" is so common. Many diseases are passed down from generation to generation, not entirely because of cells or genes, but because the same food choices, eating habits, and activities are passed down from generation to generation. Dr. Russell Blaylock provides support of this claim in his book, *Health and Nutrition Secrets.* He states that, *"Our early nutrition significantly influences our genes, affecting our health as adults. Poor nutrition leads to programming for an early onset of cardiovascular and brain degeneration and cancer."* He also mentions in the book how we can successfully turn gene cells on and off with our food choices. If we are predisposed to some type of degenerative illness, we can often avoid it entirely by eating a clean, plant-based diet and avoiding all chemicals, food additives, and low-grade foods – such as fried foods.

FOOD ADDITIVES

"Food producers are deliberately supplementing the diet with food additives of a toxic nature at the rate of over three pounds per year for every person in America." – *Viktoras Kulvinskas, Survival into the 21st Century*

The average diet consists of a variety of foods and drinks containing flours, sugars, MSG, hydrogenated oils; sodium benzoate and other health depleting preservatives; high-fructose corn syrup; salt, aspartame, artificial colors (food dyes) and flavors; milk, meat, cheese, eggs, genetically modified produce; pesticides, fungicides, miticides, defoliants, and many more toxins. This means you are not eating actual food, but rather, you are eating concoctions that consist of mixtures of many unhealthful chemicals. These chemicals are added in small enough amounts that they will not kill you immediately, but they will slowly deteriorate your organs, your skin, and your vitality, paving the way for the diseases known to the medical world as "degenerative," and "chronic."

"I understand why millions worldwide use stimulants such as tobacco, alcohol, coffee, tea, cola drinks, and 'pep pills.' They try to fight the desperate moods of fatigue and depression caused by auto-intoxication. Most people are not living; they are merely existing. They are so full of toxic poisons that living becomes an effort. Few people rise early to see the sunrise and greet the new day with eagerness and joy. I do now. Analyze your life. Improve where needed." – *Paul Bragg, ND. PhD*

One of the worst food additives is monosodium glutamate (MSG). There are many names for MSG, including: calcium cascinate, hydrolyzed vegetable protein, textured protein, monopotassium glutamate, hydrolyzed plant protein, maltodextrin, yeast extract, glutamate, autolyzed plant protein, glutamic acid, sodium caseinate, and autolyzed yeast. Each one of these coded names contains similar excitotoxin components. Excitotoxins are neurotransmitters, such as glutamate, that damage the nerve cells by means of excessive or altered stimulation. MSG is an excitotoxin that has been linked to obesity, asthma, headaches, depression, seizures, and heart disease, to list a few. When it was discovered how toxic and poisonous MSG is to the body; the food industry and pharmaceutical industry tried to sneak around the warnings and code the names. As a result, we continue to get sick from chemicals that alter nerve function. It is of utmost importance that we eliminate all foods from the diet containing MSG or any of its aliases.

"Ever read the 'nutritional' labels on food packages? They think so little of your intelligence that they list all of the stuff they put in your food that WILL kill you. You see twelve words that you cannot pronounce and you eat it anyways. All of the chemicals, preservatives, sugars, and poisons they add to food; this is not nutrition, this is behavior modification. America is the number one hoarder of money, land, natural resources, and food. We eat more food more often than any other nation, and then carry it around inside of us for seven weeks, seven months, seven years, even seventy years, while it putrefies and decays. That is why you all stink. Your armpits, your bad breath, they are telling you that you stink from what you eat. From what is rotting inside of you." – Dick Gregory, Intro to Viktoras Kulvinskas' Survival into the 21st Century

I am sure by now you have heard of trans-fats and how bad they are for your body and your health. Trans-fats are unsaturated fats that have a double carbon-carbon bond. Because of this double bond, fewer bonds connect to hydrogen, so there are fewer hydrogen atoms. During the food production process, hydrogen is added to eliminate the double bonds and create a complete or partial saturated fat. This product, known as partially-hydrogenated or hydrogenated oil, is then added to most of the common foods eaten by the average person on a Standard American Diet. These fats have been linked to increased risk of coronary heart disease in multiple medical studies.

Concurrently, I am confident many of you are not yet aware that although some regional laws have been passed banning the use of trans-fats, many of the food manufacturers still sneak them into their products. When you see a packaged food featuring the claim "zero grams of trans-fat," be sure to check the label. In the ingredients you will most likely see some type of partially-hydrogenated or hydrogenated oils. These are trans-fats. Any oil that is added to a packaged, processed food item is equivalent to trans-fat. When fats and oils are cooked, fried, sautéed, or otherwise highly heated, they become rancid. Rancid oils and rancid fats are equivalent to trans-fats. Nearly all cooked meats contains trans-fats. All dairy products, after pasteurization, contain trans-fats. Even chocolate, whether dark, or milk chocolate, contains trans-fats. This does not mean you cannot eat chocolate any more, it means you must make the conversion over to "raw chocolate." You can find recipes for "raw chocolate" all over the internet which call for the use of raw organic cacao powder or raw organic carob powder. These recipes can also be found in almost any raw food recipe book. Check out *Hooked On Raw* by Rhio, or *Ani's Raw Food Desserts* by Ani Phyo. Because cacao can be considered a neurotoxin and makes many people feel edgy, the use of carob is becoming increasingly more common. It is also important to refrain from using agave syrup.

The questions that many people start to ask now are: Why are these chemicals being added to our foods? Why have we believed that we have been eating good food when it has been poisoning us all along? The answer to why the chemicals are being added to the food is because the food companies use them to "improve" taste, add to the consistency of the food product, and increase the shelf life. Because the good omega-3 oils go rancid and decrease shelf life, they replace them with trans-fats. Meanwhile the pharmaceutical companies are investing in these food chemical companies, knowing these food additives will slowly degenerate our cells and tissues over time and lead to the development of different diseases. There are growing concerns that some of the money that has gone to cancer research and to the research of certain diseases has really been going to create food additives that will keep these sicknesses in existence. Many believe this research money just feeds the sickness.

The truth is that we have been deceived by the food industry. We have been misled by the pharmaceutical empire that controls a portion of our economy. We have been lulled into believing anything in a package is safe because it is marketed as being beneficial or enjoyable. These chemicals are keeping the massively profitable pharmaceutical industry prospering. They are a major reason why we remain sick, develop degenerative diseases, and die by the millions from unnecessary and unnatural deaths.

In 2008, the *Center for Science in the Public Interest* (CSPI) in Washington, DC, petitioned the *Food and Drug Administration* (FDA) to ban artificial food dyes because of their connection to behavioral problems in children. Two years later, a new CSPI report, *Food Dyes: A Rainbow of Risks*, further concluded that the nine artificial dyes approved in the United States likely are carcinogenic (cancer-causing), cause hypersensitivity reactions and behavioral problems, or are inadequately tested. This was published in an October 2010 issue of *Environmental Health Perspectives.* These artificial dyes are derived from petroleum and are found in thousands of foods, most commonly in breakfast cereals, candy, snacks, beverages, vitamins, and other products that are advertised to appeal to children.

If you continue to eat foods full of these additives while failing to provide your body with the nutrients it needs, just as you would need to maintain a building or a car engine, your organs will begin to fail you. Ingesting foods lacking in true nutrients, and with weak energy, toxins, and chemicals, assures that each new cell your body generates at that time will also be toxic, weak, and likely to function at a low level.

To make things worse, people feed their children this garbage and the poor kids have no other choice but to eat it. All of this is sad to watch and it is taking place in an increasing number of countries as they begin to adapt to the unhealthful American way of eating, and as GMO foods are grown more frequently and being used in the international food chain by profit-driven corporations. I have hope that together we will change this soon. We have to stop supporting the fast food industry. We have to stop consuming these chemical-laden foods. Although it may be a challenge at first, you have to decide what is more important to you: The feeling of being stuffed with low-quality food, or the feeling of being alive and in good health? Are you going to choose cheap foods that are really just stomach fillers, or will you provide your family with the foods that nurture vibrant health?

I urge you to do your own research on food additives, and when you do, read articles from the *Pesticide Action Network*, review studies from the *Organic Consumer's Association*, and look for studies published in the *Vegetarian Journal* or any sources that have not in some way been funded by the pharmaceutical, food, dairy, egg, or meat industries. Read books from credible sources such as *Excitotoxins* by Dr. Russell Blaylock, *What's In Your Food* by Bill Statham, and *Food Politics* by Marion Nestle. Remember, the commercialized food industry pays people to write false reports in order to continue misleading the consumer, so it is wise to find credible sources that are not being paid off.

"The rapid degeneration of the Australian aborigines after the adoption of the Government's modern foods provides a demonstration that should be infinitely more convincing than animal experimentation. It should be a matter not only of concern, but deep alarm that human beings can degenerate physically, so rapidly, by the use of a certain type of nutrition, particularly the dietary products used so generally by modern civilization." – Dr. Weston A. Price, Nutrition and Physical Degeneration

PROCESSED FOODS

"Millions upon millions of Americans are merrily eating away; unaware of the pain and disease they are taking into their bodies with every bite. We are ingesting nightmares for breakfast, lunch, and dinner." – John Robbins, Diet for a New America

According to Dr. Robert S. Harris in his *Nutritional Evaluation of Food Processing*, "Nutrients are destroyed when foods are processed because many nutrients are highly sensitive to heat, light, oxygen, and the pH of various substances and additives used in the process. There is no question that processing food reduces the amount of nutrients that are contained within."

Surveys conducted by the *USDA Economics Research Service* (ers.usda.gov) reveal that around seventy percent of the calories in the Standard American Diet come from processed foods. These consist of all foods that have been altered. When altered, especially with high heat, the proteins become denatured, the enzymes are inactivated, the vitamins are damaged, and the biophotons fade or vanish.

Many of these foods have been "fortified" with synthetic nutrients. These nutrients have very little, if any, positive effect on the body. Examples of foods that may be in your pantry that are fortified would be cereals, crackers, pasta, toaster pastries, and frozen microwaveable food products.

Dr. Weston A. Price did a ten-year study of fourteen indigenous cultures. The results are in his book titled, *Nutrition and Physical Degeneration.* Every primitive culture he studied that had not been exposed to the Westernized diet had virtually no disease, no sickness, perfect dental arches, very little tooth decay, and extremely high immunity when he first arrived. Only a short distance away in the port towns, where the people were introduced to the Standard American Diet of processed foods, hydrogenated oils, canned items, bleached flours, and white sugars, he immediately began noticing changes. Sickness and disease was common. In fact, the very same diseases that occur in the United States began to occur in these fourteen other regions. Dental caries appeared. Newborns had crooked teeth, deformed jaws, and smaller craniums. The IQ's in adults and children began to lower. He concluded that processed foods not only deteriorate the health of adults and children, but also degenerate the organs and body, and literally lower the intellect of those who eat them.

If you have cabinets full of processed foods, I encourage you to dispose of them and replenish your cupboard with high-quality organic foods provided by nature and free of synthetic nutrients and chemical additives.

FAST FOOD

In my world, fast food does not exist. The last time I ate fast food I was twelve years old. I am lucky because my father regularly prepared nutritious meals for our family. When I did have fast food, it tasted odd to me. I refuse to eat at fast-food restaurants. On a trip to the Florida Keys one year with my family, my sister wanted to get the sweet tea from McDonald's. During the stop I had to use the restroom and because I refuse to go into McDonald's, I walked about six minutes away to use a different restroom because I was disgusted by the smell of the place. I simply dislike all fast food chains. In my opinion, McDonald's is guilty of just about every crime possible, from human rights, to animal abuse, political corruption, environmental destruction, and causing the extinction of species. I passed one by the other day and saw their sign that displayed the wording: *"Proud to Have Served Over 99 Billion."* The sign should have read: *"Proud to Have Poisoned Over 99 Billion."*

When I go running, I often go out of my way to be sure I bypass the local Burger King. The smell of that place lingers in the air and is suffocating. When I smell it, I get an uneasy feeling. I think of the Animal Holocaust, of factory farms, and slaughterhouses. It smells like the burning flesh and the tortured souls of what were once beautiful, innocent animals that should still be roaming the Earth.

Something I learned while researching is that meat which has been seized because of contamination is often resold as what they label as class 4-D meat. This is the meat they use in fast food items. In accordance to the USDA beef grading guidelines, grade four meat is when *the carcass is usually completely covered with external fat, except that muscle is visible in the shank, outside of the flank and plate regions. Usually, there is a moderately thick layer of external fat over the inside of the round, loin, and rib, along with a thick layer of fat over the rump and sirloin. There are usually large deposits of fat in the flank, cod or udder, kidney, pelvic and heart regions.* This means the meat served is loaded with cooked fat, which is a major contributor to heart disease, obesity, heart attacks, strokes, and cancer.

In an article published in a 2008 *Obesity Reviews* journal, *researchers analyzed total fat and trans fat in seventy-nine samples of fast-food menus consisting of French fries and fried chicken (nuggets/hot wings) bought in McDonalds and KFC outlets in twenty-six countries in 2005–2006. They found that menus standardized to the total fat content in 160 g of chicken meat and 171 g of French fries (a large serving at an American McDonald outlet) varied from forty-one to sixty-five grams at McDonalds and from forty-two to seventy-four grams at KFC.* That study shows that the same product, by the same provider, can vary in fat calorie content by more than forty percent, and unknown to the consumer, may not substantially comply with recommendations for healthy food. In this case, it is possible that supposedly standardized fast food meals contribute more to an unhealthy diet than currently thought. These meals are said to be standardized, meaning they are planned in accordance to a government regulated nutritional standard.

I'm sure you have heard the statement at least a hundred times in your life, but you really are what you eat. You become what you eat because the cells which your body generates during the moments you are eating are constructed of the substances you have eaten. Fast food meat is often dyed with sodium nicotinate to keep it from appearing as its real color, which is a yellowish gray. Not many meat eaters would care to see yellowish-gray meat on their plate, but after a little coloring is added to make it appear more "flesh-like," they will devour it.

To be at an optimal level of health, fast food cannot be included in your diet. It is not okay to have it once a week. It is not okay to have it once-in-a-while. You should never consider fast food as food. I know it can be convenient to stop at a drive-thru and grab that quick and toxic stomach filler, but think about how much more convenient your good health will be if you avoid these food choices and eat only high quality foods containing real nutrients.

SUBWAY: EAT PROCESSED

There is a popular line in the movie *Braveheart* where the King of England says, *"The problem with Scotland is that it is full of Scots."* Well, I would like to borrow the tone of that lousy king with a claim of my own: *"The problem with Subway is that it is full of subs."*

A very common misconception is that Subway is a healthy eating option. Although it is a healthier option than most other fast-food establishments – because the food items contain fewer calories, this does not mean the quality of the food is beneficial to health. Millions of people indulge in Subway products believing they are nurturing their bodies. Just because a guy named Jared who was overweight decided to exercise and start moving and as a result lost some weight, it does not in any way mean he is completely healthy. Jared did a great job overcoming obesity, but I do not think standing behind a fast-food corporation to promote his weight loss sends a good message out to those others who may be trying to lose weight.

Fast food restaurants serve processed meats containing nitrites and nitrates, which have been identified as cancer-causing, as well as heterocyclic amines and other cooked meat carcinogens; breads containing bleached, refined gluten grain flours and bromide; soft drinks loaded with artificial sweeteners, chemicals, phosphoric acid, and the ever so dangerous sodium benzoate; fruits and vegetables that are often genetically modified; and dairy products that are full of growth hormones, low-quality proteins, and antibiotics. In addition, the chains promote their foods as being healthy, when they are truly hazardous combinations of all of the worst food groups that are also saturated with chemicals.

If, by being healthy, they mean eating the food will make you more likely to have a heart attack, this would be accurate advertising. Rather, their marketing is misleading. The reality behind their foods is that there are various types of unhealthful ingredients packed into one "meal." This, I must say, is the opposite of "healthy."

In independent laboratory tests conducted by the *Physician's Committee for Responsible Medicine*, it was found that KFC's grilled chicken items contain alarming amounts of PhIP, one of the most abundant heterocyclic amines in cooked meats. This carcinogen is known to bind directly to DNA, causing mutations. DNA mutation is considered by many experts to be the first step in cancer development. Although these tests were carried out to specifically target menu items from KFC, this does not single them out as the only fast-food establishment serving items containing these cancer-causing compounds. It is a widespread belief that all meats cooked at high temperatures contain some heterocyclic amines.

Do you know what the seven worst categories of foods are? They are meat, dairy, eggs, processed sugars, cooked oils, processed salts, and gluten flours. Fast food joints serve all of these and they combine each of them together in one meal. This is not proper food combining. Each of these items requires different digestive juices to be broken down and digested. When the food products are mixed, as they are with any sandwich, the digestive juices neutralize each other and the food does not digest well. This is why many people carry around extra pounds of weight and have excess plaque coating their intestinal walls. It is the sugars, gluten grains, fermentation, putrefactive bacteria, animal protein, rancid oils, and slew of toxic chemicals that lead to cancer, obesity, heart disease, diabetes, and many other diseases.

"The Western lifestyle is characterized by a highly caloric diet, rich in fat, refined carbohydrates and animal protein, combined with low physical activity, resulting in an overall energy imbalance. It is associated with a multitude of disease conditions, including obesity, diabetes, cardiovascular disease, arterial hypertension and cancer. Malignancies typical for affluent societies are cancers of the breast, colon/rectum, uterus (endometrial carcinoma), gallbladder, kidney and adenocarcinoma of the esophagus." – The World Health Organization

Have you ever seen the videos where burgers from the most popular fast food companies were left out to rot and they did not decompose? Because of the additives and preservatives, many of these foods do not break down. French fries could sit out for decades and the structure of them would not change much. Now imagine what happens when you allow these toxic items to enter your body. We cannot consider anything that will not decompose in nature to be food. Fast food "restaurants" serve plasticized food.

What people need to realize is that calories are not everything. When eating at places such as Subway because of the "low calorie" count in their menu items, or similarly, with following a diet such as Weight Watchers to count calories, one can still become unhealthy and eat their way to sickness. The problems we face in this country do not have to do with eating excessive calories as much as they do with eating garbage, additives, and GMO's. Cancer will still develop if you eat one thousand calories a day of processed, chemically laced foods before it will develop if you were to eat three thousand calories of raw, organic plant-based foods.

Heart disease is mostly attributed to poor diet. Dietary cholesterol is found only in animal-based foods. In the *China Study*, Dr. T. Colin Campbell studied the dietary effects on blood cholesterol levels and determined that *animal protein consumption by men was associated with increasing levels of "bad" blood cholesterol, whereas plant protein consumption was associated with decreasing levels of this same cholesterol.* This tells us we should avoid animal products if we want to lower our cholesterol levels and prevent heart disease. Simply restricting calories will not prevent disease from occurring.

50

The worst of the animal products are the processed meats and cheeses. *The University of Hawaii executed a study that followed nearly 200,000 men and women for seven years. The results concluded that people who consumed the most processed meats showed a sixty-percent increased risk of pancreatic cancer over those who did not consume processed meats.*

The staple of the Subway diet is processed meat. It depends on what the customer orders, but other than their veggie option, each sub they serve is piled with processed meat and offers the choice of adding cheese. Meat is a major contributor to cancer and heart disease. Cheese is a major contributor to heart disease and cancer. The flours and gluten grains used in the bread contain compounds that trigger a variety of health problems. The refined sugars, sodium benzoate, and food coloring hidden in the condiments, bread, pickles, peppers, "fresh" fruit slices, and soft drinks compromise the function of the pancreas. The margarine made from palm oil that is in the cookies, and soybean oil in the bread, both oxidize the cells and cause inflammation, leading to weakness and fatigue.

I noticed a middle aged man sitting in the Subway located inside of a local "health club." He was wearing nice clothes and most likely makes a fairly decent salary. He was drinking a PowerAde and eating a sub with white bread. Why a "health club" would sell these items to their members who are trying to make a positive lifestyle change is baffling.

Unbeknownst to him, drinking PowerAde may cause his blood sugars to fluctuate, and deplete his power. The flours, sugars, and oils also inhibit his absorption and utilization of nutrients. In this moment, he had been deceived by the power of the marketing industry. *"People may think they're doing something healthy by grabbing a bottle of PowerAde instead of a can of Coke,"* says Kara Gallagher, PhD, an assistant professor of exercise physiology at the University of Louisville, *"but at ten calories per ounce, that PowerAde is almost as bad as a can of cola, which has twelve per ounce. Unless you're exercising vigorously, you don't need sports drinks. They have a lot of empty calories, just like anything else,"* she says.

Partially because celebrities and athletes promote fast-food chains as being healthy, there is a societal epidemic of irritable bowel syndrome and diverticulitis. Because of the junk sold by fast foods corporations, we are witnessing degenerative diseases, such as obesity and diabetes, becoming increasingly common. These garbage foods also lead to cancer, heart disease, arthritis, cancer, strokes, erectile dysfunction, and emotional disorders.

If you are a stellar athlete, or someone who is well known and well respected in society, you should be ashamed of selling out to these terrible corporations selling toxic foods that rob people of good health. Do you realize how many children look up to you because you inspire them? You are misleading them into a life of illness. I urge you to end any contract you have with them and start endorsing products that truly are healthy.

SODA IS A MIXTURE OF DEADLY CHEMICALS

I will never understand why people drink soda. Do you know that for every eight ounces of soda you drink, you add so much acidity to your body that you would need anywhere from thirty to thirty-five eight ounce glasses of water simply to dilute the acidity? Think about this and then consider that many people drink multiple sodas daily. This means they are far behind in terms of catching up to their alkaline balance. Having an acidic blood pH means disaster in the body. When your blood is acidic, your body is a breeding ground for disease. You also gain extra weight, your bones weaken and become brittle, your complexion fades, and you tax your digestive organs.

In 2001, David S. Ludwig, MD, PhD, director of the obesity program at *Children's Hospital Boston,* and colleagues at the *Harvard School of Public Health,* presented the first strong evidence linking soft drink consumption to childhood obesity. *They tracked the diets of 548 teens for nineteen months and found that kids who drank sugar-sweetened beverages regularly were more likely to be overweight than those who didn't. The researchers also found that the odds of becoming obese increased sixty percent for each can or glass a day of sugar-sweetened soft drinks.*

Soda contains high amounts of phosphoric acid, which inhibits our ability to absorb calcium and magnesium. When we are consumers of these unhealthy drinks, our bodies use the calcium in our bones to buffer the acidity. This weakens our bones and leads to osteoporosis. The sugars in sodas also feed candida yeast, and trigger weight gain, even when a person is drinking diet sodas. *Researchers found that the risk for becoming overweight increases by forty-one percent with each can of daily diet soda.* These findings were a result of eight years of data collected by Sharon P. Fowler, MPH, and her colleagues at the *University of Texas Health Science Center* in San Antonio.

I often wonder who came up with the awful idea to mix a combination of deadly chemicals together, add chemical sweeteners, and then drink the concoction. This does not sound the least bit logical.

As much as it is comical to think about, it really is sad to know that some people believe drinking "diet soda" will help them lose weight. This is so far from the truth. Bone mineral density loss, compromised cellular health, and a shortened lifespan are more likely to happen for those who consume these colas and sodas, sweetened or not.

If you are still questioning my accusation that the hospitals and the medical industry are clueless about true health, and to the point that it can be concluded that they want patients to get sicker, consider this: *it was recorded by the Soft Drink Association that eighty-five percent of hospitals in America serve sodas with their patient's meals.* In addition to serving sodas, the meals they serve are loaded down with a stew of typical food additives. If they really understood health and nutrition, they would not be serving garbage foods including meat, dairy, eggs, bleached gluten grains, and processed sugars and salts that induce illnesses; the very same illnesses their staffed doctors are "treating."

Soda is ten thousand times more acidic than distilled water. If you pour soda over a piece of the flesh of an animal, the flesh will eventually deteriorate. This also happens in your body. If you drink diet soda, or any soda at all, I urge you to quit immediately. Let the habit go and watch how fast you will see improvements in your health and life.

Soft drinks are referred to as 'soft' drinks for a reason. They soften your bones, teeth, and your chances of maintaining good health. If you want to be healthy, you simply cannot drink sodas, colas, caffeine-loaded "energy" drinks, or other highly-acidic, sugary, toxic chemically-saturated beverages. No exceptions. Even many 'fruit' juices sold in stores are not healthy.

DINING OUT

It is not only fast food and packaged processed foods that sicken us. Foods served in fancy restaurants are just as bad. I know of many couples who go out to eat every evening. They might believe they are eating healthfully because they are spending an absurd amount of money on food. They all have health issues. I have observed eight reasons why people go out to eat so frequently:

TOP EIGHT REASONS FOR GOING OUT TO EAT

1.) **They are addicted to the chemicals in the food**
2.) **They are too caught up in the status quo**
3.) **For the social life**
4.) **They do not know how to prepare meals**
5.) **They think it is healthy**
6.) **It is more convenient to eat out**
7.) **They save the time of preparing meals**
8.) **Safety of meeting in public rather than at home**

Every sit down restaurant, unless it is all organic, serves food containing residues of farming chemicals, and often synthetic chemical food additives. When we eat these foods, we really do become addicted, especially to foods containing MSG-based flavor enhancers.

I served an excellent raw quinoa dish at a party one time and a guy who eats only processed foods asked me whether or not I added salt to it. Well, I did add some pink Himalayan sea salt only because I knew the people at the party were used to salt. When I prepare food for myself I never add salt. This guy could not taste the added salt because he had become so accustomed to the strong flavor of the chemical MSG, and to salty processed foods. MSG is the most common additive in restaurants. They add it so you will always crave that particular food and come back for more. This poor guy had been poisoned so much that he lost his sense of taste and the taste of real food was absent to him. If any of you ever experience that loss of taste, remember this: a zinc deficiency may be the reason for the loss of taste. The chemicals in these foods deplete minerals from your body. As you clean up your diet, include things like raw pumpkin seeds, poppy seeds, and pecans. These will help you regain your natural taste sensation.

If you are concerned about status and feel as if you want to show off how much money you have by dining out at the nicest restaurants, I advise that you choose the nicest "raw," or organic restaurants. What good is having all of the money in the world if you do not have your health? Good health and a naturally vibrant appearance are both far more admirable and represent wealth in a much better fashion than nice clothes and makeup covering an unhealthy body and blemished skin. Get over the insecurities of worrying if people think you have a lot of money. In doing so, you may find that your life becomes more enjoyable.

If I am going to spend time with people I know who are insisting on going to a venue serving foods that I will not eat, I eat healthful foods before I go. Then, when I arrive, I stay for the socializing. We talk, we have fun, and we leave. You do not have to eat or drink. If you do order food, stay away from the cooked, refined foods and avoid all animal products. Go for the salad and maybe a light appetizer or side. You will feel much better after you leave. You will also not feel paralyzed and like you want to lie down as you do so often when leaving restaurants.

If you eat out at restaurants because you simply do not know how to prepare foods, this is a perfect opportunity for you to build and add on to who you are. You could try taking a raw chef certification course. Look up Cherie Soria and her *Living Light Culinary Institute* in Fort Bragg, California. This is the very best raw culinary school. It is in a beautiful location, and the instructors are full of vibrant energy, passion, and enthusiasm. If California is not an option for you, look into the *Matthew Kenney Academy*.

You could also pick up some raw recipe books and experiment in the kitchen. Mimi Kirk has an excellent raw recipe book titled *Live Raw*. Ani Phyo has many raw recipe books; my favorite is *Ani's Raw Food Kitchen*. Jeremy Saffron also released *The Raw Truth: Second Edition*. Eric Rivkin has a raw recipe book he titled *To Live For*. You can also look up *Rawfully Tempting* online, Dara Dubinet and Jason Wrobel videos on YouTube, or Andrea Cox (healthyhaven.net) for a variety of terrific and enjoyable raw recipes.

If you are a couple and all you ever seem to do is go out to eat, making food together at home could save your relationship. In few relationships, when the couples only share favorite restaurants, at some point or another, one of the two decides they have had enough and end it. Can you blame them? To add flavor to your relationship, you could have the perfect opportunity to bond by spending time in the kitchen. Change things up a little, get into juicing, go to a yoga class, and workout together. This could save your relationship, and prevent sickness and disease.

Eating at common restaurants is not the path to excellent health. The preservatives, chemical additives, and overcooked, nutrient-deficient food you are served is degrading your health. It does not matter how much you spend, if you are eating at a place that is not vegan friendly, all organic, and/ or raw, you are not eating the best food. Break away from tradition. Get a juicer and blender, and get into physical fitness. You will be much happier and you may surprise yourself with how much extra energy you have.

IS MEAT A TOXIC FOOD?

"Meat is not man's natural food, since he is not either a carnivorous or an omnivorous animal – whatever the physiologists may say. Every argument drawn from comparative anatomy, from physiology, from chemistry, from experience, from observation and when rightly used, from common sense, as well as the arguments from agricultural, the hygienic, the ethical and humanitarian standpoints – all agree in proving that man is not a meat-eating animal and that if he does indulge in this practice, it is to his own detriment being such an unhealthful, unnatural, and abnormal habit." – Dr. Hereward Carrington

Many argue that we are omnivores, and a lot of vegans argue that we are herbivores or frugivores. The reason why we have small canine teeth is not to tear into flesh, but to tear apart the cellulose fibers in vegetables. We don't have claws that can tear into flesh, we have nails that can peel fruit. We have a very long, plant-friendly digestive tract. We were not meant to eat meat. Everything points directly to us being put here on Earth to eat fruit, some leafy green vegetables, and nothing else other than the occasional nuts, seeds, and sprouts. If you want to read a clear explanation for this, I suggest you read Graham's book, *The 80/10/10 Diet,* or McCabe's *Sunfood Diet Infusion.*

The most important fact about this argument is the realization that, whether we are omnivores or not, this is not relevant to whether we should or should not be eating meat. The truth is that no matter what we are, or no matter what we were supposedly created to eat, meat consumption is killing us. Excess animal protein, and cooked meat carcinogens – such as heterocyclic amines and polycyclic aromatic hydrocarbons – in the diet are linked to many degenerative diseases, including cardiovascular disease, macular degeneration, diabetes, osteoporosis, multiple sclerosis, alzheimer's, colon cancer, breast cancer, prostate cancer, erectile dysfunction, and cancers of the female anatomy. We can argue all day about whether or not we were put here on Earth to eat dead flesh that degrades our health, but we cannot argue the fact that meat consumption creates acidosis and forms carcinogens in the body and this results in disease. All meat is highly acidic and when we consume it, we are inviting premature aging, organ dysfunction, and an increased risk of cancer; heart attacks; and strokes.

In March of 2012, the *Archives of Internal Medicine* released the results of two studies on meat eating and mortality. This was the first large-scale prospective longitudinal study that showed *the consumption of both processed and unprocessed red meat is associated with an increased risk of premature mortality from all causes, as well as from cardiovascular disease, and cancer.*

In a video released in January 2013 on *nutrition facts.org*, Dr. Michael Greger discusses heterocyclic amines and how PhIP is one of the most abundant heterocyclic amines in cooked meat. These carcinogenic compounds are formed at high temperatures from the reaction between creatine or creatinine, amino acids, and sugar. PhIP is nearly impossible to avoid for those who indulge in animal products because it is found in many commonly consumed cooked meats, particularly chicken, beef, and fish. After absorption of PhIP, it is converted to a genotoxic metabolite in the liver, becoming more likely to cause DNA mutation, trigger cancer, and promote tumor growth. In a 2009 issue of **Mutagenesis Journal**, a study was published titled *Dietary Intake of Meat and Meat-derived Heterocyclic Aromatic Amines and Their Correlation with DNA Adducts in Female Breast Tissue.* The study found that ingestion of PhIP causes DNA mutation that may initiate tumor growth, promotes cancer due to potent estrogenic activity, and promotes the invasiveness of breast cancer cells. This may explain the high incidence of breast cancer around the world. Eating animal products could be the trigger.

In a 2005 edition of the **Chemical Research in Toxicology** journal, a study was published finding more than twenty heterocyclic amines in cooked meats, fish, and poultry prepared under common household cooking conditions. This includes baking, boiling, broiling, frying, grilling, sauteeing, and smoking. Urine samples from subjects eating meat were found to contain high levels of PhIP, and other health degrading heterocyclic compounds. Even those who refrained from eating meat, yet still included boiled eggs, or cheese, in their diet showed traces of these harmful compounds in their urine.

In a comparative risks analysis study, it was found that *one piece of grilled steak has the equivalent carcinogens as six-hundred cigarettes. This is equivalent to smoking a pack a day for thirty days each time a steak is eaten.* This comparison was based on a study that was published in *Science Journal* back in 1964. Now think about people who eat steak every day and smoke. This is why heart disease and cancer are so common among people who do so. One main source of these carcinogens in grilled meats are polycyclic aromatic hydrocarbons. These polycyclic aromatic hydrocarbons are highly carcinogenic atmospheric pollutants that are formed by incomplete combustion of carbon-containing fuels such as coal, tar, wood, fat, tobacco, and incense. When the fat and juices from the meat drip over the heat source, causing flames, these flames then adhere to the surface of the meat. Multiple studies have shown that high levels of these hydrocarbons are found in cooked foods, particularly in meats cooked at high temperatures, such as with grilling or barbecuing; and in smoked fish.

"What are we eating? We are eating the rotting carcass of a murder victim. So let's not dress it up." – Philip Wollen

In March of 2012, researchers at *Harvard Medical School* released the results of a study concluding that a diet high in red meat will shorten life expectancy. They studied over 120,000 people and found that red meat increased their risk of death from cancer and heart problems. The team analyzed data from 37,698 men between 1986 and 2008, and 83,644 women between 1980 and 2008. Their study proved that by adding an extra portion of unprocessed red meat to someone's daily diet, they would increase their risk of death by thirteen percent. They would also increase their risk of developing cardiovascular disease by eighteen percent, and cancer by ten percent. The figures for processed meat were higher, with a twenty percent overall mortality, twenty-one percent for death from heart problems, and sixteen percent for cancer mortality.

While most studies point directly to red meat and pork as being the most toxic meat sources, poultry is beginning to more recently be exposed as a serious health threat. In July 2012, *ABC News and the Food & Environment Reporting Network* carried out a joint investigation, discovering that a growing number of medical researchers are claiming that more than eight million women are at risk of contracting urinary tract infections from superbugs that are resistant to antibiotics and growing in chickens. These superbugs are being transmitted to humans in the form of E.coli and prions. Prions are infectious agents composed of proteins in a misfolded form. They are responsible for the transmissible encephalopathies found in many mammals and cannot be destroyed by means of irradiation, or any other form of pasteurization, or cooking. All known prion diseases affect the structure of the brain or other neural tissue, and are untreatable and universally fatal.

Amee Manges, epidemiologist at *McGill University* in Montreal, shared her knowledge on this issue stating, *"We are finding the same, or related E.coli in human infections and in retail meat sources, specifically chicken."* Maryn McKenna, reporter for the *Food & Environment Reporting Network*, summed this up by announcing, *"What this new research shows is, we may in fact know where it is coming from. It may be coming from antibiotics used in agriculture."*

"We've known for fourteen years that a single meal of meat, dairy, and eggs triggers an inflammatory reaction inside the body within hours of consumption. Within five or six hours, the inflammation starts to cool down, but then what happens? At that point we can whack our arteries with another load of animal products for lunch. In this routine, we may be stuck in a chronic low-grade inflammation danger zone for most of our lives. This can set us up for inflammatory diseases such as heart disease, diabetes, and certain cancers one meal at a time." – Dr. Michael Greger

Throughout life it is wise that we focus on longevity and being as healthy as we can for as long as we can; that we keep our bodies nourished, and minds active by utilizing our talents and intellect. In order to do this we must keep our organs healthy and our minds engaged. Eating meat damages our organs, drains our vitality, and voids our opportunity to experience vibrant health. The oils and cholesterol in meat slow our system, alter our ability to detox and eliminate waste, and leave residues in our tissues; laying the groundwork for the accumulation of more toxins.

"The more red meat and blood we eat, the more blood thirsty and violent we get. The more vegetarian food we eat, the more peaceful we become." – Ziggy Marley

It is safe to say that eating the flesh of dead animals is not in any way relevant to extending longevity; it is not in any way relevant to curing anything. I do not find it to be positive in any way to take the life of any creature, and I also know that the pharmaceutical industry flourishes from the consumption of meat and dairy. The pharmaceutical industry makes tremendous amounts of money from selling drugs to the animal farming industry for the livestock, and then they make more money from the people suffering from the effects of eating the chemically-saturated meat, dairy, and eggs. In the *Union of Concerned Scientists* report on antibiotic use in livestock, the author and director of their food and environment program, Dr. Margaret Mellon, reported that, *"U.S. livestock producers use about 24.6 million pounds of antibiotics annually for 'non-therapeutic' purposes (growth promotion and disease prevention) as opposed to treatment of disease. The non-therapeutic total includes about 10.3 million pounds in hogs, 10.5 million pounds in poultry and 3.7 million pounds in cattle. By contrast, humans use approximately three million pounds of antibiotics annually in the U.S."* This statement reveals to us that pharmaceutical companies make more money from selling drugs to the owners of factory farms, to inject in the animals for non-therapeutic purposes, than they do from humans purchasing them to attempt to combat their illnesses.

A step in the right direction for us is the outcome of a court case in March of 2012. In the case of the *Natural Resources Defense Council et al. v. FDA, in the U.S. District Court for the Southern District of New York, no. 11-3562,* a federal judge ruled that U.S. regulators start proceedings to withdraw approval for the use of common antibiotics in animal feed, citing concerns that overuse is endangering human health by creating antibiotic-resistant superbugs. At the time of this ruling, antibiotic-resistant infections were costing Americans more than $20 billion each year. This number was determined by a 2009 study conducted by the *Alliance for the Prudent Use of Antibiotics and Cook County Hospital.* As we awaken to the dangers behind the meat industry and begin to see that meat consumption is in no way benefiting our health, I have hope that we will be on the better side of many more court rulings.

To be safe, and assure good health, the best thing that we can do regarding this matter is choose to refrain from eating all meat.

THE PROTEIN MYTH

In the book, *Diet For A Small Planet,* Frances Moore Lappe uses the analogy, *"Eating meat to get protein is about as efficient as paddling a canoe with a chopstick."* This is not a fallacy. Meat is a very poor source for the amino acids we need to form protein.

We have known for decades that most plant-based fats are healthy, while fats from animal products are harmful. It is common to hear about bad carbohydrates from refined flours and sugars, and healthy carbohydrates coming from fresh, raw fruits. Why is it though, that we still have not been able to distinguish the good from bad proteins? Meat, dairy, and eggs do contain proteins, however this is not the protein we want as humans. This is bad protein. We want protein from edible plant matter.

The first thing that many of us need to realize is that we need amino acids, not foreign animal proteins, to form proteins. There are twenty different food-sourced amino acids from which proteins are made. When we take in animal proteins, our system breaks them down into the individual amino acids we need to make proteins of our own that we can utilize. So by eating amino acid-rich foods, we benefit more because we bypass the process of breaking down the proteins into amino acids. All plants contain the amino acids our bodies use for making protein. Because amino acids are damaged by heat, cooked meat contains damaged amino acids, and is not a good source of protein. We must go directly to the source, being plant-based foods. All raw fruits, vegetables, nuts, seeds, sprouts, and water vegetables contain the amino acids our bodies need for making proteins.

In the documentary, *A Delicate Balance*, we are introduced to an enzyme known as a *mixed function oxidase enzyme*. This enzyme acts as a natural defense mechanism, inactivating potentially harmful chemicals that enter our body, and making them harmless. Researchers discovered that only plant-based proteins will keep this enzyme active, while animal proteins inactivate the enzyme, turning the chemicals that have entered our body into carcinogens. These carcinogens then damage the genetic content of cells, and when mutated DNA is replicated, the result is cancer cell formation. The role animal protein plays in the inactivation of mixed function oxidase enzymes, explains in part how animal proteins cause our bodies to turn against us, and promote cancer progression. So not only is meat a bad source of protein for humans, the protein that is provided by meat is damaging to the human organism.

Dr. Udo Erasmus defines protein in his book, *Fats That Heal, Fats That Kill*, as, *"The main structure for the body, muscles, and cells; also for making chemistry go in the direction of life."* Protein is important. What is more important though is realizing that we do not need more than thirty-five to forty grams of protein a day in our diet, depending on our weight and height. The *World Health Organization* released a statement that suggests we not consume more than 4.5 percent of our daily caloric intake from protein. This comes out to an average of about twenty-three grams of protein per day for someone consuming around two-thousand calories a day. According to an entry in the *Journal of Clinical Nutrition*, our total calories from protein should not exceed 2.5 percent. This would only equal about thirteen grams a day.

Ideally, we should not exceed any more than eight to ten percent of our daily intake of calories from protein. Many of us are exceeding that amount and creating acidosis in our bodies. A December 2012 infographic compiled by the grocery delivery program, *Door to Door Organics*, found that Americans eat at least twelve ounces of meat daily, exceeding their "recommended" daily amount by more than fifty percent. When we have an excess amount of protein in our body, we cannot make use of it and it is stored as waste. When we metabolize the protein, we create uric acid and ammonia, in addition to several other bowel toxins.

It is nearly impossible to develop a protein deficiency eating a raw vegan diet rich in fruits and vegetables. In fact, many of us have an over abundant amount of protein in our bodies. In *Survival Into the 21st Century*, Viktoras Kulvinskas, states: *"Protein in excess of our needs is not utilized by the body. Cooking meat also destroys the amino acids that are needed for building enzymes and healthy tissues. The protein is poorly absorbed and largely unavailable to the cells. For these reasons, much of the protein we eat passes from the body or is stored in tissues as waste."* As we continue to worry that we are not receiving enough protein in our bodies, we are ingesting too much and as a result we are creating excessive amounts of waste inside of our tissues.

When people discover that I do not eat meat, dairy, or eggs, they often ask, "Where do you get your protein?" Most of the time, they follow this question by asking, "How do you keep all of that muscle on if you don't eat meat?" As much as I want to laugh at the questions they ask, I acknowledge the fact that we live in a society where myths are created and false information is spewed for the sole purpose of marketing products that range from meat to dairy to soy to pharmaceuticals – all for the sake of maximizing profits at the expense of our health and the health of our loved ones. The people who ask me these questions cannot help but believe what they were taught growing up. Often they get their nutrition education from flawed sources, such as commercials, misinformed medical professionals, and the USDA food pyramid (which was created by trade groups representing the meat, dairy, and egg industries).

As children, many of us were raised with the idea that milk will strengthen our bones, and that meat will make us stronger and help us to grow bigger. Nothing could be further from the truth. Children believe what they see, what they hear, and what they are told. When this idea is embedded in their minds throughout their childhood, they carry the misinformation with them through their lives. We need to stop this from happening to more generations, and to reverse this pattern of misinformation by teaching true, plant-based nutrition.

The best food in the world will make us more intelligent. Complete protein sources do not just make us stronger or bigger, they improve our ability to utilize our intellect. The brain runs on carbohydrates and consists of neurons that communicate by way of neurotransmitters and electrical currents. We need complete protein and the quality mineral, essential fatty acid, and enzyme sources of raw plants for these systems to run and produce serotonin, dopamine, and adrenaline.

Where do we find the best food sources that also provide complete proteins? Definitely not in animal products like milk, cream, cheese, butter, or meat. Dr. T. Colin Campbell explains in *The China Study* that, *"Foreign proteins from livestock nourish cancer cells more than they nourish our bodies."* The protein from milk, meat, or eggs, therefore, is not a good source of protein. It is natural for the animal from which it came and is a structure of amino acids formulated only for the function of that animal.

The China Study was conducted over the course of decades by researchers at Cornell and Oxford University. Over six-hundred thousand people in twenty-six different provinces were placed in groups; with one group fed a meat-based diet and the other group fed a plant based vegan diet. Only the groups that were on a meat based diet developed cancers, while not one person on the plant-based diets had any signs of cancer whatsoever. The most interesting part is that they reversed the roles, and the meat eaters who developed cancer were given a plant based diet, and their cancers soon disappeared. Concurrently, the groups who were healthy and on a plant based diet had meat introduced into their diet and they soon developed cancer. This study proves without any discrepancies that meat eating (and especially the consumption of animal protein) is directly linked to cancer.

"What protein consistently and strongly promoted cancer? Casein, which makes up eighty-seven percent of cow's milk protein, promoted all stages of the cancer process. What type of protein did not promote cancer, even at high levels of intake? The safe proteins were from plants." – Dr. T. Colin Campbell, The China Study

The main protein in milk, casein, is nourishing food for human cancer cells. Our bodies do not require this type of protein. Milk is also contaminated with a variety of chemicals and additives from the unnatural diet given to the cows. In addition, we lose our ability to digest milk in our bodies after three years of age.

When you learn about digestion, you discover that we must convert the food we eat into a liquid form, and smaller macro and micro components, in order for it to pass though the intestinal villi, get filtered through the blood, and for the nutrients to be assimilated and metabolized throughout the body. When you consider this, you have to also consider how much wear and tear you are putting on your body by forcing it to convert such heavy, toxic foods into liquids.

Eating meat, dairy, eggs, and highly heated foods require more energy to break down and digest in order to convert to liquid form than it takes to break down raw fruits and vegetables. Protein can be broken down into amino acids and delivered to the cell sites, but the protein in animal products and highly heated foods is treated differently, requiring more work for our systems to digest.

Meat contains uric acid and urea. When digesting this poor quality food, these acid by-products become difficult to metabolize. We tend to absorb them into our muscle tissues before we can excrete them from our bodies. This is what gives the highly acidic "muscle-heads" you see roaming around the gym their bulky look. With the exception of a few vegan bodybuilders, these guys and girls are not doing themselves any favors using animal protein. Most of the time they are simply rich in foreign proteins and loaded with unnatural amounts of muscle weight, not essential for their bodies to function at a healthful level.

Do you know where bad breath comes from? Do you know where body odor comes from? Bad breath and body odor come from a variety of things, including bacteria, infected tonsils and glands, cancer, yeast, and an overload of toxins and/or foreign substances including those along the alimentary tract.

Putrefactive bacteria from the meat, dairy, eggs, and other chemicals you have overloaded your body with are problematic for the eliminative and cardiovascular systems. They also leave behind a toxic residue. This residue helps to create odors and taints your vitality, slowing and dulling the systems. Even the strongest chewing gum and heaviest deodorant will not get to the root of this problem and cease the odors from returning. These residues and putrefactive bacteria can also create the environment for illness and disease.

As I got into a natural diet, I realized that my breath improved and no longer had the need for deodorants. If you are searching for a good deodorant, use essential oils as an alternative, or go for the "Crystal" deodorant. Be sure you get the fragrance-free variety. This is simply mineral salts that you roll on and they neutralize odors without all of the chemicals contained in popular deodorants that rely on chemicals.

Going back to the protein dilemma; research done by the **Max Planck Institute of Research** concludes that when we cook meat we lose at least fifty percent of the protein. Many of the amino acids are damaged, making them useless. Of the protein remaining, depending on the heat, only about forty percent is bio-available. So if we were to eat portions of meat said to have forty grams of protein, after cooking, there would only be twenty grams remaining in each. Of that remaining protein, we will only utilize around eight grams. This is equivalent to the amount of protein we would receive from just one tablespoon of organic spirulina. The protein from spirulina is also one-hundred percent bio-available. The energy wasted used to break down animal protein, converting the solids into a liquid, will leave us feeling sluggish. Then the residues of cholesterol, saturated fat, uric acid, and cooking toxins clog our systems.

Some people understand the truth about animal protein and go off in search of a replacement. This is where they often make choices that are not the best. Many of them switch to soy products. Soy protein is not a good source of protein and soy can be problematic. Soy is notably high in phytic acid – which inhibits the body's ability to absorb, deliver, and utilize many other important nutrients. Soy is known to be estrogenic and having excess estrogen will interfere with our progesterone receptor sites, our testosterone receptor sites, and may increase our body fat.

There are reasons why some vegetarians appear frail or weak. They simply do not make very good food choices, and many consume diets rich in soy, processed salts, gluten, and lots of sautéed and processed vegan foods. It is not because they do not eat meat. The reason is that they are not nourishing their bodies in the best way, and many follow diets lacking in raw fruits and vegetables, but rich in fat and salt.

Another protein believed to be more beneficial than it is happens to be whey protein. Whey is a waste product and by-product of the dairy industry.

Whey was previously discarded of by dairy farmers until a business man decided he could fool consumers into believing it is beneficial. This triggered companies to begin packaging and distributing it as a protein supplement. As with all other dairy products, whey is also high in allergens. Do yourself a favor and stay away from whey. It is not a healthful substance, it degrades health. It is not relevant how many lab studies the company marketing the product claims it has been through. The truth is that it does not work as a health generator. More and more reports of fraudulent clinical studies are appearing over time and the best bet here is to research the obvious.

"The lie that you need to eat milk, eggs, or dead animals to get protein in your diet is the lie that has built up the factory farming and slaughterhouse industries into huge environmental travesties in which billions of animals live horrible lives and die terrible deaths – with many of them being cut into and dismembered while they are still alive.

All fruits and vegetables contain the essential amino acids your body needs to make protein. You will get all of the amino acids you need by eating enough calories of fruits, vegetables, nuts, and seeds." – John McCabe, Sunfood Traveler

Raw plant protein is always easier for the body to process than animal protein, or proteins that have been heated to high temperatures. All fruits and vegetables contain an array of amino acids. When you eat enough calories of them it is impossible to develop a protein deficiency.

Another excellent source for protein is superfoods. Medicinal mushrooms such as chaga, reishi, and maitake are rich sources of protein. The best superfoods I have found to eat for complete protein are: goji berries, hemp seeds, spirulina, blue-green algae, and chlorella. Maca powder is also a reliable source; however, this is not a complete protein source because it is one amino acid short. The grain-like quinoa is high in protein and is a good replacement for rice, pasta, and other carbohydrate sources. Be sure to eat your quinoa after it has soaked for at least a couple of hours, and while it is in its raw state to preserve vitamins and other nutrients.

All fruits and vegetables contain the perfect ratio of amino acids our bodies need for forming protein. Hemp happens to be one that a lot of people say gives them some sort of feeling of completeness, and many people say that using hemp protein has helped them satisfy their ability to stay raw vegan. The body can absorb the nutrients from hemp seeds and utilize them to build strong hair, nails, skin, muscle, and connective tissues. According to John McCabe, in his book *Sunfood Living*, *"Hemp seed provides all of the essential fatty acid and amino acid nutrients in the best form and at the best ratio for the body to maintain vibrant, strong, elastic, and healthy tissues."* Hemp seeds are the only food available that contain the exact ratio of omega-3 and omega-6 essential fatty acids. Pretty cool, huh? Aside from algae, hemp seed is the highest protein food available consisting of around thirty-six percent protein by weight. Spirulina is the number one protein source by weight.

Spirulina is a fresh water alga that consists of about sixty-five to seventy percent protein. Because it is easily converted to liquid upon entering the body, we utilize this protein more efficiently than most other sources. Spirulina consists of seven to eight percent phycocyanin (blue pigment), which is one of the most important nutrient compounds to ever be discovered. Phycocyanin has been said to generate stem cell production. In addition to the high amount of protein and the phycocyanin, two to three percent of spirulina consists of chlorophyll. Chlorophyll is the blood of plants and is also a human blood builder. This makes spirulina a terrific food choice.

To maintain an optimal level of health, we must feed ourselves a diet of undamaged amino acids. To achieve this optimal level of health, meat is not necessary, soy is not necessary, dairy is not necessary, and eggs are not necessary. We can instead eat the foods grown from Earth that are mineral rich, nutrient rich, living, and full of wonderful enzymes that will replenish us, preserve our youth, make us feel alive, and boost our ability to utilize our intellect and talents.

I don't know about you, but I like to feel energized, happy, and full of positive energy after I eat. So, I hate to spoil your pig roast, but eating animal products will do the exact opposite. They will wear down your body to the point of lethargy, draining your energy. After a meal rich in raw fruits and vegetables, I'll be out elevating my mind and bursting with happiness, positive energy, and motivational thoughts.

WAIT, THOSE PLANTS ARE ALIVE!

A lot of meat-eating advocates attempt to justify the brutal torturing and slaughtering of billions of animals each year by relating the killing of living creatures to the killing of fruits and vegetables. While I agree plants are indeed living, I do not in any way think this can justify the caging, torturing, chemical fattening, and slaughtering of billions of animals.

Dr. Richard Oppenlander does a good job distinguishing the two. He states that, *"Plants are living structures with chlorophyll-containing cells. They take carbon dioxide out of the air in exchange for producing oxygen. They do not have blood, brains, organs, nervous systems, or feelings. Contrary to this, animals are living organisms that have saturated fat and cholesterol associated with all of their cells and tissues. They do have blood, organs, brains, nervous systems, and feelings."*

If you are someone who does not want to harm these living plants, you can always eat fruits, picked green leaf vegetables, seeds, nuts, and a limited amount of certain grain-like foods. You are not harming the planet, or plant, in any way by eating these foods that do not require the killing or unrooting of the plant.

I CAN EAT EGGS, RIGHT?

"How did people ever even figure out that eggs were edible? Did they see something come out of a chicken and think, 'Boy, I bet that would be tasty?' There had to be a first person who ever ate an egg. I'm sure it wasn't pleasant." – Ellen DeGeneres

The answer is, NO. Eggs are not food for humans. There is no reason for anyone to support the egg industry. Eggs are acid-forming in the body. By eating eggs we form excess mucus. In addition to acidosis, the components of eggs, including concentrated proteins, saturated fat, and cholesterol, clog our lymphatic system, intestines, and colon. The protein in eggs is a little more bioavailable than meat, yet still not nearly as bioavailable as a plant protein source. Raw egg whites contain enzyme inhibitors that require our bodies to use internal enzymes from the pancreas to digest. We always want to avoid using these enzyme reserves. To destroy these inhibitors, the egg whites require cooking, and when you cook them, you denature the amino acids that make up the protein, and harmful heterocyclic amines begin to form.

According to *PETA* (People for the Ethical Treatment of Animals), *"There are 452 million hens being used for their eggs annually. When they no longer produce eggs, they are then slaughtered and their meat is sold as food."* For those of you who consider yourselves vegetarian and still eat eggs, you may want to research this topic a little further. You are contributing to this mass-caging, abuse, and slaughtering of these animals. Additionally, billions of male chicks that cannot produce eggs and are too small to be used for flesh are thrown into "macerators" while they are still alive, or else gassed, or suffocated in trash bags to be disposed of as waste.

Aside from the myth that eggs are the most highly utilizable source of protein, many people believe we have to eat eggs in order to sustain adequate amounts of the nutrient, choline. Choline is a vitamin that aids digestion and absorption. The truth is that we can eat whole, living foods and receive more than enough protein and choline. Choline is found in abundance in foods such as broccoli, brussels sprouts, cabbage, cauliflower, chickpeas, flaxseeds, garlic, grapes, green leafy vegetables, legumes, lentils, onions, pistachio nuts, sprouts, and ripe tomatoes.

"Of all the cancers, egg consumption was most tightly correlated with breast cancer risk. Those eating more than a half an egg a day were found to have nearly 3 times the odds of breast cancer compared to those that stayed away from eggs entirely." – Michael Greger, MD, nutritionfacts.org

Eating eggs also leads to the formation of prostate cancer. In a study published in the December 2011, *Cancer Prevention Research* journal, it was found that men who consumed 2.5 or more eggs per week had an eighty-one percent increased risk of developing lethal prostate cancer, compared with men who consumed less than 0.5 eggs per week   .

In Dr. Michael Greger's 2012 presentation "Uprooting the Leading Causes of Death," he points out that in the Harvard Heath Study's competing risks analysis – which compares risks to one another – after a thirty-five year follow up, it was found that *the amount of cholesterol from consuming one egg per day will cut a woman's life short as much as smoking 5 cigarettes a day for 15 years.*

Protein is not needed in abundance. Your best sources for protein come from complete protein foods, and what is most important is that the foods you eat contain an array of amino acids. Raw fruits, vegetables, sea vegetables, and sprouts contain these amino acids. Because we create proteins from the amino acids in plants, it should be noted that we are getting enough protein when we eat fruits, vegetables, nuts, seeds, edible flowers, and seaweeds.

Soaking raw nuts and seeds increases their amino acid content and makes the nutrients in nuts and seeds more bioavailable. Knowing this, live foodists often soak their nuts and seeds. Beyond soaking the seeds, you can also let them grow into germinates, where a small root begins to appear, and further, into sprouts, which is when the leaf formation begins.

In addition to containing beneficial nutrients, edible raw plant matter, especially greens and seaweed, also helps bring the body to a more alkaline state, eliminating acidosis, and clearing up the mucus that is present and encrusted from years of eating eggs, dairy, meat, gluten, and cooked oils.

PIZZA IS DISGUISED DISEASE

"The increase in cancer, heart disease, diabetes, obesity, and asthma that has occurred in the Western world over the past century, directly correlates with the increase in dairy consumption." – Dr. Adam Meade, Chiropractor and national health advocate

Among the worst foods you can eat are cheese, meat, processed sugars, those which are rich in oil extracts and salt, and those containing gluten grains. Pizza contains all of these ingredients, and therefore is one of the most unhealthful foods. In school cafeterias, pizza is a common choice for students and faculty. Teachers, and parents, often arrange pizza parties, where groups of children will indulge in slices of this health depleting product thinking it is okay. If you want to be vibrantly healthy, do not eat pizza. If you are a parent and you care about your child's health, do not allow them to eat pizza.

The cheese and meats in pizza contribute to heart disease, osteoporosis, strokes, and cancers. The dough containing gluten grains can trigger anxiety and bi-polar-like symptoms, and can contribute to, or aggravate, irritable bowel syndrome and thyroid imbalances. The sauce is often loaded with refined sugars, which can lead to cancer, candida overgrowth, cholesterol issues, and high trigycerides, which nurture heart disease. Knowing all of these negative health consequences, why is it that so many people still choose to bake, order, and eat this poor food choice?

"Any lactating mammal excretes toxins through her milk. This includes antibiotics, pesticides, chemicals, and hormones. Also, all cows' milk contains blood. The USDA allows milk to contain from one, to one and a half million, white blood cells per milliliter. Another way to describe white cells where they don't belong would be to call them pus cells." – Robert M. Kradjian, MD, Breast Surgery Chief Division of General Surgery, Seton Medical Centre

IS CHEESE ADDICTING?

Casein is the protein found in milk. Because there is less liquid in cheese, casein is more concentrated in cheese than it is in milk. According to Dr. Neal Barnard in *Breaking the Food Seduction*, when the body attempts to digest casein, it is converted into what is known as casomorphins. These are opiates. Just like any opiate, they are highly addicting and when people try to refrain from consuming them, they can have withdrawal symptoms. Because of this process it is within reason to say that cheese is addicting.

If you are searching for the single worst food for the development of cardiovascular disease, you can stop searching at cooked cheese. Not only is it very difficult to digest and clogs the arteries with residues, it also brings with it a bad form of coagulated, inorganic minerals, leaving calcifications of plaque in the arteries.

In an April 2008 issue of the *Journal of Human Nutrition and Dietetics*, a study titled the *Association between Cheese Consumption and Cardiovascular Risk Factors among Adults* was published. The study showed that *more frequent cheese consumption was associated with less favorable body composition and an increased cardiovascular risk profile in men.*

For the production of some cheeses, rennet, an enzyme, is used to speed the coagulation and separate the milk into solid curds and liquid whey. The whey is then drained off, the curd is heated, and it is then molded and shaped into a cheese. This rennet is obtained by cutting the stomach out of a newborn calf or lamb, because adult mammals don't have the enzyme needed for its production, and newborn calves and lambs need the enzyme to help digest and absorb milk. These baby animals are the victims of the cheese industry. Almost all European cheeses still use animal rennet. This may provide fuel for any vegetarians who still eat cheese, not believing the animals are being harmed in the process, to reconsider their stance.

I have read numerous articles about American cheese containing high amounts of aluminum. The aluminum is added to make the cheese creamier. It is also a poison and is believed to be linked to many health issues, like brain cancer, autism, and Alzheimer's. One of the healthiest things you could ever do is eliminate cheese and all dairy from your diet. If you like the taste of cheese, there are raw vegan alternatives that can be made of nuts, seeds, and vegan probiotics. These can be beneficial to your health, providing essential fatty acids, enzymes, amino acids, and beneficial bacteria that improve digestion, nutrient intake, and the immune system. There is a book titled, The *Ultimate Uncheese Cookbook,* by Joanne Stepaniak, which is full of raw, dairy-free cheese recipes.

DAIRY - DO WE REALLY INGEST THE SECRETIONS FROM ANOTHER ANIMAL?

"The nine million cows in America, for the most part, are not healthy. Half the herds in America have cows affected with bovine leukemia virus, half the herds have cows infected with a disease called Crohn's disease, which is caused by a bacterium called mycobacterium paratuberculosis. Forty million Americans have been affected with irritable bowel syndrome from this bacterium. Every person with Crohn's disease tests positive for mycobacterium paratuberculosis. This was published in 1965 for the Proceedings for the National Academy of Science. We are talking about real science here, not things I'm making up. There are thousands of studies published in scientific journals, and thousands of converging lines of evidence that tell us that milk does not do the body any good. We should no longer continue to drink the body fluids from diseased animals." – Dr. Robert Cohen, *Milk: The Deadly Poison*

Human beings are the only mammals that are not completely weaned from milk at the end of infancy. Every other animal, including the cow, weans their young from milk once they have developed to the toddler stage. No other mammal drinks the secretions of another animal. Humans are the only ones who do both. Many humans drink milk from their mothers, then they continue to drink milk throughout life by getting it from other animals. This is not something we do naturally; it is something we have been manipulated into doing by one of the largest, greediest, and most profitable industries in the world – the dairy industry. It is a filthy habit that should be discontinued. The human dietary need for milk from other animals is nonexistent, as long as we are eating an array of plant-based foods.

"There is a compelling argument that today's pasteurized milk, in all its guises, has virtually no redeeming features at all, and serves only to cause disease and poor health. By simply switching from dairy to non-dairy milk we will make a dramatic and long-lasting improvement to our health." – Dr. Amy Lanou, *Physician's Committee for Responsible Medicine*

A study published by the Archives of Pediatric and Adolescent Medicine in March 2012, reports that dairy products and calcium do not prevent stress fractures. Researchers tracked the diets and physical activity of adolescent girls for seven years and found that the girls who received the most calcium from milk and dairy products more than doubled their risk of a stress fracture.

"Milk was never meant to see the light of day; it is the mother's flowing gift of life to her newborn baby – human, calf, or other mammal – and is meant to flow directly from the mother's nipple to the baby's lips. The dairy farm operation is a grim distortion of this process." – Dr. Michael Klaper, Vegan Nutrition

There is no replacement for mother's milk for infants, and once weaned from their mother's milk children should never again drink milk. A review of several studies that was published in a 2011 issue of Nutrition Reviews titled, *Consumption of Cow's Milk as a Cause of Iron Deficiency in Infants and Toddlers*, supports my claim. The conclusion of the review determined that, *"The feeding of cow's milk to infants and toddlers is strongly associated with diminished iron nutritional status and an increased risk of iron deficiency. The negative effects of cow's milk on iron nutritional status are thought to mainly result from the low iron content of the milk. Cow's milk also causes occult intestinal blood loss in many infants and contains potent inhibitors of iron absorption from the diet. The feeding of unmodified pasteurized cow's milk also places infants at high risk of severe dehydration and may increase the risk of obesity in childhood. Because of these adverse effects, unmodified cow's milk should not be fed to infants."*

When we consume dairy, we excrete strong digestive juices in the stomach, and mucus is then excreted in the throat and nose. The fatty components in dairy are responsible for the production of this congesting mucus and it becomes a breeding ground for viral invasions and bacterial infection, while blocking nutrient absorption.

Because we are not able to easily digest milk from another species, we form excess mucus and plaque. People who consume dairy are much more likely to develop colds many times throughout the year. They get sick because the sickness binds to the mucus that clogs their lymph system. This could all be prevented if they would eliminate all dairy products from their diet, including creamer, ice cream, milk, whey, cheese, salad dressings, and other foods with milk products as ingredients.

Another reason why milk from other mammals is so bad for the human body is because of the pasteurization and homogenization processes carried out prior to being sold. According to Dr. Gill Langley in the book, *Vegan Nutrition*, *"The process of heating milk in order to pasteurize it causes the proteins in cow's milk to denature. These denatured proteins are linked to atherosclerosis and heart disease."*

We should never allow our children to drink milk from other animals. The consumption of dairy is responsible for many of the weight problems we see all over the world. Obesity is spiraling out of control and dairy is a major contributor. Contrary to what some false medical studies suggest, eliminating dairy from your diet will eliminate excess mucus from the body and help you lose weight. I have had several clients who each lost at least fifteen pounds in the first month of training with me after they cut dairy from their diets and began to exercise.

Feed your kids dark leafy greens rather than dairy. If you are looking for a good way to get them to eat spinach, kale, and chard, introduce them to the classic "Popeye" cartoons. Teach them the motto, *"I'm strong to the finish, because I eat my spinach."* Greens are a much better source for calcium than milk. In fact, lots of different veggies are better sources for calcium than dairy.

If you look at the **Harvard Medical School** webpage and search for *"my healthy plate,"* you will see that they no longer include dairy on their daily food pyramid. The research has been done and the conclusion is that dairy is not a suitable food for humans. Pasteurized dairy is not even a suitable food for animals. Baby calves can die if they drink pasteurized cow's milk.

"Imagine taking five sticks of butter and molding them into a softball-sized sphere of greasy animal fat. If you are the average dairy eater living in America in 2003, you will be taking into your body this additional saturated mass weighing 1.7 pounds, which is that much more than what the average individual of 1969 ingested during each twelve-month period. A 1.7 pound glob of saturated fat multiplied by ten years of a child's life is equal to seventeen pounds. By the time a child of the 21st century turns thirty, he or she will have eaten fifty-one pounds more saturated fat than a child of the sixties." – Dr. Robert Cohen, notmilk.com

On a train ride to Chicago one day, I noticed an older man with a suit and tie who was sitting across from me. He was struggling to get his work done. Each time he started getting close to working, he had to take out a tissue to blow his nose. As he would put it away, he would cough. After he would finish coughing, within minutes he had again took out that same tissue. Is this living? Not in my world. The last time I was sick was when I turned sixteen years old. I had my wisdom teeth pulled and was forced to take terrible antibiotics. This was the last time I ever took synthetic medicine.

The reason why this man was blowing his nose so frequently is more than likely because he eats dairy products and drinks milk. I am quite certain that this is his problem. I did not ask him, and I did not see him drinking milk, I suspect this because the most common way we generate excess mucus in our bodies is from dairy. When milk is pasteurized, the enzymes are destroyed. Without the enzymes that are present in raw milk, milk cannot be digested efficiently. In fact, even with the enzymes intact, humans still are unable to process milk from other species. The body expels these foreign excretions by converting them into mucus and then we blow it out of our noses, or cough it up. Sometimes people develop boils on their skin and the mucus exits through the skin. While in the body, this mucus coats our internal organs and disrupts many of the natural processes.

"Up to a gallon of extra mucus is created in the body as a result of drinking milk and consuming dairy." – Dr. Robert Cohen, notmilk.com

When I was a child and I drank milk with every meal, and nearly every morning with my cereal, I often had problems with throat congestion. I wished there was some kind of way I could rid myself of it. I thought my condition was natural. I had no idea it was really the milk I was drinking that was triggering my body to create excess mucus. I had been tricked in school into believing milk was healthy for my bones. It was not until later in life that I realized the milk I had been drinking was not beneficial and was the real culprit behind all of the years of discomfort.

Many degenerative diseases can be linked to the consumption of milk. Along with meat and eggs, milk is a major contributor to osteoporosis. All of those stories we were fed growing up about milk being healthy for the bones turned out to be the exact opposite. They were lies.

Over the years I have listened to several people tell me stories of how their doctors have misinformed them that they need to drink milk in order to get their adequate calcium. This is not true. We can only absorb a very small fraction – roughly thirty-two percent – of the calcium in milk. In order for calcium to be assimilated in the body, it must be accompanied by magnesium. Milk does not contain magnesium. Spinach and leafy green vegetables contain both magnesium and calcium in the perfect ratio. Maybe as children we should have been watching more Popeye cartoons, or spending more time in the garden with our parents, rather than viewing so many milk commercials about milk doing our bodies good, and commercials promoting the food products containing dairy and other health-degrading ingredients.

When a problem with calcium absorption arises, chances are there is too much phosphoric acid or uric acid in the system. Uric acid comes from eating meat, and phosphoric acid comes from drinking sodas, among many other sources. These acids contribute to the development of osteoporosis. Once diagnosed, patients with osteoporosis are rarely, if ever, told they should refrain from drinking sodas or eating meat – or to avoid dairy.

The healthy bacteria known as lactobacillus and acidophilus digest some of the sugars (lactose) and proteins (casein) in milk. While you wean yourself from dairy and are cleansing the body of this waste, it may be beneficial to supplement with a vegan probiotic containing these bacterium. This will speed up the elimination process. If you are eating an all raw vegan diet, however, these are no longer necessary to take as a supplement. The body naturally produces the bacteria we need and if we eat a clean diet, we should not have a problem maintaining adequate amounts of healthy bacteria, which are also referred to as intestinal flora.

I encourage you to eliminate dairy from your diet. Give it a few weeks and watch what happens. When you rid your body of dairy products you will notice many improvements in your life. You will breathe easier, you will run faster, your endurance will improve, and you will notice that you do not get sick as often, if ever. Without the presence of excess mucus, bacteria and viruses will have no place to linger and multiply.

WE ARE EATING GLUE

Do you know what one of the main ingredients in common household glue happens to be? The answer is casein. According to Dr. T. Colin Campbell, casein is the most common protein in milk. This means we are practically drinking glue when we drink milk. If you would like more interesting facts on the dangers of dairy, access the website that Dr. Robert Cohen developed to give us more knowledge about the harmful effects of dairy (notmilk.com).

Another bit of information you may want to know is that milk sold in stores is allowed to contain over 750 million "pus" cells, also referred to as somatic cells, per liter. This is based on *US Department of Agriculture* standards. Cows are forced to produce so much excess milk that they often begin to bleed through their udders. This blood contaminates the milk. So essentially you drink blood and pus with each glass of store-purchased milk.

Parasites and candida yeast thrive in excess mucus that lingers around the body. Do yourself a favor, remove dairy from your life. You will be a much happier, healthier, and leaner person.

WHAT ABOUT FISH?

I'm not an advocate of eating foods that are high on the food chain. Why eat fish, to get nutrients? Why not eat the foods that fish eat? This is where the fish get their nutrients. There is no reason to filter nutrients through the organs of another species prior to obtaining them. We can eat algae supplements or add kelp powder or dulse flakes to our entrees instead, eliminating the dietary cholesterol contained in fish. There are wonderful varieties of seaweed and algae as well that are edible and are great compliments to many dishes. To name a few: kelp, dulse, nori, spirulina, wakame, and AFA blue-green algae are all good food choices that will provide us with a greater abundance of the nutrients we think we are obtaining from fish. The key to optimal health is to eat as low on the food chain as possible – as in edible plant matter, not animals.

The blue whale eats only phytoplankton. It also happens to be the largest mammal on the planet and remains sexually active until old age —or— the end of its life, nearly two-hundred years later. Similar to how the strongest, leanest, and most muscular land mammals such as cows, elephants, gorillas, and horses eat only plants, so do blue whales. They each eat as low on the food chain as possible. We should follow their lead and eat a plant-based diet. Doing so will nourish and strengthen our bodies.

When fish is cooked, any healthy oils that may be contained within are degraded. This means they are equivalent to trans-fats. These bad oils cause inflammation and lead to all sorts of other health issues. Because the oceans are so polluted from our waste, fish contain heavy metals, industrial pollutants, pharmaceutical drugs, and farming chemical residues. These waste products also impact the wildlife that eat fish. Some animals that eat fish, such as bears, do not eat the fish for protein. They eat the fish for the fat. Only a relatively small part of their diet is meat based. As is typical with carnivores, bears can also tolerate high amounts of cholesterol in their diet without getting heart disease.

Many people continue to believe that eating fish provides us with omega-3 fatty acids, which are critical to brain cell function, and boost levels of DHA and EPA. Many people also think that eating fish prevents cognitive decline and staves off dementia. However, we can maintain adequate amounts of these nutrients from the alpha-linoleic acids (ALA) found in raw plant oils. In a ten-year study published in the ***American Journal of Clinical Nutrition*** in 2010, researchers found that the omega-3 long-chain fatty acids found in fish oils did not lower dementia risk. Those who ate fish regularly developed dementia at the same rate as those who did not eat fish. Further research has proven that the most important foods for brain function are not fish or fish oils; they are ALA-rich foods, such as raw hemp seeds, chia seeds, flaxseeds, pumpkin seeds, walnuts, and fruits and vegetables. The ALA found in many plant oils has been shown to have direct anti-arrhythmic properties, meaning they help prevent sudden cardiac death. In the ***Neuropsychopharmacology Journal***, researchers reported that ALA actively promotes neuronal plasticity. This stimulates the growth of new nerve cells, and enhances nerve growth factors that protect against depression. This ALA is not obtained from eating fish. We are nourished with ALA from eating raw plants. To maintain happiness and achieve optimal health, our best option is to avoid all food that once had eyes, was born, had a family, and was once a living creature with a soul.

In 2007, the ***Institute of Medicine*** compiled the risks and benefits of eating fish. They stated, *"The contaminants in fish that are of most concern today are mercury, polychlorinated biphenyls (PCBs), dioxins, and pesticide residues. Very high levels of mercury can damage nerves in adults and disrupt development of the brain and nervous system in a fetus or young child. The effect of the far lower levels of mercury currently found in fish have been linked to subtle changes in nervous system development and a possible* *increased risk of cardiovascular disease."*

While many people accept the belief that eating fish is a healthy choice for losing weight and maintaining health, consider the chemical pollutants found in fish that disrupt our metabolism and may pave the way for obesity. A February 2009 study published in *Molecular and Cellular Endocrinology*, titled *Endocrine Disrupters as Obesogens*, suggests that chemical obesogens in the food supply may be contributing to the obesity epidemic. In our body we have preadipocytes (pre-fat cells), which are fibroblasts that can be stimulated to form adipocytes (fat cells). These chemical obesogens were found to stimulate the formation from preadipocyte to adipocyte. Adipocytes – also known as lipocytes or fat cells – are the cells that compose the majority of adipose tissue, and store energy as fat. We are exposed to obesogens by means of our diet, and it was determined that these chemicals are found most abundantly in fish. So, as we continue to eat sea life, we trigger the body to store more energy as fat, and this could cause weight gain.

In addition to fish being a poor food choice, shellfish are also known to contain phycotoxins, which are produced by microalgae. The November 2011 edition of *Chemical Research in Toxicology* published a study introducing cyclic imines as being a harmful phycotoxin with fast-acting toxicity. These marine biotoxins were shown to be fatal in rodents, and are said to be responsible for the high incidence of shellfish poisoning that occurs worldwide.

As we learn more about the toxins found in fish, and as we educate ourselves further on true nutrition, we begin to realize that eating fish is not necessary for health, or is it essential for a lean frame. We discover that eating seafood is more harmful than it could be beneficial. Once we see it from this perspective, then we can take it up another step and learn how the fishing industry is close to wiping out the entire population of fish in the sea.

In August 2012, the completion of a four year study conducted by an international group of ecologists and economists on 7,800 marine species around the world's ecosystems concluded that all of the world's stocks of seafood will collapse by the year 2050. This is due to the present rates of destruction by the fishing industry. Over sixty percent of the fish taken from the sea by this industry are ground up and force-fed to vegetarian livestock in the meat industry so they can be fattened and slaughtered. As Philip Wollen mentions in the St. James Ethics debate, vegetarian cows have now become the largest ocean predators. This is not natural. Access *kindnesstrust.com* to learn more. Because of factory-farmed pigs now eating fish, the captain of *Sea Shepherd* now claims pigs are the number one ocean predator.

Each product purchased from the meat industry contributes to the death of marine life. The ocean provides the majority of oxygen on Earth, and if we continue doing what we are doing, all ocean life will soon die. When ocean life dies, life on land will go with it. The solution to this problem is simple:

refrain from eating meat and all animal products and the meat industry will collapse. See the book *Extinction* by John McCabe.

SWEETS TURN OUR SPIRITS SOUR

If you type the words *sugar* and *disease* together into a Google search you will see there are fifty-four million results. The consumption of sugar is linked to obesity, diabetes, heart disease, osteoporosis, hypertension, hypoglycemia, mineral depletion, adrenal fatigue, weakened immunity, and several other negative health conditions. Sugars are often hidden in most of the food that the average person eats, with or without them knowing. Processed foods such as meat, bouillon cubes, cereals, peanut butter, sauces, soups, dressings, condiments, packaged foods, baked 'goods,' frozen dinners, and breads usually contain added sugars, to go along with other harmful food additives. Many bottled juices contain added sugars. Several medications use sugars as fillers. The fluids that are administered intravenously in hospitals also contain sugars.

Sugar comes in many forms. There are refined sugars, brown sugars, sugar crystals, cane sugar, evaporated cane juice, beet sugars, high-fructose corn syrup, glucose, sucrose, maltose, lactose, fructose, agave nectar, heated honey, and synthetic sweeteners. These sugars are deleterious to our health, unless they are eaten in their natural state, coming from raw fruits or vegetables.

Sugar is acid-forming and leads to an imbalance in the ratio of phosphorus to calcium. Sugar causes excess calcium excretion, and when we lose this calcium, the pH level in our body tilts toward acidity. Because we store alkaline minerals in our bones, we then draw calcium from them to buffer our pH level so it becomes slightly alkaline. This process weakens our bones and contributes to osteoporosis.

In his book, *The Sugar Fix: the High-Fructose Fallout That is Making You Fat and Sick*, Dr. Robert J. Johnson presents the possibility of a connection between excess sugar consumption and high uric acid levels. Uric acid is a by-product of cellular breakdown. Because sugar leads to the death of cells, RNA and DNA degrade into purines. These purines are then further broken down into uric acid. Animal proteins are another example of commonly eaten foods that break down into uric acid. Meat and sugar are staples of the standard American diet. This would explain why human uric acid levels have more than doubled since the early 1900's. Dr. Joseph Mercola believes *high uric acid levels are a more potent predictor of cardiovascular disease and overall health than high cholesterol levels.* Many doctors, however, do not see the correlation between uric acid levels and health.

Dr. Miriam Vos, a professor of pediatrics at Emory University, conducted research with a team to determine a possible link between sugar and triglyceride and cholesterol levels. The results were published in an April 2010 issue of the *Journal of the American Medical Association.*

Vos led a group of nutritionists, epidemiologists, and physicians in an analysis of data from a national health survey of more than 6,000 men and women conducted between 1999 and 2006. They interviewed each participant about what they had eaten twenty-four hours prior to the survey, and then calculated the sugar content of these foods using the government food pyramid equivalents. *On average, the respondents consumed twenty-one teaspoons of added sugar a day (which does not include sugar from natural sources), accounting for nearly sixteen percent of their total daily caloric intake.*

Those consuming twenty-five percent of their daily calories in added sugar were twice as likely to have low levels of their good HDL cholesterol (these levels should be higher). Forty-three percent of the highest sugar consumers recorded low HDL, while only twenty-two percent of the lowest sugar consumers did. Those who consumed the most added sugar also had the highest triglyceride levels. Low HDL and high triglyceride levels are two primary risk factors for heart disease.

Sucrose and glucose raise our blood sugar levels. We must produce insulin then to bring them back down. Too much insulin production is known to elevate blood pressure, cholesterol, and triglyceride levels. Insulin increases deposits of plaque in the arterial walls. Too much insulin also leads to weight gain.

By now, many of us know the dangers of high-fructose corn syrup and how it leads to obesity and many other health issues. Corn syrup damages the mucoid layer of the intestines and thus interferes with nutrient absorption. Some brands of mass-marketed honey are produced after bee farmers feed their bee's high-fructose corn syrup. The result is that the honey becomes equivalent to high-fructose corn syrup. Agave nectar is heated at a temperature high enough to degrade the enzymes and is also unhealthful. If you would like to listen to an explanation of why agave nectar is not the best alternative to sugar, search for John Kohler's YouTube video on agave.

Because many of us crave sweets, it would be difficult to completely wean ourselves from everything sweet in our diets. Fructose is an example of a sugar that does not require as much insulin to be broken down. This is the sugar found in raw fruit. Fresh, organic fruits, or dried fruits, are the only sources of sugar we should be consuming. Contrary to what many people think, eating raw fruits, especially berries, can help reverse diabetes. Truly raw dates are a source of food helpful in overcoming a craving for sweets. If you feel like you must add sweetener to your food, use Stevia or date syrup. A small amount of raw organic maple syrup is more beneficial to your health than a small amount of sugar. Remove all processed sugar from your life and your health will improve.

THE STARCH MOLECULE

"People fill themselves up with cooked starches because they are dense and give them that filled feeling that replaces the emptiness they have in their lives from the disconnection from nature and the lack of love that they may not even know they are experiencing." – **John McCabe,** *Sunfood Diet Infusion*

At times, when I go into a regular grocery store, I observe the people who shop there, and take note of what they put into their carts. Almost always, one of the most common products is bread and other cooked gluten grain products, such as bagels, cereals, cookies, crackers, and pastries. I notice many of them prefer the bleached, white bread with flour coating the top of the loaf. I look at their pasty skin which resembles the loaf. The reason they look this way is not because "they are getting older", it is because they are aging themselves by making these food choices. These poor people have been misinformed by food advertising and misguided by food labeling. If they truly want to be healthy, one of the things they must give up is food that contains flours, especially those with gluten grains, such as wheat, barley, and rye. Spelt is also a form of wheat that contains gluten. All bleached grains should be avoided.

Cooked, refined, starchy foods can be damaging to the skin because starches are not easily digested once they are denatured. They are not soluble in water, alcohol, or ether. Starch from poor food choices can contribute to the formation of stones in the gall bladder and cause an unnatural coagulation of the blood in the vessels and capillaries. This may contribute to the formation of hemorrhoids, tumors, cancers and other abnormalities. Dr. Norman Walker explains the reasoning behind this best in his book, *Become Younger.* He states: *"As the starch molecule is not soluble in water, it travels through the blood and lymph streams as a solid molecule which the cells, tissues, and glands of the body cannot utilize. Therefore the body tries to expel it. As the eliminative organs become afflicted with an accumulation of these molecules as a lining of their walls, like plaster on the walls of a room, they cannot be expelled through these channels. The next best means of exit is through the pores of the skin and so we have pimples."*

Foods that are refined of their fiber can stick to the intestines and colon, where they accumulate toxins while interfering with nutrient absorption. The ancient Egyptians used to make glue from flour and water. Flour slows the metabolism, causing weight gain, and nurturing disease.

Flour also contains a toxic by-product known as *methionine sulphoximine* (MSO) which is formed during the process of bleaching flour with nitrogen dichloride gas. This by-product, MSO, blocks the production of glutathione and glutamine in the body. The glutathione happens to be one of our most important antioxidants. Glutamine helps clear out the ammonia that is produced in the body from breaking down animal protein.

White rice and white potatoes are also less than ideal choices of foods. If you are eating brown rice or sweet potatoes you will be better off than eating flour-based foods, but one should still limit the intake. Rather than eating rice, try foods such as quinoa, millet, buckwheat, or amaranth. If you choose to eat potatoes, use yams or sweet potatoes that are organic, non-GMO, and steam them, do not bake, roast, sautee, or fry them. Applying high heat to potatoes triggers the formation of carcinogenic acrylamides. These compounds decompose non-thermally to form ammonia. An acrylamide is a known lethal neurotoxin and its formation on some cooked starchy foods was discovered in 2002. These foods include bread, cocoa powder, coffee, French fries, potato chips, Pringles, roasted almonds, and whole wheat bread. In 2005, the *Women's Lifestyle and Health Cohort* found after conducting a study on 43,404 Swedish women that the women's greatest sources of acrylamides were from coffee, fried potatoes, and crisp bread. It is wise to avoid foods that contain acrylamides.

To clarify, the carbohydrates we consume should not come from weak sources such as pasta, white rice, white potatoes, white breads, or gluten grains. It would be better to shift to consuming mostly fruits, some pseudograins, and foods such as yams and sweet potatoes to satiate your deisre for starches. These raw fruits and other foods are always good sources of carbohydrates that will help us to maintain even blood sugar throughout the day.

I suggest reading, *The Starch Solution*, by Dr. John McDougall, to learn about the benefits of eating whole food sources of starch, and to help influence your decision of which starches you will include in your diet.

COFFEE – OSTEOPOROSIS IN A CUP

A toxin can be defined as *any substance that is harmful to the body, which the body cannot use in any way for life-maintaining purposes, and which costs the body energy and nutrition to eliminate.* We create several toxins as by-products of metabolism within our own bodies (endogenous toxins), and we ingest other toxins (exogenous).

Our bodies are always working to eliminate poisons from the system and this is done through stimulation. When the metabolism is increased by a substance, it is stimulated. Caffeine is a toxic stimulant and the "high," or burst of energy some people feel after drinking coffee is really the result of the body being stimulated to eliminate the caffeine from the system. The caffeine, or any stimulant for that matter, is not responsible for the energy one may feel after ingesting it. The body increases its metabolism to remove the toxins from the system by producing adrenaline. The production of adrenaline causes the liver to release glucose into the bloodstream. The glucose is then converted into energy. This energy is used to eliminate the poisons (being the stimulants).

Caffeine stimulates the release of glucose from the liver, providing the body with a temporary blood sugar high. Many people become addicted to the feeling and they drink coffee for this temporary blood sugar high. Coffee is just as addictive as chocolate and the two may provide a similar temporary increase in energy. By simply eating raw fruit, you could receive a high, but in a more gentle and healthful manner.

Caffeine belongs to a family of alkaloids that includes caffeine, nicotine, sugar, salt, and meat, and it has no food value whatsoever. To eliminate this poison, our bodies are forced to use energy and minerals from our tissues and bones, and this stresses the adrenal glands, the liver, and the pancreas, while also increasing the production of stomach acids. The caffeine then mixes with the hydrochloric acid and forms another toxin, which some refer to as caffeine hydrochloride, and the liver reacts by producing bile and releasing it to flush this toxin from the system.

Caffeine cannot be associated with good health. It is highly acidic. When you drink coffee, the acid and caffeine leach the healthy alkaline minerals from your bones, similar to how calcium is drawn away from the bones when you eat meat, drink soda or milk, smoke cigarettes, and eat clarified sugars. The most important alkaline mineral stored in bones is calcium. An acidic diet raises acidity in the blood, which the body works to balance by relying on stores of calcium. This means that when you drink coffee, you are depleting the stores of calcium from within your bones. If you drink coffee every day, you are increasing the likelihood of experiencing osteoporosis. When you drink fluids that decrease your bone mineral density and rob you of alkaline minerals, you should not be surprised that your health is negated.

Coffee stains the teeth, laying the groundwork for dental decay and gum disease. A diet of cooked starches, clarified sugars, and coffee, accompanied by cigarette smoking is terrible for dental health.

In October 2012, a *Harvard Medical School* study published in *Ophthalmology and Visual Science*, linked heavy coffee consumption with an increased risk of developing exfoliation glaucoma, which is an eye disorder that leads to vision loss. Researchers indicated that adults who drank three or more cups of coffee per day were thirty-four percent more likely to develop exfoliation glaucoma than those abstaining from coffee.

I have never been a coffee drinker. I often seem to be the rare bird in the crowd. It seems that the majority of adults do indulge daily in lattes, cappucino, and other coffee drinks. The U.S. has over one-hundred thousand coffee cafes. Together they serve billions of cups of coffee annually.

By adding more alkalinity to your diet and shifting away from the acidifying foods, you will discover that you no longer crave these stimulants. Find yourself an organic greens superfood supplement such as **Green Vibrance** or **Fields of Greens**, both made by **Vibrant Health**, *Vitamineral Green*, or even **Infinity Greens**, and drink that in the morning to go along with eating a variety of fruits. These greens supplements most often come in a powder form, and by adding one scoop a day into a cup or shaker with four to six ounces of water, or organic juice, this will provide you with an energy boost that will last until your lunch break without the usual crash. I have had several training clients who have eliminated their coffee addictions by taking a shot of this **Green Vibrance** each morning to replace their usual cup of coffee.

THE DOWNSIDE OF SOY

My belief is that many vegans or vegetarians who appear frail and malnourished are that way because they made the unwise decision to replace meat with soy. Much of the soy being sold today and added to food products is genetically modified and highly estrogenic.

According to the *Stanford University* website, in 2011 soy was the leading genetically modifed crop globally. It occupied over 185 million acres of land. Meanwhile, as the United States and Brazil fight for the lead in the global market for soy, deforestation in the Amazon Rainforest and Brazilian Savannah continues. This means chopping down the trees that regulate our atmospheric carbon, and the killing of plant and animal species to clear more land for soy plantations. All the while these environmental travesties are taking place, it is known that genetically-modified soy is not even beneficial to our health. A study published in July 2010 by the *Institute of Ecology and Evolution of the Russian Academy of Sciences* showed the results of a two year study in which three generations of hamsters were fed genetically modified soy. By the third generation, most hamsters who were given the genetically-modified soy lost the ability to have babies. They also suffered slow growth rates and a high mortality rate amongst their newborn. Some of these hamsters even began to grow hair in their mouths as a result of eating the genetically modifed strands of soy.

In September 2010, Dr. Joseph Mercola published an article, on *mercola.com*, explaining that soy contains what are known as "anti-nutrients." These include saponins, soyatoxins, phytates, protease inhibitors, oxalates, goitrogens, and estrogens. Each of these play roles in altering the normal functioning of the body. The goitrogens may block the synthesis of thyroid hormones, interfering with iodine metabolism. Phytic acid is what inhibits our ability to assimilate and utilize many essential nutrients like zinc, magnesium, and calcium. Soy contains the highest phytic acid content of all seeds and legumes. This could be why many new vegans fail with the diet; they tend to replace meat with soy, which is a better alternative, but still not a good food choice. As a result, their body chemistry falters.

A September 2003 article published in the *Journal of Nutrition* reveals *that isotope studies have proven phytic acid to inhibit the absorption by human subjects of iron, zinc, calcium, and manganese.* Because soy is high in phytates, it is safe to conclude that soy also inhibits the absorption of these nutrients.

Some long-term vegans who are overweight can attribute that extra weight to the excess estrogen from all of the soy they have been consuming, which has contributed to their weight gain.

If you are going to include soy in your diet, which I recommend you do not, be sure it is the fermented soy such as natto, miso, or even tempeh. When soy is fermented, the phytic acid levels begin to decline and the nutrients are less likely to be inhibited. Natto is also rich in vitamin K2, which is beneficial for dental health.

If you are drinking soy milk, it is a good idea to stop now and convert to almond milk, hemp milk, sunflower milk, or even coconut milk. It is simple to make non-dairy milk in a blender. By adding almonds, or hemp seeds, with a few dates, a little vanilla, and maybe a banana, to some water, you will have a great tasting milk that costs less, is rich in nutrients, and is devoid of all of the sugars, such as rice syrup or evaporated cane juice, that are often found in packaged, non-dairy milks. You will also avoid the chemicals found in the packaging, and reduce pollution by not purchasing packaged non-dairy milks. While soy does contain some nutrients, it is better off avoided. Homemade non-dairy milks are nutritionally superior to the packaged ones. The marketing and selling of soy and soy products is just another way for people to make money by deceiving the consumer. Soy milk is also rich in acrylamides.

I'm sure many know by now that under the guidance of Dr. Dean Ornish and Dr. Caldwell Esselstyn, the former President, Bill Clinton, converted to a vegan diet and is successfully reversing his heart disease. It is great to have such a well-known person promote the vegan diet. I think his transformation has been incredible. I still think he has room for improvement though. While many people may not agree with me in the standard American world, I think the former president may be eating too much soy.

It is a very good thing to eliminate meat and dairy from the diet, however, replacing them with soy is not the best choice. While I am a very strong advocate of the vegan diet and I admire the work of Dr. Dean Ornish, I believe he should not be recommending soy. I also believe the elimination of soy should be an addition to the "vegan manifesto." If a "true vegan" cannot eat bee pollen granules, then they should also not be eating soy.

WHAT IS GLUTEN?

The phrase–or–term "gluten free" is becoming more common in society as people are finally beginning to understand the negatives of gluten on health. Gluten is a protein contained in rye, wheat, and barley, and these three grains are not necessary in our diet. Gluten contains two toxic protein fractions known as gliadins and glutenins. Gliadin has been shown to cause inflammatory bowel disease. Glutenin is not easily digestible. They both contribute to diverticulitis, celiac disease, and dermatitis herpetiformis. They break down the ileum to the point where problems with absorption start to occur. Gluten grains are also high in lectins and when the lectins bind to insulin receptors, they interfere with glucose metabolism. They cause intestinal damage and protein and carbohydrate malabsorption. Gluten has been linked to several symptoms, including fatigue, headache, arthritis, irritability, depression, ADD, bi-polar disorder, and inflammation in the liver, kidneys, heart, and blood vessels.

While wheat has been a staple of the American diet for many years, it is finally dawning on us that we should not be eating it. The only occasion when we should ever use wheat is when we are sprouting the berries to make wheatgrass. Another instance would be soaking sprouted wheat berries and using the fermented liquid to make what is called "rejuvelac." This is a very healthy and refreshing beverage that is loaded with B-complex vitamins and amino acids. After being soaked, we can then allow the berries to sprout into wheatgrass. Aside from the sprouts, wheatgrass, and rejuvelac, we do not need wheat in our diet.

I have often been asked about what type of foods we can use to replace gluten grains. The answer is that we should not substitute anything for the foods because gluten grains are not vital foods for our health. Many people develop allergies from eating gluten grains. Skin irritations, such as eczema, are linked to eating gluten grains. It is best, and highly advisable, for all gluten grains to be eliminated from the diet.

If you are looking for a good way to eliminate gluten, go for sprouted grains. With a dehydrator and a few simple ingredients, you can make your own sprouted grain breads that contain no gluten grains. The website *rawfullytempting.com* will provide you with a few recipes. By making sprouted non-gluten breads, it will help to eliminate flour from your diet. Additionally, start using quinoa, millet, buckwheat, and amaranth. These foods are known as pseudograins, and are a staple food for the *Thrive diet,* which was formulated by vegan tri-athlete Brendan Brazier. Despite its name, buckwheat does not contain wheat. Amaranth is a seed that comes from a leafy plant. These foods are not acid-forming, as many grains tend to be. It is not difficult to eat a well-balanced diet while refraining from gluten grains.

IS PEANUT BUTTER OKAY?

I cannot count how many people I have consulted with who are struggling to lose weight, and think they are eating well, but are adding peanut butter to their smoothies or their foods. Eating peanut butter makes it difficult to drop weight. Almost all peanut butter is roasted. This means that the fats have become unhealthful.

It is disturbing to read the labels on the jars of different peanut butters marketed toward children. They all contain refined sugar products like high-fructose corn syrup, hydrogenated oils, palm oils, and processed salt. Some even contain synthetic dyes and flavors. If you are an avid peanut butter eater, or if you like your PB & J sandwiches, try replacing peanut butter with raw almond butter or raw walnut butter. If you make it yourself at home in a food processor, it is much more cost-efficient. Start by finding truly raw nuts, and then soak them in water overnight. After soaking simply dump them into a food processor or nut butter grinder. Within minutes you will have fresh raw nut butter. Additionally, be sure to use flourless bread that is free of gluten grains with your sandwich. From these simple replacements alone, it is likely that you will drop weight and gain extra energy.

Peanuts contain high amounts of aflatoxin, which can be harmful to some people, and in rare cases, can be fatal. Even organic peanuts may contain this fungus. This explains why so many people have peanut allergies. There is one type of peanut that does not contain aflatoxin, and that is the jungle peanut. This peanut is also high in vitamin B3.

I urge you to stop allowing your children to consume peanut butter. There is a reason why so many places do not allow peanuts or peanut butter near their premises. If you are going to eat peanut butter, be sure it is organic and raw with no oils or sugars added. A better choice, as I've stated, would be the raw jungle peanuts, raw almonds, raw pecans, or raw walnuts. Remember to soak the raw nuts for several hours before eating them or using them in recipes. As Karyn Calabrese mentions in her book, *Soak Your Nuts*, nuts contain enzyme inhibitors and when you soak them, they are released, making the nutrients more readily available, and the digestion process easier.

WHY COOKED OILS ARE BAD

I have had several clients that have had acne issues. Acne can result from consuming cooked oils, coffee, chocolate, clarified sugars like agave and corn syrup; hormones from animal products; and gluten grains. Although this is something that is not always easy to mention to those who may be self-conscious about their skin troubles, I always find ways to get the point across to them that they must stop eating foods that contain cooked oils, dairy, and other unhealthy foods. Cooked oils are some of the most likely substances to contribute to bad skin. They are not capable of mixing with water. Since we are a water-based life form, this makes it difficult to metabolize cooked oil. Cooked oil is sticky. If you have ever tried to scrub the cooked oil residues from the surface of a pot or pan, you should know that the process is not easy. These oils stick to our organs in the same way. They cause inflammation in the tissues, slow metabolism, and end up on cell membranes where they interfere with nutrient absorption and cell waste elimination. They also harm the cardiovascular system, slow nerve processes, and accelerate the aging process.

Because cooked oils negatively affect our skin's health and help trigger the formation of acne, I always feel it is necessary to inform those people I know, or those who I consult with, who have acne, of exactly how they can eliminate these problems without seeing a dermatologist, taking medications, or treating their skin with harsh chemicals.

When oil is cooked under pressure, highly toxic trans-fatty acids are created and they end up on, and are absorbed into, the cell membranes. This causes them to become blocked and alters the immune system. We have to eliminate them from the body somehow and because the skin is our largest eliminative organ, we tend to excrete oils through our skin.

All raw fruits and vegetables contain essential fatty acids. There is no need to add oil to the diet. The only reason is for taste sensation. But all bottled oils, including olive oil, can contribute to heart disease. A study published in the *Journal of the American College of Cardiology* revealed that cardiovascular system "dilation was worse" after twenty-four people, twelve who were healthy and twelve who had high cholesterol levels, consumed olive oil. The Director of Nutrition at the *Pritikin Longevity Center*, Jeffrey Novick, MS, RD, explains that *olive oil is not heart-healthy.* He admits that foods rich in monounsaturated fats, like olive oil, are healthier than foods which are full of saturated and trans-fats, but he also clarifies that *just because something is "healthier," it does not mean it is good for you.*

I HEARD FAT WAS HEALTHY

Some fats are healthy and optimal for our well-being. It is important to ingest these good fats. They should come from plant-based foods such as: coconuts, avocado, raw olives, nuts, and seeds – particularly hemp seeds and chia seeds. Although it is not advisable to add oils to your diet, if you are going to, or would like to, use raw coconut oil or hemp oil. Hemp oil is a better choice than flax because hemp contains more omega-3's, which are essential fatty acids needed for optimal health. The consumption of oil slows blood flow. When blood samples are taken from people who have recently consumed an oily meal, the oil will float on top of the blood sample. For this reason, I avoid adding oils to my foods.

Because certain nutrients in the body are transported by way of fats, eating good fats will help deliver them to the cells for proper and efficient utilization. It is only when we cook these fats that they become damaging to our tissues and systems.

All processed foods and anything cooked from restaurants have some kind of rancid fat or oils in them. The amount of oils and food additives you get when eating at restaurants, other than truly raw vegan cuisine, is detrimental to your health. All cooked oils are degraded, and not only do they suppress the immune system, but they are also a major cause of free radical damage and this contributes to premature aging and disease. Heavy metals, chemicals, and other toxins also accumulate in fat, especially sticky, cooked fats.

A common myth is that extra virgin olive oil is the best oil to cook with. While I agree that olive oil is a better choice than many of the other oils, such as canola and palm oil, which should always be avoided, this is completely erroneous information if you do not include the fact that olive oil should only be used when it is raw. Even raw, olive oil is not a healthy choice. All oils are degraded when they are exposed to high heat. If you are going to heat oil, at least use organic virgin unrefined coconut oil. It will sustain temperatures up to two-hundred eighty degrees Fahrenheit and still keep from going rancid. You will, however, still denature the enzymes and damage any oils in the plants you are cooking.

To experience vibrant health, cooked oils should be avoided. Even fish contains rancid oils that are equivalent to trans-fats when cooked. This is one reason why a vegan diet is important for maintaining the best of health. We can get our nutrients from other foods. We do not need meat, dairy, or eggs.

It is important to note that all fat in excess causes sugar to store in the body longer and this raises our blood sugar levels while feeding candida yeast and cancer cells. I will cover this more in a later chapter. Additionally, Dr. Michael Greger states that, *"A single fatty meal can paralyze the arteries for five to six hours from the inflammation that is induced."*

I also want to mention that canola oil is a poor choice of oil because it is often retrieved from genetically modified plants. It is over sixty percent erucic acid, which is an unhealthful monounsaturated fat. Even organic canola oil is not a good choice for those wanting to experience the best of health.

Palm oil should also be avoided, not only because it is harmful, but as McCabe explains in his book, *Sunfood Diet Infusion*, orangutans are being killed off, and their habitats demolished, to plant and expand oil palm plantations to create this product. The entire story behind it is extremely sad. Palm oil is an example of oil that becomes damaging to health when it is heated. *In an analysis of country-level data from 1980-1997 derived from the World Health Organization's Mortality Database, U.S. Department of Agriculture international estimates, and the World Bank (234 annual observations; twenty-three countries), it was determined that increased palm oil consumption is related to higher ischemic heart disease mortality rates in developing countries.* The results were published in the December 2011 *Global Health* journal. Please do not consume food products containing palm oil, or support the companies which add it to their products. Palm oil is not good.

ARE YOU DRINKING GOOD QUALITY WATER?

There have been, and always will be, disagreements and varying opinions on which water we should be drinking, as well as how we should store our water. I personally detect varying levels of energy from different sources of water I drink and this is what has led me to include this section.

Regarding to the source of the water, the safest water for us to drink is distilled water. While some believe drinking distilled water will remove nutrients from the body, the opposite has been confirmed as being true. Distilled water can draw the inorganic minerals out from the body, helping to remove excess calcium deposits that are causing plaque to buildup in our joints and arteries.

If possible, I strongly encourage you to check the count of *Total Dissolved Solvents* (TDS) in the water you drink. I even check the count on the water I use to bathe. Dissolved solvents affect everything that consumes, lives in, or uses water. They comprise the total amount of mobile charged ions in water. This includes minerals or metals dissolved in a given volume of water. The TDS reading includes any inorganic element present other than the pure water, water molecule (H_2O), and suspended solids. We want a lower TDS level in the water we drink as well as the water we use to wash our bodies. The lower the TDS level, the more efficiently our body cells will be hydrated. When their is a high TDS count in your water, you are most likely being exposed to contaminants that can pose health risks and even hinder the absorption of water. This may contribute to several ailments including bloating, upset stomach, arthritis, and fibromyalgia. When we shower in water with a high TDS count, we become a filter for that water because the heat opens our pores and then we absorb some of the contaminants. This makes it important for us to filter all of our water sources in our homes (showers, faucets, and fridge).

The *U.S. Environmental Protection Agency* (EPA) places a limit on the contaminant level for consumption of water at five-hundred before it is labeled as a biohazard. For drinking water, I recommend you not exceed a level of ten.

Anything from zero to ten is the range I stay within. You can be sure the level of water is safe by performing a test on it.

So how do you test for TDS? It is simple. You can purchase a TDS water testing meter on Amazon or a site you prefer for around $30 (USD) and simply fill separate glasses with the water from all the water sources in your home. I recommend you test your shower, your faucets, and especially your drinking water. If you have a fridge with filtered water, be sure to test it.

I have a friend whose water we recently tested from his fridge and the reading came back at 384. That is toxic water. He was having an issue with his ankles and joints bothering him and the source of his problem could very well have been a bad water source. The excess calcium and minerals in the water supply may have been leading to calcification of his joints. Calcification of the joints is arthritis. The spout that was pumping the water out of his fridge was nearly closed with plaque. This is what happens in the body. The arteries and joints get blocked with this plaque as well. It is amazing how simply adding a filter to your water, or changing your water filter on time can have an enormous impact on your health.

To make things easier for all of you, determined to find the very best water available in my region, I purchased several brands of bottled waters and tested them. While I still do not believe I have found the best water, I have a better idea of which waters can be considered safe for my health. Here are the results of my testing:

Whole Foods brand spring water in big bottle: 027

Whole Foods spring water small, individual bottles: 105

Valley Springs "Something special from Wisconsin":   198

Ice mountain in a small bottle: 183

Fiji Water in small bottle: 125

Smart Water: 026

Hinckley Springs: 011

Wal-Mart Drinking Water: 002*

Wal-Mart Distilled Water: 000*

Dasani (owned by Coca-Cola):   022*

   *All bottled water is bad news. Bottling water adds a tremendous amount of pollution to the planet. Everything from the drilling, processing, and shipping of the petroleum, to the creation of the bottles, to the shipping of the water, and the trash created by all of the billions upon billions of water bottles adds to plastic and petroleum pollution that is ravaging Earth.
   * I do not encourage consumers to shop at corporate stores such as Wal-Mart, nor do I enjoy contributing to their profits, however, because many consumers purchase their food products and beverages from Wal-Mart, I took a special trip for this purpose.
   * Although Dasani has a low count of 022, keep in mind that this is not pure water. There is a small list of ingredients on the Dasani water label. They include: Water, magnesium sulfate, potassium chloride and refined salt. Refined salt is not healthful and can cause damage to capillaries, including the vascular system in the kidneys and eyes. This makes me wonder why Dasani is the only water offered at many amusement parks, arenas, theaters, and other venues. Why is Dasani being sold at schools as the only source of water for our children to consume? Could it be because of the kickbacks paid to schools? Children, and all humans, should not be drinking bottled water in plastic bottles. Prior to the 1970's, they did not.
   I also decided to purchase two of the bottled gallons of water for infants and young children at Wal-Mart. I noticed that one brand includes fluoride and calcium chloride "for taste." Both of these contribute to health problems. The results of the two bottled waters for infants:

Since 1948 Nursery Purified w/added minerals: 024

Gerber pure purified water: 087*

   *The label on the bottle recommends adding the purified water to baby formulas and cereals. This is not the brightest idea. Adding this water with harmful contaminants to your baby's formula, which already consists of many chemicals and toxins, and additionally, adding the water to cereals containing high-fructose corn syrup and other harmful substances, such as farming chemical residues from non-organic farms will only degrade the health of your child. When considering how many additives and chemical residues are in mass-marketed infant and children's foods, it is no wonder why so many infants are sick and being taken to medical doctors. It is no wonder why the juvenile-onset diabetes (type 1) rates are rising; and why our children are developing leukemia and other cancers. The additives and chemical residues, including those that leach from the packaging, are likely doing the damage.

Finally, I decided to test the water in my home and also my friend's home. The results left me with two must-dos: I had to put filters on all of my water sources, and I needed to change the filters that were already there. Here are the results:

Kitchen sink w/ no filter: 217

Kitchen sink w/ filter that needs to be replaced: 233

Shower w/ no filter: 256

Shower w/ filter that needs to be replaced: 277

Well water bathroom faucet: 430

Well water kitchen sink: 406

Well water fridge water w/ filter: 384

My testing for the level of TDS in water raised my awareness to a few things. There is a need for us all to put filters on all of our water sources and change them regularly, or else have a reverse osmosis system installed. It would be of value for us to test the water we drink for the TDS level prior to continuing to drink that water. We should all consider bottling our drinking water in glass rather than plastic, and solarizing it by letting the glass bottles sit in the sun for a day or two.

Dr. Fereydoon Batmanghelidj was able to successfully cure several patients in his lifetime by having them incorporate clean water into their diet. He helped them reverse conditions from peptic ulcer to constipation to asthma to allergies and many more ailments, simply by having them drink pure water. He is the author of the book, *Your Body's Many Cries for Water*.

I consider it essential for everyone to try to drink up to two quarts of clean water every day. I personally aim to drink a gallon of distilled water daily. Sodas and colas do not replace water in the system. Neither does coffee or tea. Juice is not an alternative unless water is not available. Fresh fruit also becomes an option in this instance. Juices should be fresh and unpasteurized. The purest water is the living water we get from eating organic raw fruits and raw vegetables. Always keep in mind that fruits and vegetables are the best water purifiers in existence. By converting to a raw food diet, we also receive clean water in the fresh produce we consume.

YOUR NUTRIENTS SOOTHE ME

I finally found you.

From beneath the ground you sprouted your gifts and blossomed.

Your nutrients soothe me from pharmaceutical nuisance.
You give me love, laughter, and joy in the most natural way.

Each day you share your enzymes and I give back to nature with the good intention you instill in me from eating your roots.

You are all of Mother Earth's fruits, you are kale, and you are the superfoods of the world.

Your cures never fail.
I fell in love with the way your doses are so potent.

I blend you up in smoothies every day.
I eat you raw and absorb you into me.

You give me hope that all of the world's sickness will cease to exist.

This organic lifestyle you have given me is everyday bliss!

Now that you know the truth about the common foods you have been eating, it becomes obvious that it is time to change the way you eat. Unless you desire sickness or you enjoy being overweight, this is a perfect opportunity for you to change.

For some it is easy to make the transition right away and go completely raw. For others you may find it easier to take baby steps. Baby steps are okay as long as you do not baby yourself for too long. Aim to make improvements weekly and it should take you no longer than a month to start eating most of your diet raw.

In today's world where cancer, heart disease, and diabetes are more common than smiles, happiness, and laughter, there is a need for change. Being aware of what you are eating is the best way to address this need for change.

Chapter 3: WHND

"We have, however in the first place, the need for a strength of character and will-power, such that will make us use the things our bodies require, rather than only the foods we like. Another problem arises from the fact that our modern sedentary lives call for so little energy that many people will not eat enough, even of a good food, to provide for both growth and repair, since hunger appeals are for energy only, the source of heat and power, and not for body-building minerals and other chemicals." – **Dr. Weston A. Price, *Nutrition and Physical Degeneration***

In a society where so many people are consuming health-robbing foods, the questions being asked seem as though they would be about what foods we should avoid, rather than what foods are safe for us to eat. We must start by eliminating all unhealthful substances from the diet. This means no fast foods, no fried foods, no processed foods, no meat, no dairy, no eggs, no sugars, no gluten flours, no cooked oils, and nothing with synthetic chemical additives.

I know this list seems to be a lot, but it is simpler than it appears in words. You can start by purchasing only fresh foods that are not packaged. If you feel you must have packaged foods, at least purchase organic, non-GMO foods so you know you are not getting all of the chemical residues.

We are only hungry when our body craves nutrients. If we feel hungry, it does not mean we need to fill ourselves until we cannot eat anymore. All this does is disrupt the natural processes of the body and tax the organs. When we fill our bellies with nutrient-deficient foods, like so many of us do, once the stomach starts to find more room we find ourselves hungry again. This is because we are starving our body of nutrients and filling it with non-foods that are not much other than stuffing. When we repeat this process over and over, not only are we not being wise with our food choices, but we establish the foundation for an assortment of illnesses. By eating wholesome, raw, organic, non-GMO foods, we provide our tissues with the nutrients they need and find that we are no longer hungry.

It may take some time for your body to get used to being satiated while still not having an overstuffed belly, but over time you will adapt and figure out a way that works for you. During the transformation phase, many people tend to overeat, even when the food is raw. This is because they do not yet understand the difference between having a full stomach and being fully satiated. The best approach to solve this problem is to continue eating a low fat, high-nutrient diet rich in raw fruits and vegetables, until you find that connection between your mind and the rest of your body once again, just like you had at birth.

I always have my clients start the first phase of their diets by eliminating all packaged foods that contain: partially-hydrogenated or hydrogenated oils, palm oil, canola oil, high-fructose corn syrup, bleached flours, artificial sweeteners, food coloring, monosodium glutamate (MSG), hydrolyzed proteins of any sort, gluten grains, refined sugar, regular salt, and sodium benzoate and other preservatives. I also advise eliminating all red meat and pork from the diet in addition to all dairy products, sodas, and eggs.

This allows them to continue eating foods with unrefined flours that are not bleached, unrefined cane sugars or organic evaporated cane juice, and sea salt in the first phase of their program. I do not believe these foods are healthy, but I find this to be a healthier option for them to make the transition than some of the foods they were previously eating.

During this time, they also add juicing to their diets. They begin juicing with green juices. This helps to regenerate their production of hydrochloric acid, which makes it easier to break down the roughage from the raw foods they will soon be ingesting regularly.

Once they get this under control, I make sure they eliminate all animal products from the diet. This includes all beef, pork, chicken, fish, and other meat or meat extracts (broth, gelatin, jello), and all dairy products (milk, cream, creamer, cheese, ice cream, butter, yogurt, whey, and casein). To help them get a visual of why it is important that they refrain from eating animal products, I suggest that they watch the documentaries: *Forks Over Knives, Earthlings, Meet Your Meat, The Future of Food, King Corn, Fat, Sick, and Nearly Dead,* and *May I Be Frank.*

In this second phase of their program, they should be comfortable enough to make the complete transition to a vegan diet. During this time, they are introducing raw foods and still lightly cooking some foods, such as by boiling or steaming: wild rice, brown rice, lentils, millet, quinoa, beans, and root vegetables. This should be no more than three weeks into the program.

After they are comfortable with this phase, I have them incorporate more raw foods into their diet until their diet is mostly or entirely raw, whichever they prefer. In this process of no more than two months, I have had clients who have lost anywhere from twenty to one-hundred pounds.

To give you a better picture, I have made two separate grocery lists. Do not purchase anything from the unhealthy side, and only purchase foods from the healthy side, and I assure you that you will have a much more healthful and enjoyable life.

HEALTHY GROCERY LIST

Organic fruits (bananas, avocados, tomatoes, apples, citrus, peaches, pomegranates, cucumbers, bell peppers, berries, etc)
Organic vegetables (leafy greens, celery, yellow vegetables, etc)
Organic root vegetables (turmeric, ginger, radishes, beets, carrots, sweet potatoes, etc)
Organic herbs (parsley, purslane, cilantro, basil, etc)
Organic grains (quinoa, millet, buckwheat, amaranth, oats)
Raw organic nuts and seeds (almonds, Brazil nuts sparingly, pecans, pistachios, walnuts, sunflower seeds, pumpkin seeds, flax seeds, chia seeds, hemp seeds)
Raw organic superfoods (goji berries, carob powder, fenugreek, maca powder, aloe vera)
Organic water veggies (blue-green algae, chlorella, spirulina, kelp, dulse, nori, wakame, etc)
Organic sprouting seeds (mung beans, broccoli seeds, radish seeds, alfalfa, sunflower, etc)
Organic virgin unrefined coconut oil & organic coconut
Organic cold-pressed extra-virgin olive oil (for your hair)
Organic sprouted whole-grain grain breads/wraps - unleavened
Organic sweetener (stevia, dates, maple syrup, coconut sap crystals)
Organic dried fruits (dates, figs, currants, raisins, Turkish apricots)
Organic hummus made fresh with zucchini instead of garbanzos
Distilled, pure water in glass jars
Organic spices for flavor (black pepper, cayenne pepper, curry, cumin, coriander, herbs, chili powder)
Organic peppers (chilies, cayenne, Serranos, habaneros, fresnos, Jalapenos, bell peppers, sweet peppers, etc)
Green Vibrance, Infinity Greens, Vitamineral Green, or Field of Greens supplementation
Organic fermented foods (kombucha, Kim-Chi, sauerkraut, etc)

UNHEALTHY GROCERY LIST

Pop Tarts (regular and generic)
Microwaveable frozen dinners
Hot Pockets (all frozen packaged foods)
Frozen pizzas (any type)
Colas and Sodas (Coca-Cola, Diet Coke, Sprite, etc)
Milk (pasteurized milk is indigestible)
Cheese (all cheese is unhealthful, fat-free, organic, or not)
Meat (beef, chicken, pork, lunch meat, fish, reptiles, crustaceans)
All chips, including baked
Cheetos (regular and flaming hot)
Donuts (Krispy Kreme, Entenmann's)
Bread (Any bread that contains flour and/or gluten grains)
Sugar (Any type of refined sugar, including corn syrup and agave)
Pastries (breakfast strudels)
Canned soups (MSG laden and full of chemicals leached from the cans)
Popcorn
Coffee (regular or decaf)
Juice cocktails (Sugary drinks)
V8 (very little nutrients and chemicals leached from the can)
Beer (regular, dark, or light)
Alcohol (Any type of liquor should be avoided)
Medicine (Aspirin, Tylenol, Advil)
Condiments (Ketchup, mayonnaise, Worcestershire)
Processed Meats (Sausage, Bologna, lunch meats, etc)
Ice Cream (All brands and types)
Freezer Pops (Popsicles, Frozen sugar)
Candy (Chocolate, bars, candies)

THE FOUR BASIC FOOD GROUPS

In school we were taught to follow the four basic food groups – meats, dairy, fruits/veggies, and grains. By following these four basic food groups from a young age, and especially non-organic, processed varieties of them, we are laying the groundwork for illness. This style of diet is used to plan meals in hospitals, school cafeterias, juvenile detention centers, the military, and prisons. This is why those people who visit hospitals continue to go back, and could be part of the reason why those who are incarcerated continue to commit crimes.

In his book, *Vegan Nutrition*, Dr. Michael Klaper presents an interesting tidbit about what a nutritious day of eating would look like if you were to follow the guidelines of the basic four food groups. A "nutritious" day of eating would include: a breakfast of bacon or sausage with eggs, and toast with sugary jam and/or butter, washed down with a glass of milk. Lunch could be something like a cheeseburger or chicken sandwich with French fries and a milkshake. Dinner would be a steak or fried chicken most likely with a baked potato that is loaded with salt, butter, and/or sour cream. The fruits and vegetables would be the lettuce and tomato on the sandwich and the remnants of fruit in the milkshake or the jam on the toast. Ice cream would be an ideal dessert and potato chips, or maybe a piece of fruit, would be the snack of choice in between meals. By eating these meals, you can expect an array of different illnesses mixed with slothful energy.

We cannot follow these basic four food groups and expect to experience vibrant health. To experience and maintain the best of health, we need to eat raw, organic and fresh produce every day – and eliminate all processed foods, meats, eggs, and dairy from our diets while remaining physically active.

A much better plan would be the "*Basic Nine*", consisting of fruits and vegetables, leafy green vegetables, sprouts, nuts and seeds, grasses, algae, sprouted non-gluten grains, herbs, and maybe some superfoods mixed into our meals, juices, smoothies, and snacks, such as hemp seeds, chia seeds, and freshly ground flax and/or fenugreek.

What the USDA has done is created nutritional guidelines for the sole purpose of selling meat and dairy to the consumers for profit. The USDA functions as a trade group for the meat, dairy, egg, and grain industries. It is all a part of their carefully designed business strategy. They wanted to sell all of their crops and products so they infiltrated the educational, military, medical, jail, and prison institutions and sold them on the USDA food pyramid's "*nutritional guidelines.*"

John Robbins' landmark book, *Diet for a New America,* was chief in educating people about the lies of the USDA food pyramid. In the book, John mentions that the concept of the "*basic four*" food groups was promoted by the

National Egg Board, the *National Dairy Council*, and the *National Livestock and Meat Board*. He also goes on to explain how the *National Dairy Council* is the foremost supplier of "*nutritional education*" materials to classrooms in the United States. This is why we were deceived for so many years into believing animal products are somehow beneficial to our health. The truth has been revealed that they are not in any way contributors to good health and we should soon see a gradual shift away from this deadly advice.

As more of us research and discover the truth, and as more of us protest against the teachings of the USDA and FDA and their false nutritional scams, we can hope that the guidelines will begin to disappear.

THE REAL FOOD PYRAMID

The food pyramid below is what we should have been following all of our lives. As children we should have learned to follow this pyramid rather than the disease-promoting food pyramid we were deceived into following by the USDA. This pyramid suggests that we eat abundant amounts of leafy greens and fruits. We should moderate our intake of protein-dominant foods, and they should be sourced only from live food choices like dark greens, and also sprouts, seeds, and nuts. We should understand that all fruits, and all vegetables contain the amino acids our bodies use to build protein, and that there is no need to consume problematic animal protein that induces disease. All of the medicinal foods such as wheatgrass and seaweed should be eaten sparingly when needed. By observing this pyramid, you will see that the unnecessary grains and animal products are not included. I found this chart on the website **vegan-raw-diet.com**. The site also provides a lot of helpful information. By following this chart, we can be assured we will ingest the nutrients our bodies need for experiencing optimal levels of health.

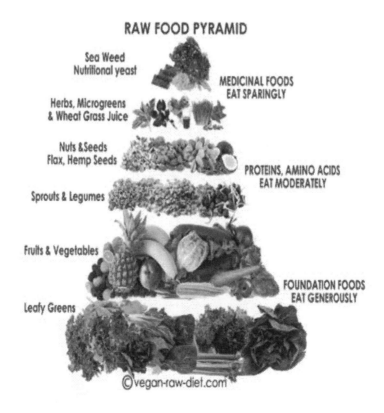

THE FOOD PYRAMID OF DISEASE

The food pyramid that was created by the USDA (below from usda.gov), which we have been manipulated into following since elementary school, is misleading and can infuse our bodies with common degenerative and chronic diseases. If you compare the two charts, you will notice that the real food pyramid advises the consumption of healthful, lively foods and the USDA food pyramid is full of dead foods. By following this "dead food" pyramid, we are basically inviting sickness, disease, and premature death. You notice that it suggests breads, starches, and cereals in the most abundant amount without clarifying which of the grains and other starches are healthful, and which, like gluten grains and bleached grains, are unhealthful. Making your diet consist so abundantly of these food choices is bad advice, and can trigger health problems. The chart also suggests that meats, dairy, and eggs, which are the leading inducers of heart attacks, strokes, diabetes, arthritis, Alzheimer's, osteoporosis, and certain types of cancer, including colon and breast cancer, to be heavily present in the diet.

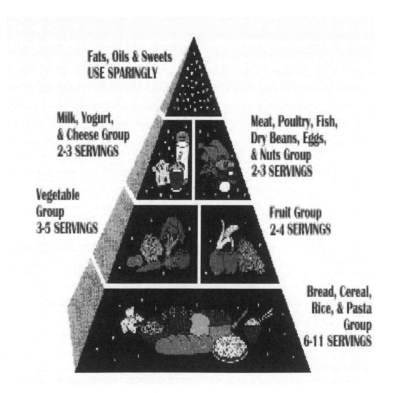

BALANCING YOUR pH

"The pH level of our internal fluids affects every cell in our bodies. The entire metabolic process depends on an alkaline environment. Chronic over-acidity corrodes body tissue, and if left unchecked will interrupt all cellular activities and functions, from the beating of your heart to the neural firing of your brain. In other words, over-acidity interferes with life itself. It is at the root of all sickness and disease. – Dr. Robert Young, *The pH Miracle*

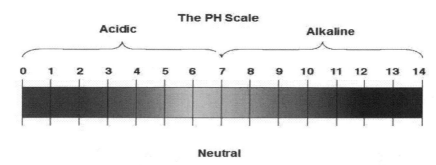

It is highly important that we understand the acid/alkaline balance in our bodies. Alkalizing foods are those that are rich in calcium, magnesium, sodium, potassium, and iron. Acid-forming foods are foods rich in sulphur, phosphorus, iodine, and chlorine.

Flesh foods (meat), grains (except for millet and buckwheat), and peanuts are all acid-forming because they have a greater concentration of one type of mineral. By eating leafy green vegetables and organic fruits, sprouts, spirulina, chlorella, and some seaweed, we will gain alkalinity in our bodies.

The human body is constantly fighting to maintain an optimal pH of 7.365. When our body becomes too acidic, we leach calcium and alkaline minerals from our bones and other tissues to buffer the blood. It is important for your system to maintain this slightly alkaline pH level. To be at the best of health, your pH level should be between 7.35-7.40. The problem is that many people have levels as low as 6.3. When your blood becomes this acidic, you are likely to develop acidosis. For your body to function properly and to be in congruence with every other part of your body, you have to be at 7.0 or above.

The pH level of your body is one way to determine the level of your health. By following a raw, plant-rich alkaline diet and getting regular exercise, you will be less likely to experience stress, will sleep better, and will find contentment. You will lose extra belly fat, you will become more alert, and you will notice a lot of other positive changes in your life. You may even begin to feel happier, less sluggish, and more energized.

Acidosis conditions nurture heart disease, cancer, arthritis, osteoporosis, and other degenerative conditions. This condition is caused by deficiencies of minerals such as calcium and magnesium, combined with a deficiency of vitamin D and residues of unhealthful food additives and farming chemicals.

While it is possible to create a temporary alkaline state by drinking carrot and parsley juice, a permanent alkaline state can be reached by adhering to an alkaline diet. Once you become alkaline, you will start to feel whole again and you will look better, feel more vibrant, and live much more efficiently because your system, including your brain and other organs, will function better.

Be sure to regularly check your pH level. Systematic acidity is one of the major contributors of cancer. PH strips (litmus paper) are sold at pharmacies for fewer than five dollars. Dr. Robert Barefoot uses pH strips as "ice-breakers" to open his seminars. He has everyone test their pH. Before they reveal their results to him, he often guesses accurately their pH simply by observing the shape of their bodies, the tone of their skin, and the complexion of their faces.

Being acidic inhibits the ability of the body to reach the highest state of excellent health. It makes you more likely to experience stress, putrefaction, and anger, and to suffer physical injuries. It draws down the body and mood, and increases the likelihood of weight gain and hormonal imbalances.

The following is a list of acid-forming and alkaline-forming foods. Always eat more alkaline than acidic by eating about eighty-to-ninety percent alkaline foods and ten-to-twenty percent acid foods.

ALKALINE FOODS

To feel radiantly alive and to function at a high level wherein you can fully express your talents and intellect, follow an alkaline diet. Most alkaline foods are safe for human consumption. The foods I am listing in this segment are healthy alkaline foods.

Fruits: apples, apricots, bananas, blackberries, blueberries, cantaloupe, cherries, coconuts, currants, dates, dried fruits, figs, grapefruit, grapes, guava, honeydew melons, kiwis, lemons, limes, lychees, mangos, nectarines, oranges, passion fruit, papaya, pears, peaches, persimmons, pineapple, pomegranates, raisins, strawberries, tangerines, and watermelon.

Vegetables: alfalfa, artichokes, asparagus, avocados, basil, bean sprouts, beets, bell peppers, broccoli, broccoli leaf, Brussels sprouts, cabbage, carrots, celery, cauliflower, cauliflower leaf, chard, chives, cilantro, collards, cucumber, dandelion, dill, eggplant, fennel stalk, garlic, green beans, kale, leeks, lettuce, mung bean sprouts, okra, olives, onions, parsley, parsnips, peas, pumpkin, radishes, sauerkraut (raw, not canned), spinach, sprouts, squash, sweet potatoes, tomatoes, turnips, watercress, yams, and zucchini.

Various others: almonds, amaranth, apple cider vinegar, chestnuts, dulse, herbal tea, kelp, millet, miso, molasses, organic spices, seaweeds, and various algae.

ACID-FORMING FOODS

Acid-forming foods create acidosis in the body. Acidosis conditions nurture stress disorders, stress injuries, and inflammation. We always want to avoid an acidic body condition. This does not mean we have to avoid all acid-forming foods. I have listed the acid-forming foods to always avoid and the ones that are necessary for properly balancing the pH level in your body.

Acid foods to avoid: alcohol, artificial coloring, artificial flavoring, aspirin, barley, breads, cakes, candy, canned foods, cereals, cheeses, chocolate, coffee, condiments, cooked corn, corn starch, crackers, custards, dairy products, diet sodas, dressings, doughnuts, egg whites, eggs, flours and flour-based foods, gelatin, gravies, grits, ice cream, jams, jellies, ketchup, mayonnaise, meats, gluten grains, pasta, pastries, processed oils, peanuts, rice cakes, rice, rice vinegar, salt, sodas, soybeans, soy products, spaghetti, sugars, tapioca, tea (conventional), vinegar, yogurt

Acid foods in moderation: cranberries, dried beans, garbanzo beans, lentils, mustard, oatmeal, nuts, plums, prunes, seeds

LIVING FOODS

"Keeping your body healthy is an expression of gratitude to the whole cosmos — the trees, the clouds, everything." – Thich Nhat Hanh

When you eat food, you become drawn to the source of the food. So by choosing to eat fruits, vegetables, and other plant based foods, you are drawn to nature, the origin of that food. The living energy reunites you with more of life. When you eat meat (dead flesh) and other processed foods that lack living energy, you begin to require synthetic entertainment to stimulate an undernourished and understimulated mind. The dead energy from the food sucks you into TV, celebrity gossip, mainstream media, and being an observer rather than a participant in the things you enjoy. Ultimately, you change the course of your evolution.

The enzymes in live foods aid digestion. Living foods contain life within them. A sprout is a perfect example of a living food. All of the nutrients in sprouts are unharmed and they are ready to provide the body with nutrients. Other living foods are raw fruits and raw vegetables. Fresh, unpasteurized green juices and smoothies are also considered "living."

By eating and drinking more living foods, we liven up, gain more energy, and tend to have more charisma. If we are sick and we introduce living foods, we notice almost immediately that we start to feel better. Living foods are for living people. If you want to be alive, I suggest you eat foods that are alive.

Meat, dairy, eggs, bread, and grilled, fried, baked, and other highly-heated foods are not *lively* choices. They will give you negative energy and nurture frustration, sadness, dissatisfaction, stress, slothfulness, and anxiety.

EASILY DIGESTED FOODS

It is important that we eat foods that are easy to digest. This conserves energy and allows our body to function at its peak level. These foods require less energy to break down; therefore, we can use that energy to perform other tasks, such as repairing damaged cells and tissues, detoxifying our organs, filtering our blood, and especially, providing fuel to our brain so we can be mentally alert. Therefore, we always want to avoid heavy foods. Examples of heavy foods are: meat, eggs, dairy, sugar, breads and gluten grains, and cooked, fried, and sauteed oils.

When foods are light, and easily digestible, the proteins are easily broken down into amino acids, the carbohydrates are broken down into simple sugars, and the fats are broken down into fatty acids and glycerol, thereby allowing each of these substances to be assimilated regularly. This takes a burden off of our digestive system and relieves our pancreas of laboring unnecessarily.

These foods that are easy to digest include: raw fruits and leafy vegetables, green juices, and sprouts. You can sprout many types of seeds and beans and they will turn out delicious. Some of my favorite sprouts are mung bean, radish, broccoli, alfalfa, sunflower, fenugreek, adzuki, and mustard.

Sprouts are very simple to grow. All you have to do is put about a half of a cup of mung beans or other seeds in a sprouting jar. Then soak them over night in filtered water. Strain the water the next day and let the jar lay on its side in a cabinet where it is dark. Pour some clean water in there and swish them around twice a day so they get rinsed and do not dry out. In three to six days you will have a jar full of sprouts.

For those of you who enjoy bread, some companies make breads that are made out of sprouted grains. Essene bread and Manna bread are two good options. Ezekiel makes sprouted bread, but they add gluten to it, making it a poor choice. If they were to remove the gluten grain I would endorse their product. You can find these breads at many grocers that offer organic foods. Sprouted grain breads are a good choice of food for those of you going through the transition to maintaining a cleaner diet. They can help wean you from eating bread altogether. A better option would be to make your own flourless sprouted bread in a dehydrator. Victoria Boutenko's book, *Raw Family Signature Dishes* has bread recipes. So does Kristen Suzanne's book, *EASY Raw Vegan Dehydrating*.

ORGANIC FOODS

It is smart that we buy our produce organic, and if we can, maintain an organic garden. As I mentioned in the first chapter, organically grown foods are higher in mineral, vitamin, and antioxidant content. They are also free of pesticides and safe from being genetically modified.

A review published by *the Organic Center*, a nonprofit food research outfit, in March of 2008, and titled, *New Evidence Confirms the Nutritional Superiority of Plant-Based Organic Foods,* found that *total phenolics, vitamin E, vitamin C, quercetin, and total antioxidant capacity of organics exceeded that of conventionally grown produce – in the case of total antioxidant capacity, by eighty percent. Conventional products had higher levels of potassium, phosphorous, and total protein, all basic constituents of conventional fertilizers.* Nutrition scientist Denis Lairon reported similar findings in a review published in 2009 in *Agronomy for Sustainable Development.* In addition to the nutritional superiority of organic foods, they are not exposed to the chemicals which conventional crops are.

A young lady once sought my advice about fruit allergies. After observing her situation, I realized that all of the fruits she had reactions from were the ones containing the highest amounts of pesticides, herbicides, fertilizers, miticides, and fungicides. One particular food she had allergic reactions to was strawberries. Her problem was not the fruit itself, but the farming chemicals used on the fruit. All she had to do was switch from conventional strawberries to organic strawberries and she was fine. Strawberries have tiny holes on the surface and they absorb more farming chemicals than nearly any other fruit.

The produce that you should always buy organic is: apples, bell peppers, celery, cherries, cucumbers, grapes, lettuce, peaches, pears, spinach, strawberries, and tomatoes. This does not mean that I am encouraging you to purchase your other produce conventional, I am telling you to refrain from purchasing these particular foods conventional. I always urge everyone to buy all of their produce organic and to support local farmer's markets.

If you are lucky enough to be in the Houston, TX area, become familiar with Kristina Carrillo-Bucaram and her *Rawfully Organic Coop (fullyraw.com)*. I dream that one day she will be able to spread her concept of "*organic goodness*" in other cities and towns across the country, and around the world.

CHLOROPHYLL

Grasses contain enough nutrients for us to survive on them alone. We do not, however, want to eat grasses all day. The blood of plants, and the liquid from these grasses, is known as chlorophyll. Chlorophyll is a pre-cursor to vitamin A, a natural detoxifying agent, and a deodorizer. It is very similar in molecular structure to that of hemoglobin, or human blood. Hemoglobin is centered on the iron atom, while chlorophyll is centered on the magnesium atom. This is the main difference between the two substances. If you read the book, *Biological Transmutations,* by C.L. Kervran, he explains how the human body is capable of transmuting certain minerals into other minerals once inside the body, as they are needed. He states that silicon can be converted into calcium, and that magnesium is converted into iron as it is needed.

If magnesium is converted into iron as it is needed in our bodies, there is no reason why any one of us should develop anemia or have iron deficiencies. If we do develop anemia or an iron deficiency, we cannot easily supplement with iron because it can be toxic to our liver. The solution then could be eating foods rich in chlorophyll.

What many do not know about magnesium is that a blood test could come back indicating sufficient amounts in the blood and the person could still have a magnesium deficiency. This is because we store magnesium in the tissues, not the blood. When we have low magnesium in the tissues, many problems arise in the body.

Wheatgrass is among the best sources for chlorophyll. Many grasses and greens contain chlorophyll. The fresh water alga, spirulina, is rich in chlorophyll as well. Therefore it is beneficial to drink wheatgrass shots and include green juices full of leafy greens and other alkaline vegetables in your diet each day to provide your tissues with sufficient amounts of magnesium.

It is possible to rebuild your blood supply in seven days by doing a seven day wheatgrass juice fast. The chlorophyll in wheatgrass is so powerful that it can inhibit the growth of leukemia cells. A study that was published in the *Turkish Journal of Medical Science* in 2011 titled, *Antiproliferative, apoptotic and antioxidant activities of wheatgrass,* found that *plant-based diet supplements help the prevention and therapy of several kinds of cancer because they contain micronutrients, a class of substances that have been shown to exhibit chemopreventive and chemotherapeutic activities. In the study, the effects and oxidant/antioxidant status of aqueous and ethanol extracts of wheatgrass were tested in human chronic myeloid leukemia CML (K562) cell line. K562 cell lines were treated with ten percent (w/v) concentration of aqueous and ethanol wheatgrass extracts. Both preparations inhibited the growth of leukemia cells in a time-dependent manner. It was* concluded from the study that wheatgrass extract has an antioxidant activity, inhibits proliferation of leukemia cells, and induces apoptosis.

FRESH JUICES

Juice that you make at home in a juicer or that you buy fresh from a juice bar is far superior to the juice sold in bottles. Unless labeled otherwise, the bottled juices are always pasteurized. The pasteurization process degrades certain nutrients, including biophotons and enzymes. Leaving fresh juice out for more than a few hours will also deplete it of some nutrients.

According to Dr. Michael Greger, up to ninety percent of the nutritional value is lost when we choose fruit juice rather than whole fruit. This is based on the Oxygen Radical Absorbance Capacity (ORAC) of fruits compared to fruit juices. Foods listed as "rich in antioxidants" should have an ORAC level of at least 1,000 per 100 grams. The study, titled, *Pressing Effects on Yield, Quality, and Nutraceutical Content of Juice, Seeds, and Skins from Black Beauty and Sunbelt Grapes*, found that up to ninety percent of nutrients were being thrown in the trash. The pasteurized juices had less total phenolics, total anthocyanins, and ORAC levels than the whole grapes.

To make it easier to keep fresh juice in your diet, purchase a juicer, such as a Champion, Green Star, Jack LaLanne, or Breville. You may be able to find used juicers for sale on craigslist.org or ebay.com, or at a thrift store.

Juices are high in electrolytes, which are necessary for vibrant health. Green juices contain chlorophyll, which is, as I just mentioned, an incredible substance. Fresh juices also contain a good balance of minerals like calcium, magnesium, potassium, and sodium. The magnesium combined with the calcium makes the calcium more readily absorbed and is excellent for bone health. The potassium balances out the sodium as well, helping your body maintain homeostasis. Drinking fresh juices will give your kidneys and liver a rejuvenating boost.

In a review of government data, researchers from Baylor College of Medicine found that *children between the ages of two and eleven who consumed an average of 4.1 fluid ounces of one-hundred percent fruit juice daily had significantly higher intake levels of vitamin C, vitamin B, potassium, riboflavin, magnesium, iron, and folate, than non-juice drinkers, who, on average, did not meet the recommended intake levels for many of these essential nutrients. In addition, the fruit-juice-drinking group was found to consume significantly more whole fruits, and fewer added sugars and fats.* In a separate study, researchers from Louisiana State University found similar findings of higher intake levels of nutrients from fresh juice in children between the ages of twelve and eighteen. You can juice with combinations of multiple juices or simply stick to one or two that you like. I like to use at least three vegetables in each juice I make. No matter what you decide, you will always gain energy when you drink fresh juices.

For your homemade juice, pick a combination of any of these: asparagus, beets, beet leaf, broccoli leaf, cabbage, carrots, cauliflower leaf, celery, chard, collard leaf, cranberries (whole and fresh), cucumber, dandelion, fennel stalks, ginger, green apples, kale, lettuce, parsley, peppers, purslane, spinach, sprouts, tomato, wheatgrass, wild greens, or yellow squash. See Sergei Boutenko's videos on YouTube to learn more about wild greens.

If there is an edible green that is not on the list, you can still juice it. Get creative. A nutrient-rich energy boosting juice that I recommend is a combination of carrot, celery, beet, and parsley. Carrot is usually a good base and cucumbers produce a lot of juice. Green apples provide a good tart sweetness. Get creative with it. You can also add spirulina or chlorella. There are plenty of recipe books out there for fresh juice blends if you need some extra guidance. A reliable and affordable book is Jay Kordich's, *The Juiceman's Power of Juicing*. You may also want to purchase *The Big Book of Juices* by Natalie Savona or *The Juicing Bible* by Pat Crocker.

BLENDED DRINKS

I like to have at least two blended drinks a day. Purchasing a high powered blender such as a *Blend Tec,* or *Vita Mix,* can be advantageous because they can be used to blend any food at a high speed without leaving large remnants of seeds or fibers in the drink. If you cannot afford a high powered blender at this time, that is perfectly okay. You will get by just fine with an inexpensive blender from the thrift store, or you could purchase one online.

While it is important to drink fresh organic juices daily, be sure to also include whole fruit smoothies. As I mentioned, juices can contain less total phenolics, anthocyanins, and ORAC levels than whole fruits. A 2007 edition of *Food and Chemical Toxicology* found that there are anti-cancer properties in phenolics that were retrieved from apple waste being discarded after juicing. Phenols are chemical compounds that are found in plants that protect the plant from bacterial and fungal infections, as well as from UV radiation damage. They are known to have high antioxidant profiles and are found mostly in the skin and seeds of raw fruits and vegetables. Juices are often void of these compounds, as well as anthocyanins, so it is necessary to eat whole fruits, or drink smoothies containing the skin, seeds, and pulp of fruits in addition to juicing. Anthocyanins protect cells from high light damage by absorbing blue-green and ultraviolet light. They are powerful antioxidants found in red, purple, and blue plant matter and are stored in all tissues of higher plants, including leaves, stems, roots, flowers, and fruits. Foods rich in anthocyanins include, berries, cherries, currants, eggplant peel, grapes, purple rice, and red cabbage. The January 2012 edition of *Molecular Nutrition and Food Research* published a study on dietary anthocyanin-rich plants, showing a role in obesity control, diabetes control, cardiovascular disease prevention, and improvement of visual and brain functions.

My morning smoothies always consist of all organic ingredients and contain the following: two or three frozen bananas, a handful of fresh or frozen berries (blackberries, blueberries, raspberries, and strawberries) and cherries, a tablespoon of ground flax, a tablespoon of spirulina, a tablespoon of dulse, a tablespoon of fenugreek seed powder, two tablespoons of chia seeds, a teaspoon of maca powder, two or three tablespoons of hemp seeds, about two-to-three cups of fresh chard, kale, or spinach, a dash of vanilla bean powder, and the rest of the blender filled nearly to the top with distilled water or coconut water.

What I have found is that bananas do well as a base for any smoothie. Their consistency holds the drink together and they also provide just enough sweetness to perfectly compliment the taste of the greens. It is important that you get organic bananas, as the chemicals used on non-organic bananas have caused many health problems for farmers, including severe birth deformities in their children. If you live in a large city, it is likely that you can purchase cases of bananas from a fruit wholesaler at a discounted price. Let them ripen until they freckle, peel, and then freeze them for later use in smoothies. When bananas are not available, other options may be apples, peaches, mango, or fresh-squeezed orange juice.

If you have a high powered blender, you can try throwing an avocado pit in your drink. These contain high amounts of soluble fibers. The most important thing is to get creative with it, have fun, and discover for yourself which combinations satisfy your taste.

WHERE DO I GET MY CARBOHYDRATES?

One diet that I would never recommend is one that is low carb. Any diet that is high in protein or high in fat is also not a good idea, no matter what your condition may be. In a 2009 study published in the *New England Journal of Medicine,* titled, *A look at the low-carbohydrate diet,* it was determined that *high-fat, high-protein, low-carbohydrate diets (which are usually high in red meat, such as the Atkins and Paleolithic diets) may accelerate atherosclerosis through mechanisms that are unrelated to the classic cardiovascular risk factors.* Carbohydrates are vital for our well-being. While some who follow the Paleo-style diet may experience weight loss, they are not improving their health by eating this way.

Humans have long, plant-friendly digestive tracts, and we are born to eat diets consisting mainly, or completely of fruits and vegetables. We receive our fats and our proteins from eating sprouts, nuts, grains, and seeds in the amounts they are needed. Where many people go wrong is in eating the wrong carbohydrates, such as baked goods and refined sugars. Fruits are healthy, and are the ideal carbohydrate.

I'm sure you have heard the terms complex and simple carbs, well, I do not resort to those definitions or labels. The simple approach is to cut out all refined sugars (white sugar, brown sugar, sugar in the raw, agave, and corn syrup) and all flours and baked goods (such as doughnuts and cookies) from your diet. This suddenly cuts your food options down to only a few choices. Fruits, vegetables, soaked raw oats, carrots, beets, pseudograins, and sprouted grains are the only foods you should consume for carbohydrates. If you like pasta, you can wean yourself off of pasta by replacing wheat pasta noodles with organic quinoa or brown rice pasta. Be sure the pasta has two ingredients in it. Those two ingredients should be organic brown rice and water, or organic quinoa and water. If the pasta contains brown rice flour it is no good. Brown rice and quinoa pasta taste similar to the unhealthful ones. Many say that quinoa pasta is the best tasting of all. While brown rice and quinoa pasta are still a cooked food, they are a much better choice than pastas made of wheat, spelt, or other ingredients.   Boiling them also avoids acrylamide formation.

Spaghetti squash is another option, and has the added bonus of some beneficial natural plant chemicals. When boiled or heated it has an interior that shreds into pasta-like strands. My advice is to purchase a vegetable spiralizer and make raw pasta from zucchini, sweet potato, or yellow squash. A spiralizer is a piece of kitchen equipment that is used to make noodle-like strands from vegetables. You can purchase them online and they are usually less than fifty dollars.

The best choice of carbohydrate is fresh, ripe organic fruit. Green leafy vegetables are another good choice. If you feel you must eat grains, go for the pseudograins. Soak quinoa, millet, buckwheat, oats, or amaranth, and try making some dishes with those. Sprouted grain bread could be used for weaning yourself from bread, if you are a heavy bread eater. Your goal should be to get away from bread and gluten grain pasta altogether.

WHERE DO I GET MY PROTEIN?

As I mentioned in chapter two, animal protein is not a healthful food for humans. Proteins are made of amino acids, which are in all fruits and vegetables, sprouts, nuts, and seeds. You can get all of your amino acids in sufficient amounts by eating a plant based diet. As long as you eat enough calories from fruits and vegetables, you automatically, and easily, get enough of the amino acids your body uses to create proteins.

How many people do you know with a protein deficiency today? I am guessing zero. People do not easily or commonly get protein deficiencies. What happens to those who become frail or sick is they have a vitamin or mineral deficiency, a deficiency in omega 3 fatty acids, a lack of raw fruits and vegetables in their diet, and an overload of toxins in their body.

Always remember that excess animal protein is linked to disease, and when we take in more protein than we need, we cannot utilize this protein, so we store the excess in our organs, where they putrefy, laying the groundwork for illness.

Protein makes up the bones, muscles, skin, cartilage, and tendons and fascia that hold us together. It creates the enzymes, hormones, mucus, digestive fluids, blood, lymph, and other fluids that assure our organs function. We create proteins from amino acids in the food we eat.

In an interview with Dr. T. Colin Campbell that was published in the *May/June 2011 issue of the Vibrant Life* journal, Dr. Campbell addresses how much protein we really need in our bodies. He states, *"Protein only needs to be about ten percent of our diet, even for growing children. For adult men, that's about fifty-six grams of protein per day. Adult women need around forty-six grams daily, and children need considerably less."* He explains this further by saying, *"Many Americans believe they must eat lots of meat to provide their bodies with sufficient amounts of protein. As a result, the average American eats around 222 pounds of meat each year, taking in seventy to one-hundred grams of protein every day. Along with this excess protein comes extra fat and cholesterol. This creates an environment that nurtures cancer cells, heart disease, and a host of chronic illnesses. The good news is, plants have protein, too. It is present in sufficient amounts in plants to supply all the protein our bodies need."*

My best advice would be to stop worrying about protein. We will always provide our bodies with a sufficient amount by eating amino acid-rich foods, which is what raw fruits and vegetables are.

HOW DO I GET THE RIGHT FATS IN MY SYSTEM?

The best sources for your lipids and essential fats come from: blue-green algae, chia, coconuts, flaxseeds, hemp seeds, olives, avocado, sunflower seeds, almonds, pumpkin seeds, durian fruit, and raw, green leafy vegetables. You can also sprout nuts and seeds and obtain good fats from eating those sprouts.

While fats are essential to our health, we must make sure we do not ingest too many fats. High fat diets are linked to degenerative conditions. Most high protein foods eaten today by the standard American are also high in fat. All raw fruit and all raw veggies contain essential fatty acids in every cell. There is no need to add oil to foods, or to eat oil-rich foods. Even lemons are rich in essential fatty acids. I strongly encourage following a lower fat diet closer to the "80/10/10" approach. Dr. Douglas Graham has written an excellent book that is very easy to follow titled, *The 80/10/10 Diet.* John McCabe also covers this issue in his books, *Sunfood Traveler,* and *Sunfood Diet Infusion.*

VITAMINS, SUPPLEMENTS, AND MINERAL RICH FOODS

With thousands of essential identified nutrients coming from food in various combinations, the food you take in should be rich in vitamins, minerals, and phytochemicals. All of these essential nutrients are required in different amounts to reach a level of homeostasis where your body is balanced. There are sixty-five known minerals, and of these, twenty-two are essential to the normal functions of the body. Because we cannot produce minerals ourselves, it is imperative that we eat mineral rich foods.

If you experience symptoms of frequent colds, flu, or eye, ear, nose, or throat infections, low energy, swollen glands, digestive problems, blood disorders, nervousness, sleep problems, irritability, anxiety, or even weight problems, chances are you might have nutrient deficiencies.

Vitamins, minerals, enzymes, essential fatty acids, and other nutrients work synergistically. Even foods that contain an abundance of other minerals cannot be utilized without an adequate quantity of fat-soluble vitamins. Therefore it is important to make sure we get a sufficient amount of these fats in our diet. Raw fruits and veggies contain adequate amounts of fats and vitamins, so by following this diet you have no need to be concerned.

We can get sufficient amounts of these fat soluble vitamins A, D, E, and K from eating a variety of fruits and vegetables. It is not necessary to supplement any of these by taking vitamin and mineral pills, and is definitely not necessary to eat animals or their by-prodcuts.

Vitamin A: apples, apricots, asparagus, avocados, broccoli, carrots, chia sprouts, endive, kale, papaya, prunes, pumpkin, spinach, squash, sunflower green sprouts, tomatoes, turnip greens, watermelon, yams.

Vitamin D: alfalfa, arame, blue-green algae, clover sprouts, mushrooms, olives, sunflower seeds, and of course, sunlight (the rays of the sun help to synthesize Vitamin D on our skin and then we absorb it into our system).

Vitamin E: asparagus, avocado, soaked or germinated almonds or hazelnuts, pine nuts, romaine lettuce, spinach, sunflower green sprouts.

Vitamin K: alfalfa sprouts, asparagus, broccoli sprouts, cabbage, carrots, chlorophyll, kale, kelp, spinach, tomatoes, turnip greens.

As you can see, these fat soluble nutrients can be easily obtained from eating nourishing foods. There is no reason to eat animals, or their eggs, or drink their milk in order to provide your body with sufficient nutrients. Many vitamins and minerals are dependent on the other for proper assimilation throughout the body. Vitamin A works very well with vitamin B2, for example, to keep the gastro-intestinal tract healthy. Iron needs to be accompanied by vitamin C for absorption. Calcium must be accompanied by magnesium for absorption. There are many combinations of vitamins and minerals that need each other. For this reason I am going to provide you with a list of essential vitamins and minerals and the best food sources containing them. Be sure to eat a variety.

Vitamin B1: beets, brazil nuts, green leafy vegetables, okra, oranges, raw sauerkraut, sprouted lentils, sprouted peas, sunflower seeds, wheatgrass juice.

Vitamin B2: almonds, avocado, bananas, brussels sprouts, carrots, coconut, grapefruits, kamut grass, kelp, raw corn, sunflower seeds.

Vitamin B3: almonds, Amazonian jungle peanuts, dulse, green vegetables, kelp, sunflower seeds.

Vitamin B5: apples, apricot seeds, avocado, bananas, broccoli, collard greens, oranges, pecans, soaked or germinated sesame seeds.

Vitamin B6: avocado, brussels sprouts, cabbage, cantaloupe, green leafy vegetables, green peppers, prunes, sunflower seeds, walnuts, wheatgrass juice.

Vitamin B9: asparagus, avocado, bananas, beets, broccoli, brussels sprouts, cantaloupe, dates, leafy green vegetables, lima beans, mushrooms, spinach.

Vitamin B12: bananas, concord grapes, kelp, nutritional yeast, sunflower seeds, unwashed root vegetables, white button mushrooms.

Vitamin B17: apricot kernels, blackberries, cherry seeds, cranberries, flax seeds, germinated garbanzos, mung bean sprouts, peach and plum pits, raspberries, sprouted lima beans.

Vitamin B17 is known for its ability to destroy cancer cells. If you were to combine extracted B17 with isolated cancer cells, the B17 would kill the cancer cells. This does not mean by simply eating mung bean sprouts you will kill all of the cancer cells in your body. However, our internal environment works much better to assimilate nutrients when we follow a clean, plant-based diet. Consider someone following an unhealthful diet, rich in toxins, and who has cancer. Under such toxic conditions, mung bean sprouts alone will not be as effective as if they were following a clean diet.

The intestinal flora (good bacteria) synthesize B-vitamins in our body. If you give a person on antibiotics mung bean sprouts, this will do very little for them – that goes for any medicine. The medicine and antibiotics kill good bacteria and as a result we become deficient in B-complex vitamins.

This is why it is important for anyone with cancer to do internal cleansing, follow a clean, plant-based diet, restore intestinal flora by using a vegan probiotic supplement, eliminate cooked, chemical-laden, processed foods from his diet, introduce raw, organic foods, and gradually improve his health to be weaned off of medications. As the internal environment becomes less toxic and a person starts hosting a higher ratio of healthy bacteria, these mung bean sprouts will have a much greater impact. The body will be able to assimilate and utilize the nutrients from the food, and the vitamin B17 will have freedom to attack those cancer cells.

Choline: broccoli sprouts, cabbage, cauliflower, grapes, green leafy vegetables, lentils, onion sprouts, ripe tomatoes.

Vitamin C: apples, avocados, bananas, bell peppers, blackberries, black currants, broccoli, camu camu berries, cauliflower, cherries, citrus fruits, dandelion, green leafy vegetables, kale, kiwi, papayas, parsley, persimmons, rose hips, spinach, strawberries, tomatoes, wheatgrass juice.

Vitamin H (Biotin): almonds, bananas, green peas, hazelnuts, hemp seeds, mushrooms, raw sesame tahini, tomatoes, walnuts.

Vitamin P (Bioflavonoids): apricots, bell peppers, black currants, cherries, citrus fruits, flaxseeds, grapes, mung beans, prunes, strawberries.

Bioflavonoids protect the vitamin C in your body. Vitamin C is necessary to metabolize iron. In his book, *Eco-Eating,* Sapoty Brook suggests that *eating vitamin C-rich foods with iron-rich greens helps to transform the iron from fruits and vegetables to a more readily absorbable form.* This readily absorbable iron is much better than the iron from any meat source. Broccoli, dandelion, and wheatgrass juice are great sources of both vitamin C and iron. I like to eat raw sunflower seeds mixed with black currants. The seeds contain iron and the currants contain vitamin C. You can also eat strawberries with the leaves; an easy way to accomplish this is by blending them into your smoothie.

Many people lack B vitamins, as well as vitamins A and C, in addition to a common lack of useable calcium, iron, and magnesium. Therefore, be sure you are getting adequate amounts of these vitamins and minerals in the food you eat. You should do this by eating a variety of the foods I have listed. Because the B vitamins are synthesized by our intestinal flora, we must not introduce harmful bacteria from dairy, meat, and eggs into our bodies, as it will alter the process of synthesizing these vitamins.

In order to get the minerals we need, we should eat a variety of raw fruits and vegetables. They contain a vast array of minerals that work synergistically to keep your body functioning at an optimal level. The following is a list of minerals and foods that are rich in them.

Calcium: brazil nuts, broccoli, carrots, dried figs, green beans, green leafy vegetables, kelp, oranges, papaya, sprouts, sunflower seeds, unhulled sesame seeds, walnuts, wild greens.

Iron: algae, apricot seeds, arame, cucumber, dandelions, dulse, kale, leafy greens, raisins, sesame seeds, spinach, wheatgrass juice, wild greens.

Magnesium: broccoli leaves, chlorophyll-rich foods, dandelion, leafy greens, pine nuts, pumpkin seeds, spinach, spirulina, sunflower green sprouts, wheatgrass juice, wild greens.

Manganese: almonds, coconut water, hazelnuts, macadamia nuts, oats, pineapple, pumpkin seeds, spinach.

Phosphorus: almonds, bananas, blue-green algae, carrots, chlorella, corn, dates, dulse, legumes, mushrooms, nori, pecans, pistachios, quinoa, sunflower seeds.

Potassium: avocados, bananas, broccoli, brussels sprouts, celery, dandelion, dulse, figs, green juices, green leafy vegetables, kelp, mushrooms, papaya, parsnip greens, radishes, raisins, red peppers, seeds, spinach, sprouts, watermelon, wild greens.

Silicon: alfalfa, alfalfa sprouts, apples, beet greens, cucumbers, dandelion, dark leafy green vegetables, figs, flaxseed, grapes, horsetail, kamut and spelt grass, nettle, oatstraw, onions, strawberries, sunflower seeds, tomatoes.

Sodium: apples, asparagus, beets, carrots, cauliflower, celery, cucumbers, dandelion greens, dulse, kale, kelp, olives, pumpkin, spinach, strawberries, Swiss chard, watermelon, wheatgrass juice.

Sulfur: arugula, broccoli, broccoli sprouts, brussels sprouts, cabbage, dandelion, garlic, kale, kelp, lettuce, onions, radishes, raspberries, wild greens.

Zinc: broccoli sprouts, brussels sprouts, dulse, garlic sprouts, green leafy vegetables, kelp, mushrooms, onions, onion sprouts, pecans, poppy seeds, pumpkin seeds

All of these minerals are essential to our health and well-being. The processes in the body are dependent on the presence of a variety of minerals in a synergistic way. Many medical doctors will misinform their patients that they need meat or milk for iron or calcium. As you can clearly see from the list of foods containing these minerals, their suggestions are false and misleading. For calcium to be absorbed, it must be accompanied by magnesium. Milk does not contain magnesium. For iron to be absorbed, it must be accompanied by vitamin C. Meat does not contain vitamin C. By eating a variety of fruits and vegetables and some raw nuts, seeds, and seaweeds, you will be assured that you are receiving the nutrients your body needs in the correct ratio, and are maintaining good health.

BALANCING MINERALS

"The beginning of all chronic degenerative disease is the loss of potassium from the cells and the invasion of sodium (tissue damage syndrome)." – Dr. Max Gerson, A Cancer Therapy

With that being said, this does not mean you should overload on potassium. Nor should you completely cut "sodium" out of your diet. Organic sodium is good for your body. Salt is not.

By keeping a good balance between sodium/potassium, and calcium/phosphorus, you will thrive at an optimal level of health. Eating a clean diet will assure the proper balance.

In *Eco-Eating*, Sapoty Brook includes a chart which he refers to as the *CaPNaK chart*. You can purchase this chart at *eco-eating.com*. Though it looks confusing at first glance, once you figure it out, the chart is quite simple to follow. The foods are listed on a chart where you can easily identify how to balance each of the four minerals and feel great always. I found this chart to be helpful for me on my journey to optimal health.

FOOD COMBINING

Abiding by the food combining guidelines can be tough and can easily drift into fanaticism. To begin, starches should only be combined with greens and green salads. They should not be mixed with protein-heavy foods or fruit. This gets confusing because greens happen to be protein-rich, and can have more bio-available amino acids than meat. A mistake the standard eater makes is that he tends to mix bread with meat constantly. Because they both require different digestive juices, the two offset each other, the food takes longer to digest, and even then it digests inadequately. The result is that they ferment and decay in the bowel, causing flatulence, discomfort, bloating, and weight gain. For this reason, the common sandwich should be avoided. The cooked gluten grains, which are rich in acrylamides from being baked should be reason enough to avoid the sandwich. If the meat is processed, it likely contains nitrates, which are known carcinogens, and the meat, processed or not, is rich in health-degrading free radicals.

Green leafy vegetables can be combined with just about any other food. They are easily digested and do not seem to interfere with the digestion of other foods.

Sweet fruits, like bananas, raisins, and dates, go well with celery, spinach, lettuce, and avocado. Sub-acid fruits, like apples, grapes, and pears, go well with either sweet fruits, or citrus fruits, but not necessarily with both. They also go well with avocado, spinach, and celery. Acid or citrus fruits go well with sub-acid fruits, but not sweet fruits. They are also good with avocado,

116

spinach, lettuce, and celery. Under food combining guidelines, melon should always be eaten alone. It does not combine well with other foods.

All proteins from nuts, seeds, algae, and other sources, are not advised to be combined with sugars or starches because combining them can result in excessive flatulence and discomfort. For some people this is not the case, so it may be best to experiment yourself and see which variations of foods work best for you. I find that eating a few celery stalks eases my stomach after mixing nuts with dried fruits.

If you do not combine your food properly, fermentation could take place in the bowels and this often leads to excessive gas or flatulence. Combining grains with fruit often triggers this. The fructose present in the intestines mixes with the incompletely digested carbohydrates from the grain, and your intestines move the fructose-rich mixture through too quickly for absorption. These unabsorbed carbohydrates from the grains then ferment and this could result in flatulence or discomfort.

I like to eat a lot of dates. I also love bananas. Whenever I eat too many of the two combined without eating foods rich in sodium however, I feel weak, and my abdomen sometimes feels bloated. I found that eating a few stalks of celery makes this go away. The reason, I discovered, is because I was absorbing too much potassium from the bananas, and mostly from the dates, and not enough sodium. The celery provided me with the sodium. When you have too much potassium and not enough sodium, your intestines do not contract as they should, or absorb water into the extracellular fluids, so your stools become loose and watery. At this time, partially digested food starts to ferment in the bowels, resulting in gas. Your body starts conserving sodium so your urine becomes concentrated. Adding organic sodium in the form of celery or chard will balance this.

Fruit should never be eaten with or immediately following anything other than fruit or green leafy vegetables.

If you would like to learn more about food combining I recommend you read Dr. Herbert Shelton's book, *Food Combining Made Easy*. I would not necessarily say he made it easy, but he does thoroughly explain the concept. I do not follow it perfectly, but it is a good guide.

EAT THE SEEDS

If you eat an avocado, and you bury the pit in the ground, chances are, if in the right climate, that pit might grow into an avocado tree. If you eat an apple, and you bury the seeds in the ground, chances are you could expect an apple tree to emerge from the ground. When you eat these foods, and include the seeds, you nourish your body with that same life-force energy that could have eventually sprouted into a tree, or plant. Contrary to this, if you bury a cow, or a pig, or especially the remains of a dead cow or pig, or any other animal by-product, it decays. Rather than gain life force energy from this food choice, you are given the burden of sluggish energy.

The majority of us eat fruits and we throw away the part that contains many phytonutrients. Phytonutrients are compounds found in plants that have health-promoting properties, including anti-inflammatory, antioxidant, and liver-health promoting activities. An apple is a perfect example of one of these fruits. It may be helpful to eat the core of the apple along with the seeds to receive maximum nutrition. This is the part of the apple that is rich in phenols and anthocyanins – both powerful antioxidants. Some people do get stomach pains when they eat apple seeds, so this is something you may have to experiment with to determine whether your body can handle them.

Apricot kernels also contain beneficial nutrients. The apricot kernel tastes like an almond, is a good source of fat, and contains certain compounds that work to repair the prostate. Anyone with any type of prostate issue may want to begin eating apricot kernels, and also eliminate all animal products from their diet.

According to Jeff Primack, in his book *Conquering Any Disease, many of the seeds from fruits contain cyanide derivatives that turn into hydrogen cyanide in the body. This form of cyanide is healthy and has been documented to kill cancer cells, fungi, bacteria, and viruses without damaging your healthy cells.* So the rumor that you may have heard about seeds containing cyanide does hold up to be true, but only to a certain extent.

Do not fear the seeds. You can always blend them up in a Vita Mix or Blend Tec as part of a smoothie or juice, and you will not even know they are there.

LET'S TALK ABOUT SUPPLEMENTS

"Why do we have so many vitamin stores and calcium and protein supplements if we get all of the vitamins and minerals we need from meat, cheese, dairy, and eggs? The truth is we don't. There is no fiber, there is little calcium, and there is nothing good in these animal-based foods." – Gary Yourofsky, Heroic Animal Rights Activist

I never shop at vitamin stores. No matter which of these synthetic, chemical nutrient havens may be convenient for me to shop at, I prefer not to contribute to their profits and see no need for their products. I also do not agree with the use of the great majority of supplements. I do not think they are necessary for adding muscle, retaining muscle, or for optimal health. While there are a few supplements sold in these stores that can be beneficial, like organic green superfood powders and some food-grade vitamins, for those with compromised health situations this does not take away from the fact that the products are often overpriced, misleading, and unnecessary. You can find each item on various websites for a fraction of the prices charged in the stores.

What motivated me to write about this topic was an experience I had in a Vitamin Shoppe. Although I do not care to shop at these stores, I had a ten dollar gift certificate. I debated giving it away to a client, but thought maybe I would find a book on their clearance rack that may be of use to me as references of some sort. I had no luck. I used it on some of Dr. Bronner's organic hand soap instead. While I was in the store, I observed something disturbing. A somewhat jolly and overweight man asked the store manager what supplements he would recommend to help him gain energy and lose weight. This manager suggested that the customer take creatine. I could not believe what I had heard. Creatine is an organic acid that is naturally produced in the human body from amino acids primarily in the kidneys and liver. While it can supply energy to the muscles, it is also known to cause kidney damage and is often contaminated with heterocyclic amines, such as PhIP.

I was bothered by this so much that I approached the man immediately after, directly in front of the manager, and I informed him that taking creatine would be an awful idea. The man smelled like an ashtray and appeared to be in poor health. I told him: "If you want to change your life and you want to be healthy and you want more energy, the very first thing you need to do is quit smoking. You then need to add more alkalinity to your body. You ask for a good supplement, well, start by taking a good greens superfood powder. Green Vibrance is right there on that shelf. That will provide you with an array of excellent nutrients that will not only give you this energy you desire, but will help you lose weight, and could very possibly decrease your craving for cigarettes. If you want to know how to gain more unwanted weight and lose your fight to gain your health back, take his advice and get creatine."

The results of a 2001 study regarding creatine supplementation and its effects on the kidneys and renal function were published in the *American Journal of Kidney Diseases*. The study found *that creatine supplementation resulted in greater cyst growth and worsened renal function. The results indicated that creatine supplements may exacerbate disease progression of cystic renal disease.*

My encounter in the vitamin store was not an isolated situation. This type of bad advice to sickly people is being given in these types of stores wherever they exist. They fill their shelves with synthetic chemical nutrients and urge customers to buy anything they can con them into buying. I can guarantee that this store manager has not the faintest clue of what optimal nutrition is. He most likely had fast food for lunch. He is not someone who should be giving nutritional or supplemental recommendations to anybody.

I was near a GNC store a while back and watched the sales clerk walk outside and light up a cigarette and smoke it in front of the store. Imagine walking up to that store to purchase what you think are healthy supplements and having to breathe in a cloud of smoke on your way in. What a disaster.

In addition to the misinformed employees working in many of these stores, nearly all of the supplements they sell are not necessary for maintaining or experiencing vibrant health. What is the number one supplement purchased from these stores? I would have to say protein powders, followed by multi-vitamins. This is a common mistake. The misconception that protein will help you lose weight has grown so common that someone needs to step up and put it to a halt.

If you are a bodybuilder, or an athlete, and you are looking to put on weight, sure, keep taking your protein powder, but at least make sure it is coming from a good source. Go for the vegan plant based protein. *Garden of Life* has a protein called *Raw Protein* and although I do not take it because I do not take any protein supplements, it is still better than any type of whey, milk, or egg protein products. There is also Thor Bayler's *Raw Power*. All plant based proteins are one hundred percent bio-available to the body. Whey protein and all of these other synthetic protein supplements are below fifty percent. Many of them are created in laboratories and should have no place in our bodies to begin with. Rather than helping to fuel the body, they create acidity in our system. Because we store alkaline minerals in our bones, all of the acidity from these toxic supplements tends to absorb into our muscle tissues. Sometimes this makes the muscles appear more solid. This may come off as a good sign to muscle-heads or bodybuilders, but when I look at someone who is all muscled like that, they don't appear healthy to me, only acidic. Having an acidic blood pH is not something to be proud of.

In a review of *Issues of Dietary Protein Intake* that was published in the *International Journal of Sport Nutrition and Exercise Metabolism* in 2006, it was documented that *dangers of excessive protein, defined as when protein constitutes greater than thirty-five percent of total energy intake, include hyperaminoacidemia, hyperammonemia, hyperinsulinemia, nausea, diarrhea, and even death (the "rabbit starvation syndrome").*

The truth about protein is that we can obtain all of the essential amino acids for building our proteins by following a vegan diet rich in raw fruits and vegetables. It is impossible to have a protein deficiency when you follow this type of diet. It also provides an array of vitamins, minerals, antioxidants, and other nutrients, making multi-vitamins unnecessary.

These supplements are inorganic to our bodies. When a vitamin, or any supplement, is created synthetically, it is of little to no use to the body. We cannot efficiently utilize or assimilate these synthetic versions and they often end up as sediment in the tissues, contributing to disease, or they are excreted out of the body after putting a burden on the kidneys and other eliminative organs. While some synthetic nutrients can be of use to the body, it is always best to get nutrients from whole foods, which contain a variety of components that synthetic nutrients could never provide. If you eat poorly and you feel like you must take a multi vitamin, then please do, but make sure it is a food grade vitamin. This means the vitamin must come from natural food sources and not be synthetically created in a laboratory. The vitamin should also be organic because there are food grade vitamins out there that do come from fruits and vegetables, yet they may be genetically modified, and this pretty much could equal synthetically made, or worse – as they may contain concentrated amounts of farming chemicals and other health-degrading substances.

Too often we think what we are doing is healthy, claim that we are healthy, and then refuse to accept that we are wrong once we discover that we are just that, wrong. I too, have been guilty of this behavior.

All throughout high school I thought I was extremely healthy because I was following an organic diet. In college, I thought I was even healthier because I was competing in bodybuilding competitions and extreme dieting. What worked for me was keeping my mind open. What I learned over the years is that I may have been healthier than ninety percent of the rest of the population because I was eating organic, refusing to eat red meat, taking my multi-vitamins, and exercising regularly, but I was still unhealthy. It was not until a few years ago that I realized what optimal nutrition really consists of.

One of the best ways to reach an optimal level of health is to avoid all things that are synthetic. Just like unnatural milk (the milk sold in grocery stores that is from drugged animals following an unnatural diet, and that has been pasteurized) has very little, if any, benefit to a baby cow or calf because it will get sick shortly after drinking it; a synthetic vitamin, or source of protein, has little, if any, benefit to the human body. Just like a synthetic bee pollen granule, which has been replicated to the exact same identical molecular structure as a bee pollen granule from nature, cannot be of any benefit to the bees because they could die after eating them; thus, a synthetic weight loss pill cannot be of any benefit to the human body.

If you want to be smart about nutrition, get your nutrients from eating a raw, plant-based diet. If you feel like you need supplements, make sure they are not synthetically made. Make sure they are organic. The label should mention that the product is "food-grade," and organic. Do not listen to the store managers in these chemical vitamin havens. If you do, you may fall victim to the same type of scenario the jolly little overweight man I encountered was.

Follow the advice of a raw nutritionist or holistic health coach. Remember, good marketing can sell anything, but the truth always prevails in the end. I cannot tell you how many times I have heard people trying to sell supplements claiming they are the best in the world. Guess what? There cannot be thousands of the "best" synthetic products when they basically are the same. Each synthetic product you are presented with is similar to the next.

They are all garbage. Be smart. Be good to your body. You can all win the fight to gain your health back. It is rightfully yours!

WHAT ABOUT VITAMIN B12?

Another popular topic of discussion in regards to supplementation is vitamin B12. This vitamin is important and essential for growth, production, and regeneration of red blood cells. A good amount of people develop B12 deficiencies over time. The speculation revolving around B12 deficiency is that it is most prevalent in the vegan community. This is not the truth. In reality, more meat eaters have B12 deficiencies than vegans. The reason why the whole B12 scare took place was because it was really the only thing the media could find that could possibly be perceived as a negative about a vegan diet, so they quickly jumped all over it and created unnecessary concern and worry. This stress, and this anxiety itself, may even be causing a decrease in B12 levels.

In the book, *Nutritional Evaluation of Food Processing*, Dr. Robert S. Harris and Dr. Endel Karmas state that *B12 is stable to heat in neutral solution if pure, but is destroyed when heated in alkaline or acid media in crude preparations, as in foodstuffs.* This means that cooked meat is not an efficient source of B12. This is not just a vegetarian's dilemma.

We develop B12 deficiencies by creating them for ourselves. As long as we are at an optimal level of health and our bodies are functioning properly there is no reason why we should not naturally produce enough B12. Fermentation from starches, and endotoxic toxemia from endotoxins in meat and other animal-based foods that survive cooking and stomach acids, deplete our B12. The consumption of alcohol depletes levels as well. Cooked food will destroy the production of B12 that occurs in the mouth. The use of processed soy products, such as meat replacements and tofu, may also deplete our levels of B12. Because B12 is created from bacteria, we need to make sure we are getting vegan probiotics in our diet. This will help to regenerate the natural bacterial flora which manufacture different B vitamins and synthesize other vitamins and nutrients in the body.

B12 is only available from bacterial production. It is not made by plants or animals. It is the intestinal flora, and our healthy bacteria that create B12 in our bodies. When people eat meat, the harmful endotoxins play a role in wiping out the good bacteria that would otherwise produce B12, and when people take antibiotics, the good bacteria are also killed off.

Meat is thought to be a good source for B12 because animals have more bacteria growing in them. The problem is that this bacterium is of little use after the animals are slaughtered and cooked, and the dead flesh is ingested into the human body. Much of the B12 present in these animals turns out to be

B12 analogues, which appear as B12 in animals but have no benefit to humans.

Many different experts claim we only need from 0.2-0.5 micrograms of B12 daily. In his book, *Conscious Eating,* Dr. Gabriel Cousens presents studies that were done by Doctors Thrash and Thrash which estimate that *the microorganisms in the mouth (between the teeth and gums, around the tonsils, in the tissue at the base of the tongue) and in the nasopharyngeal passages produce about 0.5 micrograms per day.* In order to maintain this, it is important to eat raw foods, because cooked food residues can alter this process.

Other experts have proven that there are bacteria which produce utilizable B12 in the small intestine. Colon bacteria is said to produce all the way up to 5 micrograms of utilizable B12 a day, however, we cannot absorb B12 from the colon. Our main source of B12 absorption comes from the absorption in the small intestine, and it comes from the high quantities of B12 secreted by the liver into the bile. This number ranges from 1 microgram all the way to 10 micrograms a day as long as we keep our eliminative organs healthy.

Just as meat eaters develop B12 deficiencies from their poor food choices, vegans and vegetarians who develop B12 deficiency are in most cases the ones who still believe they need excess protein and resort to either overloading on protein supplements, or replacing meat with soy proteins and soy products, which may alter their natural production of B12.

If you have developed a B12 deficiency and you believe supplementation will help, by all means go for it. Be sure to look out for extra ingredients that may be added. Always go organic when you do use B12, and make sure the label says it is a vegetarian product. Many supplements come in capsules that are made out of gelatin, which is derived from a variety of substances, including cows and pork. You may also want to add vegan probiotics to increase intestinal flora. These can be added to foods. Be sure to compost your organic food scraps, grow an organic garden of your own, and support farms that polycrop organically. The intensive monocropping methods of growing are known to deplete cobalt levels in the soil, which is also decreasing levels of B12 in the crops.

THE DANGERS OF INORGANIC CALCIUM

Unfortunately, calcium from calcium supplements and dairy is not easily absorbed. Instead, the calcium builds and accumulates in the body causing kidney stones, cataracts, calcification of the coronary artery (heart disease), calcification of the joints (arthritis), and calcification in the mouth from cooked starches, especially cooked sugar and dairy – which leads to cavities and tooth decay. This calcification also leads to inflammation, which then leads to numerous other symptoms.

A study published in the *American Journal of Clinical Nutrition*, titled *The Effect of Milk Supplements on Calcium Metabolism, Bone Metabolism, and calcium Balance*, found that *women who consumed three or more eight-ounce glasses of milk per day still lost calcium from their bodies, and remained in negative calcium balance, even after a year of consuming almost 1,500 mg of calcium daily, with milk being the source of this calcium.* This study reveals that we do not obtain the adequate calcium we need from drinking cow's milk.

In April 2011, the *British Medical Journal* provided a study showing that calcium supplements increase the risk of heart attack and stroke. Researchers followed 16,718 post-menopausal women in the Women's Health Initiative and found that calcium supplements increased heart health risk by thirteen to twenty-two percent.

The very best way to get sufficient calcium is to eat green leafy vegetables. As I mentioned previously, calcium needs magnesium to be absorbed in the body. Leafy greens contain the perfect ratio of calcium and magnesium. Kelp and sesame seeds are also excellent sources of calcium. Because silicon can be transmuted into calcium, it is also helpful to eat silicon-rich foods, such as, alfalfa, apples, beets, bell peppers, cabbage, carrots, cherries, cucumbers, leafy green vegetables, onions, oranges, raisins, sprouts, and wild greens. Wild grasses (whether you juice them or chew them) and teas with herbs such as nettle, horsetail, and oatstraw are also sources of silicon.

Calcium carbonate is an example of the calcium you want to avoid. This is calcium that basically comes from rocks and is not assimilated by the body. Calcium citrate, which comes from citrus fruits, is beneficial calcium. Synthetic calcium citrate pills are to be avoided. They are made synthetically. Nothing synthetic is wholesome for the human body.

Many misled people eat antacid calcium tablets with the belief that they are going to maintain good levels of calcium in their bones by doing so. By eating these tablets, they are inadvertently begging to develop poor health conditions. My suggestion would be: never eat antacid calcium tablets. Do not even consider them. It is also advisable not to consume anything else with added calcium that we cannot digest or absorb and to educate anyone and everyone you care about to do the same.

If you do ingest a calcium supplement, be careful of added ingredients. While reading the label of a popular brand of doctor-recommended calcium pills I noticed the ingredients. They include – calcium carbonate, corn syrup solid, talc, and less than two-percent of polysorbate 80, polyvinyl alcohol, titanium dioxide, polyethylene glycol 3350, corn starch, dl-alfa tocopherol, cholecalciferol (vitamin D3), sodium starch glycolate, sucrose, gelatin, calcium stearate, propylparaben and methylparaben (preservatives).

The gelatin in these calcium pills is derived from slaughtered animals. The sucrose and corn syrup solids are acid forming, leading to the inhibition of proper calcium absorption and weakening of the bones. They also add parabens, which have been proven in medical studies to be a main cause of breast cancer. I include a study in chapter seven when I mention parabens in beauty products. So now when those who ingest these calcium pills that their doctors have recommended for them to take, not only are they not strengthening their bones, but they are weakening their bones, adding acidity to their blood, and increasing their risk of developing breast cancer. This does not seem logical to me.

THE CHEMICAL FREE SOLUTION

"Until man duplicates a blade of grass, nature can laugh at his so-called scientific knowledge. Remedies from chemicals will never stand in favor compared with the products of nature, the living cell of the plant, the final result of the rays of the sun, the mother of all life." – Thomas Edison

The belief in the paradigm of synthetic medicine curing disease is wrong. The belief that fortifying processed foods makes them nutritious is false. The truth is that, to experience vibrant health, we should avoid all pills and chemical food additives.

If there was any diet out there that would be simple and easy to follow, it would be a chemical free diet. Simply avoid all chemicals in your food and avoid synthetic drugs, cigarettes, and alcohol, and your life will improve in every aspect.

When you consider the fact that chemical food additives and synthetic chemical drugs cause health problems, it should be no surprise why I am providing this view and giving this advice. The very best diet is to eat all raw organic food and to avoid ingesting synthetic chemicals.

I know there are some things one cannot always avoid, such as the chemicals in the air or in tap water, but you can avoid chemicals in the food you eat and the substances you choose to put into your body.

For more vibrant health, avoid the following items:

a.) Refined sugars and any artificial, chemical sweeteners. The only sweetness in our lives should come from fruits, from our significant others, and from keeping our children happy.

b.) Partially-hydrogenated or hydrogenated oils and trans-fatty oils. Any type of oil cooked at a high temperature, including in sautéed foods, becomes trans-fatty, even extra virgin olive oil. One of the most common myths here is that cooking with olive oil is the most beneficial to our health. But, what is true is that when you cook these oils over 150 degrees Fahrenheit, they become rancid and equivalent to trans-fats. It is best, and advisable, not to use any oils, cooked or raw, with the exception of organic virgin unrefined coconut oil.

c.) Monosodium glutamate (MSG), sodium benzoate, other harmful preservatives, and chemical flavor enhancers. These are also referred to as enhanced flavoring agents and they are so poisonous they can be deadly in high doses.

d.) Bleached flours and refined flours. By eating these, you are depleting your body of A vitamins and therefore your skin becomes pale and pasty and you accelerate aging. Over a prolonged period of time, eating these foods, and being deficient in vitamin A, can lead to skin cancers, skin ailments, and other diseases associated with the skin.

e.) All types of meat, be it mammal, bird, fish, reptile, or amphibian.

f.) Dairy products including whey, casein, ice cream, creamer, yogurt, butter, milk, or cheese.

g.) Eggs and foods containing eggs.

h.) Sodas and colas. These weaken your bones and your complexion and make you prone to depression, osteoporosis, diabetes, cancer, and obesity.

When you choose to eat processed foods such as those listed above, you degrade your health and set the pace toward illness, even if it takes years for these symptoms to show. When taking into consideration that they are also patterns that can be difficult to break, eating sugary, salty, oily, and fast and junk foods are also addictions. When you eat these things, you are not feeding your body nutrients, you are feeding addictions. Just as heroin, cocaine, and prescription drugs alter body chemistry and brain function, so do toxic foods.

By improving your diet, your health improves, and you gradually shift to a healthier overall lifestyle. If you are only eating fresh, organic raw foods, you will not have to worry about synthetic chemical additives and farming chemical residues. This makes things a lot easier and eliminates the need to check labels so frequently.

SUPERFOODS

There is definitely a "superfood craze" going on out there in the world today. Many natural foods have been identified as carriers of antioxidants and other natural plant chemicals (phytochemicals) that are greatly beneficial to human health. This does not mean we need to eat them daily. Many people abused the discovery of the foods and exploited them, through hyped-up marketing, being driven by profits. Some are substances that would best be used sparingly whenever you need an energy boost, when you need something to overcome sickness, or for specific health needs – such as using valerian root as a sleeping aid, or maca powder for reproductive health.

Some of these superfoods include: acai, aloe vera, bee pollen, blueberries, blue-green algae, broccoli sprouts, cacao, chlorella, coconut, goji berries, hemp seeds, maca, mangosteen, marine phytoplankton, pumpkin seeds, spirulina, stone fruit pits, and the list goes on. While some may be readily available to you, and even common in your diet, which is fine, others can be expensive and really unnecessary. Only the hyper-marketing can make you believe that you must have them. But, the biggest benefit can really be to the pockets of those who sell them.

Many of these foods have excellent nutritional balance and prove to hold a variety of benefits. The key is moderation. If you are suckered into buying mass amounts of different superfoods, do not eat them every day. I bought into the marketing nonsense being spewed about cacao. While cacao does contain high amounts of nutrients and antioxidants, it is also addictive and acts as a stimulant on the body. Ingesting excessive amounts of cacao often results in adrenal fatigue and insomnia.

When I was first introduced to superfoods, I combined them all together into big smoothie concoctions and would drink them daily. I felt a burst of energy. But after doing this for a while, I felt as if my adrenals were being worn down, or was having what is known as *adrenal fatigue*. Just like any other stimulant, over consuming certain superfoods can wear you down and cause you to crash. They also make you "spacey" and lead you to confusion and numbness. You lose sensation to feeling. By cutting back on my intake of cacao and maca, these symptoms went away.

Before you jump into the pool of superfoods, take some time to educate yourself and be sure to limit your intake. There is no need to over do it with anything in life.

By now, I hope you have a more clear understanding of what food is and how it works. I also assume you have a better idea of what foods you should be eating. Now you have to make it happen. Now it is time to change your lifestyle entirely, and tune into health.

Do not let yourself get discouraged when things go wrong. The fact that you are educated about real food is more than what a high percentage of other people can claim. Now you can use this education to combine a new level of health and find what works best for you.

Remember that old antagonist, failure? It seems to take delight in trying to take you down right when you are about to succeed. If failure approaches you, be ready to counter with strength from within. You no longer have room for failure, fatigue, or weakness in your life. Do not clear out a space to let them back in.

Chapter 4: EAT YOUR WAY TO OPTIMAL HEALTH

"One immediately wonders if there is not something in the life-giving vitamins and minerals of the food, that builds not only great physical structures within which their souls reside, but builds minds and hearts capable of a higher type of manhood in which the material values of life are made secondary to individual character." – Dr. Weston A. Price, observation on behalf of the indigenous tribes of the world

PUTTING IT ALL TOGETHER

"We are living in a world of convenience. We can easily pick up what passes for food everywhere we go. We can eat it as we walk down the street, grab a bite at our desks, or snack while driving our cars. We can bring it home and pop it into the microwave. We can certainly satisfy our immediate hunger; but there is a deeper hunger that prevails. And that is the hunger for a pain-free body, for endless energy to do whatever we have to do or want to do, without fatigue. It is the yearning deep within our souls for exuberance and vitality and youthfulness. And this hunger will not be satisfied with fast foods, junk foods and foodless foods. In our quest for 'convenience,' we overlook the fact that feeling ill or down or depressed is not convenient. Instead, we take it as a matter of course." – Rhio, Hooked On Raw

A common complaint I hear is that this "raw" diet may cost too much. This is only a myth. Think about how much meat, dairy, eggs, and packaged, processed foods cost. The well-known author, John McCabe, mentioned to me in an e-mail how, *"The meat, milk, and eggs of these modern days of toxic agriculture are not the meat, milk, and eggs of fifty years ago, before the world wars and development of chemical warfare, which influenced the development of toxic farming chemicals."* These are not foods we should be eating. By eliminating them from your diet, you will be able to purchase fresh, organic foods and spend less money. Also consider the medical costs related to eating low-grade foods that you will be clearing from your life. Think about how much your triple bypass surgery would have cost you had you continued to eat foods that cause cardiovascular disease.

It may not be as convenient for you to prepare your own meals and change the way you eat, but you have to ask yourself a series of questions. Do I want to feel good after I eat, or feel lethargic? Do I want to be more vibrant and have more positive energy, or do I want low energy and to feel down and sleepy all the time? Do I want to live a long, enjoyable life, or do I want to take years off of my life by eating poorly? Do I want to fit into the clothes I like, or do I want to keep shopping for XXL clothing?

All of the food items you are finding difficult to stop eating are items I do not consider food. The reason why you cannot stop eating them is because of the addictive chemicals that are being added to these foods. Once you break away from unhealthful foods and realize how unreal, and toxic they are, and how much they are limiting you from experiencing the bliss of life, you will not want to go back to them.

By cleansing your body and then following it up with a raw, organic plant-based diet, you are more likely to experience the lifestyle change you have been waiting for. This is your chance to wake up and break away from the destructive habits that have done nothing but bring you down, day after day, year after year. It is time to experience real food and live the best life you could ever imagine.

WHAT DO I NEED TO GET STARTED

You have to start with discipline. You have to be strong enough to make a commitment to yourself that you are going to improve your nutrition and raise your vibe. A great start would be to get rid of your microwave. Next, you should remove all of the unhealthy food from your cabinets and your fridge, and start from scratch. Take that healthy grocery list I provided you with from the last chapter and fill your cart with the best food in the world. Plant a garden, or simply grow a plant or two, and support local organic farmers. Visit the website of *Mercy for Animals* (mercyforanimals.org) and request their free vegetarian starter kit. They will mail you information to help you make the transition to a plant-based diet. There is a documentary titled, *May I Be Frank*, that is highly motivating and may give you the encouragement you need to get yourself going. You can find it online at *mayibefrankmovie.com.* Check out YouTube videos of Andrea Cox, Kristina Carrillo-Bucaram, Chef BeLive, Koya Webb, and Jason Wrobel for recipes and advice on how to prepare foods.

I advise that you have a good juicer and blender. If you do not have one, you can find them rather cheap online, at used stores, at garage sales, or on the community board at your local natural foods store. Of the two, purchasing a blender is more of a priority.

Juices and blended drinks assist in bringing you to an optimal level of health. The Blend Tec and the Vita Mix are considered to be the best blenders out there, but they are a little expensive. There are some other new blenders by other companies that also show promise. If you cannot afford to purchase a high-powered blender at this time, do not be discouraged. Simply purchase a blender that is less costly and will get you by for the time being. I used a forty dollar blender for years and it worked just fine for me. But a high-speed blender certainly works much better.

With a quality juicer, a strong blender, some good motivation, and great discipline, you will make the transition to a more healthful diet with ease.

130

To be sure you are getting sufficient nourishment, I suggest considering a labwork-consultation with Dr. Rick and Dr. Karin Dina. You can access their website at *rawfoodeducation.com*. Rick and Karin also offer a raw food nutrition educator course at the *Living Light Culinary Institute* in Fort Bragg, CA. If you want to equip yourself with the nutritional knowledge necessary to thrive in life,this is the course for you. Additionally, you can become certified as a raw food chef while you are there.

IS THERE A PARTICULAR DIET I CAN FOLLOW?

It is important to experiment with foods and do what feels best for you. Because I am not a "dietitian," I cannot legally prescribe a diet here in this book for you. When I coach people, I do advise sample diets that are clean, plant-based, vegan, and free of health-depleting substances. I also discuss food and health issues on my Facebook group page, *The Raw Cure*.

I do not believe in fad diets. I consider them to be *gimmicks*. The only diets that I believe in are those that are low-fat raw vegan and rich in truly raw fruits and vegetables. When you reach an optimal level of health these diets are wonderful as a base for your food choices. *Sunfood Diet Infusion* by John McCabe, The *80/10/10 Diet* by Dr. Douglas Graham, and the *World Peace Diet* by Will Tuttle each clarify many issues relating to the raw vegan diet.

The combination of a fruitarian diet, rich in raw fruits, with an adequate amount of greens, and other plant-based foods such as sprouts, nuts, seeds, and seaweed, is the best way to live according to nature, and in doing so, you will find positive energy, reach your ideal weight, and obtain optimal health. Six months after becoming a fruitarian, the great leader, Mahatma Gandhi, had this to say about his state of being:

"During this period I have been able to keep well where others have been attacked by disease, and my physical, as well as mental powers, are now greater than before. I may not be able to lift heavy loads, but I can do hard labor for a much longer time without fatigue. I can also do more mental work and with better persistence and resoluteness. I have tried a fruit diet on many sickly people, invariably with great advantage. My own experience, as well as my study of the subject, has confirmed me in the conviction that a fruit diet is the best one for us."

There is speculation that some may not be ready for this type of diet. Well, the human body is always ready for a plant-based diet. A diet rich in raw fruits and vegetables is a diet for everybody, though it is important to prepare for it smartly. You have to create balance in your body. It took time, and lots of trial and error before I started to eat all raw. But now I feel better than ever. I am sure to eat a variety of vegetables and fruit daily.

Don Robertson, *Director of EarthSave Baltimore* (earthsave.org), made this statement about a plant-based diet that is highly motivating: *"There's a growing acceptance, and appreciation of the tremendous value, both practical and spiritual, of a simple shift toward a whole food, plant-based diet. We've seen many indications of this increased awareness in recent years: A 2006 UN report pointed to livestock production as the number one source of climate changing greenhouse gases; The staff of Oprah Winfrey's TV show went vegan for a week for a special program on veganism and animal welfare, resulting in the decision of Oprah's life partner, Stedman Graham, to go to a vegan diet; Dr. Oz putting people who are at high risk for a heart attack or stroke on a vegan diet; President Clinton going to a vegan diet in order to reverse severe coronary artery disease; The coolest person on the planet, Ellen Degeneres, going vegan out of concern for animals; Gary Yourofsky's amazing YouTube video, The Best Speech You Will Ever Hear, on veganism and farmed animal protection; The outstanding Forks Over Knives documentary showing the powerful scientific evidence for the health benefits of a plant-based diet; The widespread availability of vegan specialty foods; Will Tuttle's book, The World Peace Diet, hitting number one on Amazon; and the recent report by Harvard School of Public Health stating that dairy products are not part of a healthy diet."*

THE TYPICAL VEGAN'S DILEMMA

"It seems that many people are simply uncomfortable with the unfamiliar – even if the unfamiliar is more healthful. They might consider that eating only fruits and vegetables, sprouts, nuts, and seeds, and so forth is 'weird.' But perhaps they should consider how it looks to be consuming milk from cow breasts and eating bird eggs, which are essentially bird periods. Maybe they should consider the barbaric practice of slaughtering animals, draining their blood, slicing them up, cooking them and eating them – and using a tremendous amount of land, water, and fossil fuels to feed that habit. They'd benefit from learning what the meat, egg, and dairy diet does to their health as well as to the environment." – John McCabe, Sunfood Diet Infusion

Often times, people transition to a vegan diet without having much of any education about it. They tend to replace meat products with soy and heavy, bread-containing foods. While a plant-based diet is better than one containing animal protein, there are better choices than following a soy and bread-heavy diet. Most processed soy products are full of preservatives, and hydrolyzed soy protein is equivalent to monosodium glutamate. They are also rich in acrylamides, which are not healthful. What you need to understand is that we do not need to have a meat replacement. Meat is not a good food choice. Are you really that infatuated with having the remnants of the carcass of some

132

poor dead animal on your plate? We are shifting to a higher level of consciousness now where we must accept animals as living creatures and respect them as we would respect our elders. Animals are not food for humans.

When you convert to a vegan diet, be sure to educate yourself about wise food choices. If you do not have the funds to hire a raw organic nutritionist or holistic health coach to pave the way for you, find a good book to help get you started, or watch YouTube videos. Do not just go in blindly. Dara Dubinet has a YouTube channel that is precise, informative, and educational. She also has a Facebook fan page. Andrea Cox also has a YouTube channel, facebook page, and website (healthyhaven.net) that are informative. Jason Wrobel launched his television show, *How to Live to 100*, on the Food Network. Jason is a graduate of the *Living Light Culinary Institute*, which is the prime destination for learning how to pepare raw foods, as well as for getting educated on the science behind raw nutrition. The Durian Rider brings a different energy to raw food education. He can be a little mouthy, and come off as being a bit wild, however, he is passionate about his lifestyle and does good convincing others to eat similarly, engage in exercise, and shift away from unwise choices. He has a YouTube channel as well with many educational videos. *The Banana Girl Diet* by Freelee Frugivore, *Becoming Raw* by Brenda Davis, *Hooked on Raw* by Rhio, *12 Steps to Raw* by Victoria Boutenko, and *The Simply Raw Living Foods Detox Manual* by Natasha Kyssa, are all good books that will educate you on making the conversion to a raw, vegan diet. *Raw Food for Dummies*, by Dan Laderman and Cherie Soria, will guide you through the transition to a raw vegan diet. You could also search for a book about organic gardening or research ways online to plant your own organic garden. The more self-sufficient you are, the easier your transition will be.

Please avoid making the transition and eating raw junk and vegan junk foods that are processed and loaded with unhealthful ingredients. These are commonly meat replacements, and packaged products containing agave, salt, soy, and namu shoyu. Rather, eat truly raw foods – raw fruits and veggies. Those who eat raw junk foods and vegan junk foods fail with the diet and convert back to eating meat, declaring that the vegan approach does not work, simply because they are misinformed or haven't accessed quality information.

"Animals do not belong to us. They are not commodities. They are not inanimate, stupid objects that cannot think and feel." – Gary Yourofsky

VEGAN ENDURANCE

There was an interesting medical study done at Yale in 1907 by a man named Irving Fisher. He tested three groups of people for strength and stamina: meat eating athletes, vegetarian athletes, and sedentary vegetarians. After testing them for their levels of endurance, he discovered that the vegetarians scored double on their tests. Even the sedentary vegetarians showed higher levels of endurance than the meat eating athletes. This reveals to us that beef DOES NOT give us strength or endurance as we have been manipulated into believing since we were children. Eating meat has done the opposite by depleting our strength and stamina.

In the July 2000 issue of the *British Journal of Cancer*, a study was published that clearly indicates vegans have higher levels of testosterone. This contradicts the myth that meat eaters have more stamina. The study measured testosterone levels in 696 men at Oxford University. Of the men, 233 were vegan, 237 were vegetarian, and 237 were meat-eaters who followed the Standard American Diet. The results showed that the vegans had higher testosterone levels than both the vegetarian and meat-eating men.

Dr. Ioteyko from the *Academy of Medicine in Paris* did a study that proved vegetarians have nearly three times more stamina than meat-eaters and only take one-fifth of the time to recover after testing.

John Robbins mentions a study in his book, *Diet for a New America,* which was conducted by a team of Danish researchers. The team measured the strength and endurance of three groups on a stationary bicycle; one group was fed a mixed diet of meat and vegetables, one was fed a diet high in meat, milk, and eggs, and the other was fed a strict vegan diet. What they found was that the group with the mixed diet of meat and veggies was able to pedal on the bicycle for one-hundred fourteen minutes before muscle failure. The group fed meat, milk, and eggs continued to pedal for only fifty-seven minutes before complete muscle failure. Not surprisingly, the group that consumed a strict vegan diet lasted an impressive one-hundred and sixty-seven minutes, almost tripling the outcome of the group eating animal products.

Endothelial cells are a thin layer of cells that line the interior surface of blood and lymphatic vessels. Those cells in direct contact with blood are called vascular endothelial cells, while those in direct contact with lymph fluid are called lymphatic endothelial cells. Vascular endothelial cells line the circulatory system, from the heart to the tiny capillaries. These cells use nitric oxide for vasodilation and increased blood flow. Endothelial dysfunction is a precursor for vascular diseases, especially atherosclerosis. Eating meat, dairy, eggs, and processed salts each contribute to the loss of endothelial function, disrupting the production of nitric oxide. A low-fat, raw vegan diet improves the function of the endothelial cells, increasing blood flow and stamina. This partially explains the conclusions from each of the studies pertaining to vegan endurance.

For any of you who may still consider meat as nourishing food, I recommend watching the documentaries *Forks Over Knives* and *Earthlings,* and reading *The Food Revolution,* by John Robbins. You should also read *The Ethics of What We Eat,* by Peter Singer. You may also want to search for

Philip Wollen's speech at the *St. James Ethics Debate* on YouTube.

Dr. John McDougall is a well-known and well-respected doctor who uses the nutritional approach to help heal his patients. In one of his published articles, he wrote of the Tarahumara Indians. This culture of Indians is known as "*The Running Indians*," because their entire culture revolves around running. They can run from sun up to sun down without tiring and many of them are ultra marathoners. Their methods of breathing, similar to that of lymphasizing, and their diets, are attributed to their extreme levels of endurance. After reading further about their diet, I found they eat virtually no meat and get about eighty percent of their calories from complex carbohydrates, ten percent from fats, and ten percent from protein. This ratio of nutrients eaten resembles a similar ratio advocated by Dr. Douglas Graham in his book, *The 80/10/10 Diet.*

By removing meat and other animal-based foods from our diet, and adding more nutrient-rich raw fruits and vegetables, we can greatly improve our endurance. Beets contain compounds that may reduce the oxygen cost of exercise while improving athletic performance. Check out Dr. Greger's video on *Beet Doping* to learn more (nutritionfacts.org).

CELLULAR REGENERATION

"Do animals know something that humans don't know? The answer is no. To the contrary, humans know something that animals do not: we know how to take natural food and make it more unnatural, we even know how to take unnatural food and make it more unnatural, all the while making it delightful to eat – without, however, realizing that it strains our digestive organs and pollutes our blood. We know how to flavor food with salt and condiments, and how to wash it all down with wine, beer, coffee, and tea. In short, we have elevated the practice of eating to an intensely pleasurable art form, in which eating is encouraged as much by a craving for addictive tastes, such as sugar and salt, as it is by genuine hunger, so leading to the over-indulgence that overloads our vital organs, pollutes our blood, and diminishes our vitality. Our cells get sick and we get sick." – Ross Horne, Cancerproof Your Body

Our bodies build around two-hundred thousand new immune cells every second of our lives. We are made up of trillions of cells. Each one of these cells is an individual living organism. Only after its own survival, the cell's main concerns are protecting and contributing to the health of other cells. Our cells keep us alive and we should do our best to nourish them for the span of time they live inside of us. When we fail to nourish our cells, they fail to provide us with optimal health.

Think of owning a business. You have a group of employees working for you. In order to keep them happy, you must pay them. Now, say you stop paying them and keep making them work. How long do you think that will last? Think of your cells as your employees that are battling to keep your business intact and their form of payment is good, nourishing food. Make sure you pay them well.

Even the cells of the healthiest people in the world die off at some point. Every minute their bodies are generating millions of new cells. These cells are constructed from the energy and substances that are present in their bodies at that particular time. Because of this, it is obligatory that we eat richly nourishing food. When we cheat and eat poor quality foods, we pay for it sooner or later.

Those people who eat fast food, processed food, meat, dairy, eggs, clarified sugars, cooked oils, synthetic chemicals, and all of that other garbage that is not really food, while also drinking soda or alcohol, have bodies that are constructed of trillions of weak cells that are prone to disease. Their bones are also likely being depleted of nourishment, and their organ tissues are accumulating the residues of the unhealthy foods. Those following such unhealthful diets end up being visibly unhealthy with complexions lacking the vibrancy they would have had they nurtured their bodies with truly healthy foods.

Often I hear people advising others, *"Oh its okay to cheat once-in-a-while."* But once-in-a-while often turns into regular binges. It is as if continuing to eat the lousiest foods is perfectly fine. Continuing to moderately follow a horrible diet will not bring you the best of health, or bring you to the best you can be. You would not bathe in garbage once-in-a-while, so why force your cells to bathe in it? The resolution is to permanently eliminate damaging foods.

If you like sweets, I guarantee you can find an amazing "raw" recipe that could be your new favorite, and will taste much better than your usual sweets, while containing not one health-damaging ingredient. For every food you enjoy that is killing you, there are creative recipes for healthier versions of that food which contain nutritious ingredients. You simply have to get out and explore. Chris Kendall wrote the book *101 Frickin' Raw Recipes* (therawadvantage.com). Any of Megan Elizabeth's books are recommended (meganelizabeth.com). None of her recipes require agave and each are low-fat, raw vegan. She has one titled, *Easy to be Raw Desserts*. Tiziana Tamborra and Matthew Rogers, both master dessert chefs at Café Gratitude in San Francisco, CA, wrote a book titled, *Sweet Gratitude: A New World of Raw Desserts,* and it contains several delicious raw dessert recipes. Ani Phyo also wrote a book titled *Ani's Raw Food Desserts.* My advice to you is to replace agave with organic date syrup, made simply by blending dates with water until it is the consistency you prefer for it to be.

When we eat the best food in the world, consisting largely of raw fruits, raw vegetables, and other plant-based foods, we develop the healthiest cells, and our body functions at the most optimal level. Our energy levels remain at a constant high. We bulletproof our bodies and we greatly reduce the chances of sickness taking over our lives.

TOO MUCH OF A GOOD THING IS NOT THAT GOOD

Overeating is a huge problem that many struggle with. I have been guilty of this myself over the years. When I experience the best tasting raw cuisine, I am tempted to stuff myself with it. It is beneficial to recognize and respect our cut off point. In *Eat to Live*, Dr. Joel Fuhrman states, *"It is the stretch of your stomach walls that lets you know when you are full, so people who eat lots of vegetables tend to eat fewer calories, feel fuller, and are better nourished, whereas people who eat lots of oil-rich foods eat many more calories, feel less full, and consume fewer essential micronutrients and phytonutrients."*

In the documentary *Forks Over Knives*, Dr. Doug Lisle explains how we have receptors in our stomach, which he refers to as *stretch receptors* and *density receptors*. Five-hundred calories of natural plant food will fill the stomach completely, triggering both our stretch and density receptors to signal our brain that we have had enough to eat. Contrary to this, eating five-hundred calories of processed foods will only partially fill the stomach and deceive the brain into thinking we need more food. Five-hundred calories of oils and fats do not fill the stomach at all and will trigger no response. This is why so many Americans, and those who eat oil-rich diets tend to overeat.

I discovered a scale that helped me overcome my problem with overeating while I was reading a Deepak Chopra book titled, *Perfect Weight*. Deepak refers to this chart as a satisfaction meter. Think of it like a scale that goes from empty to full and is numbered from one to eight. In a way you could look at it like a gas tank.

Whenever that tank is between levels zero and one, this means your stomach is ready for some fuel.

From levels two to four on the chart, it is suggested that you should be eating comfortably, or else comfortably digesting the food you have fairly recently finished eating.

At level five you should be feeling about satisfied. You will have provided your body with a good amount of nutrients that will hold you over until your next light meal.

Level six is when you are at the point of maximum comfort. If you eat any more, you will exceed the amount you can comfortably hold in your stomach. At this point, you feel no discomfort. Your stomach is about three-quarters of the way full and there is no reason to consume more food.

If you have gone past level six, you are more likely to feel heavy, bloated, and uncomfortable. Quite often, people go overboard and they fill the tank. This stretches the stomach and places pressure on other organs. When you frequently overeat, not only are you more prone to becoming obese, but you are prone to developing diabetes, cancer, and irritable bowel syndrome. It is best to find your cut off point. This satisfaction meter helped for me, and I hope it will also help you.

SUNLIGHT IS IN OUR FOOD

"Keep your face always toward the sunshine and shadows will always fall behind you." – Walt Whitman

Phototropism is the term used to define growth towards a light source. Many plants, and some other organisms such as fungi, exhibit this tendency to grow towards light. This would explain the concept of plants leaning around walls to reach the sunlight. Plant hormones called auxins trigger cellular changes and swelling inside of the plant, causing it to move towards the light. Humans benefit from this sunlight that is stored in the plants, known as biophotons.

"The spectrums of botanical pigments existing inside plant cells contain molecules that absorb specific wavelengths of sunlight and energy. In turn, the cells of the plant store and carry different levels of vibrational energy fields, including tiny specs of light called biophotons. These frequencies contained in the unheated substances of plants have a function when a person consumes them. There are photoreceptor proteins in the brain that are similar to those in the eyes, and they also exist throughout the body. The biophotons that exist within all living cells are part of the cellular communication system. Some people refer to biophotons as our life force energy." – John McCabe, Sunfood Diet Infusion.

In Conscious Eating, Dr. Gabriel Cousens explains how food is grown under the context of Mother Nature's energies of the sun, wind, soil, and rain. He has a beautiful way of expressing his true thoughts of nature's food. After reading his views, I respect food at a much higher level. He describes that, as he eats foods from the Earth, he, *"Sees the sun shining on them, the rain nourishing them, the wind caressing them, the Earth giving them nutrients and acting as their home."* He goes on to say, *"Forces of stored sunlight are released by the plants that they have stored through the process of photosynthesis. During the process of assimilation, the light is released from the plant into our own systems. By this process, one increases their inner strength. Heavy meat eaters become deprived of this light simulation because the light is released in the animal."*

138

When we re-factor what we consider as food, and follow a diet rich in raw plant matter, we will become aware of the energy that is in our food. The sun is our greatest source of energy. When we take the time to appreciate our food and we understand the depth of what our food contains, the act of eating becomes much more enjoyable and these living foods infuse the magic of health into our tissues and life.

A MEAT EATER'S STORY

"On May 7, 1976, After the fact was established that eating meat and ingesting other animal products is indeed, the #1 cause of cancer, especially colon, breast, ovarian, cervical, and prostate cancer, John Morgan, the President of Riverside Meat Packers had this to say: 'We shouldn't jump to any conclusions and do something foolish just because some study seems to say something that we know from common sense is not true. Beef is the backbone of the American diet and it always has been. To think that meat of all things causes cancer is ridiculous.'" — John Robbins, Diet for a New America

On March 13, 1982, John Morgan died from cancer of the colon...

This is a major problem within our country. Meat is the backbone of our diet and this is why we have gone from among the healthiest of nations seventy years ago to now being dead last among all of the largest countries in terms of health and disease. In the past century, we have doubled our meat consumption per person. We also have more than doubled our incidence of cancer, heart disease, and osteoporosis.

No matter what the meat and dairy industries do or say regarding their products, they cannot hide the truth. The truth is getting out, in books like this one, on web sites, on radio and TV shows – including *Raw Vegan Radio* and *How to Live to 100*, in magazines and newspapers – such as *VegWorld Magazine*, and in the documentaries, *A Delicate Balance*; *Forks over Knives*; *Farmageddon*; *Planeat*; *Vegucated*; *Hungry for Change*; and *Earthlings*.

THERE IS A PLACE FOR YOU HERE

In the raw food world we have a place for everybody. We welcome everyone with open arms. You do not have to pass an exam or look a certain way. It does not matter what your background may be. As long as you respect Earth, yourself, and others around you while abiding by nature's laws, you will be approved.

This means you simply refrain from eating meat, dairy, and eggs, along with extracts of them. You must give up processed foods. You should aim to eliminate all of the things from your life that are depleting from your vitality.

When you eat poor quality foods, you do not show respect for yourself. When you eat meat and consume eggs and/or dairy, you do not show respect for Earth, or the other creatures who live on it.

Be good to yourself, be honest with yourself, and always be true to yourself, and you will find a perfect place to fit in amongst others in the raw food world.

THE SECOND LESSON:

WE ARE BEING DECEIVED

We have been learning all sorts of things about food and health, and about what we should be eating. Now I want to explain to you a little about how we started to eat poorly. I want to share with you the truth behind why we are developing sickness and disease.

I have seen too many people die from cancer. I have heard too many stories of deaths from heart attacks. I know too many people with diabetes, suffering from obesity, and other diseases directly related to bad food choices. All of this is unnecessary and can be prevented.

When we understand the driving force behind foods that induce illness, and we are aware of the profits that are being made in the sickness industry, we can then discover the root cause for all of it, and not only prevent it, but reverse what has already happened.

Chapter 5: WHAT WE THE PEOPLE FAIL TO SEE

"Many times we hear only what others want us to hear. This is particularly true when facts have been discovered regarding a sensitive topic that is being sheltered for one reason or another by large business or our government." – Dr. Richard Oppenlander, Comfortably Unaware

Many of us carry on our lives as a reflection of someone else. We live as fractions of what nature intended for us to be. We grew up watching and observing what our parents did. We repeated the words our parents spoke most frequently. We ate the food our parents ate. We have become products of our environment. We believed what our parents told us and we assumed they were correct. It is in our nature to be trusting of those we love; however it is not in our nature to deceive those who have placed their love in us. Many parents have broken that natural trust and take advantage of their child's love. Through their own trust in a broken system, they have failed us.

As children, we are placed in a school system that forces us to learn the things our government wants to teach. We are taught to follow a Food Pyramid that wrongfully informs us to eat meat, eggs, dairy, and gluten grains. We are provided with school lunches that are lacking in true nutrition. These school lunch programs are saturated with corporate greed.

Through fictional history books and standardized testing, we learn little about the most important things in life. We are not taught about true nutrition, we are not taught about love, we are not taught about sickness or disease, instead we are misinformed by inaccurate textbooks, miseducated teachers, and a system that is a failure. We are taught the least relevant pieces of history, and the basics of mathematics, science, and language. We are misled into believing we need medicine after we eat the wrong foods and feel sick. We are disciplined when we express our individuality and this limits our ambitions. We are judged heavily by these "authority" figures that are often burned out by the system that also fails them. We never learn to love and we drift away from being our true selves, not connecting with our intellect and talents, or the essence of our being.

"Of what is significant in one's own existence one is hardly aware, and it certainly should not bother the other fellow. What does a fish know about the water in which he swims all his life?" – Albert Einstein

The government has recently placed spending cuts on school art programs, and in sports, yet they still have not done anything to change the school lunch programs, and they continue to increase funding for prisons.

"The U.S. spends more on jails and prisons than it does on education. Throughout the decade, starting in 2000, in California, the state government has been cutting funding to parks, cutting funding for children's programs, and cutting funding for schools, education services, and libraries, while increasing funding for prison construction, for prison guards, and for increasing the number of police officers. This is in a state where, by 2007, about $6,000 was being spent on each school student while about $40,000 was being spent on each prisoner." – *John McCabe, Igniting Your Life*

Only nature can teach us the way to live, yet in school we do not climb trees, we are not taught how to grow food, we do not learn anything about wild foods, and we do not interact with the other living creatures. We are confined inside of big buildings with brick walls and windows. The schools look more like prisons and are surrounded with blacktop pavement where gardens and nature should be. We are bullied, we are oppressed, we are confused, we are taught government propaganda, and we are being "dumbed down" to keep the economy of our country thriving while being graded on tests that are lies.

From the moment we are born, we are already being deceived. Rather than being embraced by nature, we are welcomed into the world inside of chemical drug dens known as hospitals. We are injected with disease-inducing vaccinations and immunizations that pave the way for a future of sickness and degenerative disease. Many of us are deprived of our only real source of nourishment, breast milk, and instead are given baby formulas that are laced with MSG, refined sugars, acrylamides, and fluoride. We are not given a fair opportunity to feel pure. We are denied our right to a healthy immune system by parents who lack education, are misinformed, often overwhelmed, who have not yet found ways to love themselves, and have little or no awareness of what their passions are in life as they are stuck in "the system."

As we are introduced to solid foods, rather than being given what nature provides for us to eat, such as fruits, vegetables, sprouts, nuts, and seeds, we are instead poisoned with dairy, meat, eggs, and chemically-saturated foods. Even after rejecting these deleterious food choices, parents continue to feed these unhealthful concoctions into the mouths of their children (behind the belief that these poisons are necessities for optimal nourishment) until they are conditioned to like them. What we are doing is not only destructive to their health, but is also poisoning their brains, interfering with neural activity, and disrupting their natural flow of life. Now we are not only deprived of nature and not given the opportunity to interact and enjoy the beauty of the other living creatures on Earth, but we are forced to eat them. We are fattened and diseased with their milk and mistakenly manipulated into believing it will make us strong, so no matter how bad it tastes, we continue to drink this unhealthful food. Then we get sick.

Once we develop sickness, we are forced to see a medical doctor. We are fooled into thinking we contracted sickness from germs after forgetting to wash our hands, or after playing with other kids who may be sick. We are not told the truth that this sickness comes from consuming dairy products and other animal-based foods. To a child, the doctor is often considered to be a magical person who can fix any problem and make things all better so we will no longer be sick. The problem with this fairy-tale is that the doctor is also relying on a flawed system, and is a graduate of a medical school strongly influenced by pharmaceutical and medical technology companies. An article published in the 2010 *Circulation* journal titled *Controversies in Cardiovascular Medicine*, explains how these industries fund medical education. The article states, *"The industry funds continuing medical education (CME) providers such as, physician organizations, publication and education companies, medical schools, and hospitals, many of which derive substantial profit. Support from pharmaceutical and medical device manufacturers for CME has quadrupled over the past decade and accounts for more than half of the $2.4 billion that is spent annually on CME. 'Medical education companies' were established to act as intermediaries between physicians and industry, accepting funding from drug or device manufacturers, and passing it along to physicians, medical schools, hospitals, or other organizations that offer lectures or educational programs. Although this arm's-length 'third-party' status is said to eliminate the manufacturer's influence over the educational content of these programs, the fact that most medical education companies are heavily dependent on industry for their revenue raises questions about the adequacy of this separation."*

When we visit the doctor he feeds us more chemicals known as medicine. This medicine only buries the sickness deeper inside of us so that it becomes a part of our cells and tissues and continues to accumulate and become more toxic. Once this sickness is buried deep within, we think we feel better, but something is always wrong. Our intuition may be trying to speak to us and tell us there really is something wrong, that is not being "fixed" by these drugs. We are assured that whatever it is happens to be normal and that "everything is okay." So we carry on with our everyday routine. We continue to eat nutrient deficient and chemically saturated foods, as we live indoors without nature, using chemical soaps to cleanse us and our surroundings, and learn mostly useless information that has nothing to do with self-sufficiency, and does not utilize our true talents and intellect.

After long days away from home, often we are welcomed after school with a brief moment of affection from one or both of our parents and then placed in front of the television to watch IQ-depleting shows that teach us everything that is wrong with the world. We are fed dinners from frozen packages and that are lacking in the nutrients we need. We are poisoned. The cycle continues, and with each passing generation, it gets worse, with more chemically-laced food and more animal protein.

"It is easier to fool people than to convince them that they have been fooled." – **Mark Twain**

The documentary *Forks Over Knives* informs us that, *Americans were eating around 120 pounds of meat per person annually at the beginning of the twentieth century. By 2007, that number had risen to 222 pounds per person annually. This shows us our meat consumption has nearly doubled in the last one-hundred years. As for dairy, Americans ate an average of 294 pounds of dairy annually in 1909 and by 2006, the average consumption per person rose to 605 pounds annually.* The cycle continues to grow out of control and as a result, the obesity rates continue to rise and the deaths from cardiovascular disease, diabetes, and cancer grow in number each year.

What we are not seeing is that we are failing as a civilization. We are allowing ourselves to crumble by means of our own ignorance and terrible food choices. We have detached from our most basic needs, and have become reliant on stores and restaurants feeding us toxic foods. We are allowing doctors to misdiagnose us and prescribe us poison for every ailment. We are surrendering to chemotherapy thinking it will cure our cancer when really it is killing us. We are quietly watching as our water supply is polluted with cancer causing chemicals. We are using toxic chemicals to "clean" ourselves, our homes, and our clothes. We are paying corporations as they add chemicals to our food supply while we ingest the foods and get sicker each day. We are paving the way for our children to develop disease by giving in to the lies that have been strategically constructed by the most profitable industries in the world. We are failing to love ourselves, and to love and protect our children.

"Love is the food of the soul, but you have been starved. Your soul has not received love at all, so you don't know the taste." – Osho

146

Without reading the side effects warnings on the label, we do not realize that every time we give our children medicine we may increase their chances of developing an illness worse than that we are attempting to cure. We also may fail to notice the stuff we call food has no food in it because real food contains nutrients that are beyond fat, carbohydrates, protein, and a few inorganic vitamins or minerals. Many do not seem to realize that they are poisoning their children every time they provide them with fast food, processed sweets, microwaved meals, and sodas, colas, energy drinks, and other junk beverages.

We may fail to see all of this, because we never knew to begin with. We were fooled when we were growing up. We were tainted by the tradition of eating low-quality foods. Now we live in this bubble of our deceived selves and call it the world and we do not know what exists beyond our misunderstanding of things. For some of us, we escape and marvel at the beauties previously unknown to us, and for others, this bubble gradually thickens and becomes a shell which we never hatch our way out of. Over time, this shell becomes our ending. In which of these scenarios do we exist? That is our own decision.

"Don't ever take things personal. Nothing anyone does is because of you; it is because of something that is going on in their lives. If someone is attacking me, they are attacking the part of me that they don't want to look at in themselves. If they didn't have it in them, they wouldn't be able to see it in me." – Dan McDonald, the Life Regenerator

These shells we may build around us can keep us contained in prisons of failure, poor health, anger, depression, and ignorance. We become so lost and confused that we do not know what is going on inside of our bubble, we cannot determine what may be knocking at the walls of our shells. We may not realize when opportunities come our way, so they pass us by. We have not prepared for, or conceptualized, the possibility of better opportunities being presented to us. We also may be sedated by poor quality foods, unfortunate choices of what we use for treating health problems, and by our patterns of thinking that are stuck at a certain level. What is scary is that many of those who have become trapped behind these shells of ignorance are also raising children. Then they raise their kids the same way they were raised. These shells are created for them as well. They feed into the system of despair, sickness, greed, misinformation, and suffering, and bring their innocent spirits along with them on their ride through a sedated life in a cloud of chemical-laced foods, chemical medications, and chemically-saturated homes.

It is time for us all to climb out of these bubbles that entangle our visions. It is time to crack these shells of ignorance with exploratory thoughts. We need to wake up and realize we do not have to be living far below our potential. We need to discover what real food is. We need to stop contributing to the profits of the pharmaceutical industry, processed foods industry, and overpriced and hollow education systems. We need to be available for our children, remove television from their lives, and teach them about love, optimal nutrition, and the importance of nature and their talents.

"The greatest gifts you can give your children are the roots of responsibility and the wings of independence." – Denis Waitley, Success Coach

This is our time to take back our world from the corporate greed that has saturated our lives. We need to break away from infusing ourselves with synthetic foods and drugs, and to eat truly healthy food, which consists of edible plant matter. This in turn will shut down the animal farming industry, the slaughterhouse industry, and the branches of the medical industry focused on treating patients suffering from diseases related to eating animals, dairy, eggs, and other health-degrading foods. We need to educate school children with the truth. We need to provide them with truly nutritious school lunches. We must stop giving in to these lies we have been conditioned to believe all of our lives. We must break away from our tradition of low-quality food choices, toxic medications, and sedated potential. We cannot afford to fail any longer; we must succeed with transforming society. It is time to start a new chapter of civilization, the chapter where the diseased are freed, and the medical industry admits its failures and gives in to defeat.

PHARMACEUTICAL LIES AND MARKETING SCHEMES

"A truth's initial commotion is directly proportional to how deeply the lie was believed. When a well-packaged web of lies has been sold to the masses over generations, the truth will seem utterly preposterous and its speaker a raving lunatic." – Dresden James

We have spent decades, and billions of dollars, on this so-called medical research, to advance so-called medical science. For the most part it has proven year after year, decade after decade, to be a failure. In the 1970's, around 225,000 people died annually from cancer, and now, a few decades and billions of dollars later, we are seeing nearly a million deaths a year as a result of cancer. In 2010, the *National Cancer Institute* reported their budget to be at $5.1 billion. That is a lot of research money to go into drugs that have never proven to be effective. In addition, our doctor visits have become more frequent and degenerative diseases are far more common than ever.

We have two choices to make in regards to our health: We can choose to eat right, and by doing so, completely eliminate having to make the decision of whether or not we should take medications, because sickness will not be a part of our lives; or we can choose to eat the way the typical American eats, and as a result, continue to welcome these viruses, harmful bacteria, and degenerative and chronic diseases into our lives.

There is nothing fanatical about the truth. To continue to support the failures of medicine, and support the greed of the pharmaceutical, dairy, egg, and meat industries, is what I would consider not only fanatical, but also ignorant and dangerous.

The last time I ingested anything medicine related was on my sixteenth birthday after having my wisdom teeth removed. I was given an antibiotic to make sure my mouth did not get infected. I felt horrible, and poisoned, and vowed to never again take a single pill. As a result, I have not been sick, not even a common cold, in over eleven years. This leads me to believe there is a correlation between ingesting chemical pills and being sick.

The pharmaceutical industry lies and does whatever it takes to cover up anything that may conflict with their profits. They also pay to have false and misleading medical studies released. In 2005, Dr. John Ioannidis published a paper in the journal *PLoS Medicine* that laid out detailed mathematical proof that researchers will come up with wrong findings most of the time they conduct studies. His model predicted that *eighty percent of non-randomized studies, twenty-five percent of so-called gold-standard randomized trials, and up to ten percent of the platinum-standard large randomized trials turned out to be wrong.*

Medical professionals prescribe antibiotics for viral infections and hand out painkiller prescriptions like they are candy. In November 2011, the *Substance Abuse and Mental Health Services Administration* reported that, every day, 5,500 people begin abusing painkillers. Dr. Thomas Frieden, director of *Centers for Disease Control and Prevention*, states that, "*We are in the middle of an epidemic. Every day, narcotics prescribed by physicians kill over forty people.*" This number is equivalent to that released by the *Centers for Disease Control* in 2011, which reported that *prescription painkiller medications kill around 15,000 people each year.*

Painkillers are among the most addictive medications, and their use can cause a variety of health problems. The only time one should allow these chemicals into their system is in an emergency situation, when surgery is indeed necessary, when there are burns, and in other situations where they are truly a relief.

"To boost the sale of regularly and heavily advertised products, not only do highly paid medical representatives present their sales pitch, but doctors are also enticed into promoting the drugs by the perks offered. Patients continue to use them because they are not cured. They are not supposed to be cured. They can only be treated. This is the ideal way that commercialism in medicine can thrive." – Dr. Fereydoon Batmanghelidj, The Bodies Many Cries for Water

DRUGS THAT DO NOT WORK

"The rule to determine whether a substance has a normal or abnormal relation to the living organism – whether it is a food or a poison – is simply this: If it usable in the normal processes – if it is convertible into tissue – it is food; if not, it is abnormal and poisonous." – Dr. Russell T. Trall, Water Cure for the Millions

Drugs, chemicals, and synthetic pills do not work to cure sickness or disease. I cannot put it in more simple terms. Many people have bought into the deception that they can eat whatever they want, then, if they get sick, run to the doctor to get better. But, the reality is, health does not work that way. If we get sick and see the doctor, chances are we are going to be treated with synthetic drugs, because that is what the doctor is trained to do. This can make us worse, bringing on other problems.

Common side effects from prescription drugs and antidepressants include sexual dysfunction, weight gain, sleep disturbance, nausea, headache, nervousness, and insomnia. Many antidepressants also increase the risk of suicide. In a January 2010 issue of the *Journal of the American Medical Association*, a study was published showing that *antidepressants are no better than placebo pills for those who suffer from depression.*

You may argue that some drugs provide temporary relief, but when you are sick again in just a few days or a few weeks you may start to wonder why that is. It is likely your body would have recovered without the chemical prescription drugs, and especially if you stopped eating garbage foods, drank more water, and got adequate rest.

You may also wonder why someone such as myself, or many of my other friends who eat a raw, plant-based diet, have not been sick in years. We rarely or ever get sick, and certainly do so far less than the average American. Life is much more enjoyable this way. You can live like this as well if you end your dependence on chemical drugs, and eliminate poor food choices from your life.

"To give drugs is adding to the cause of disease; for drugs always produce disease. Indeed they are believed to cure one disease, if they cure at all, but only by producing others. Can causes cure causes? Can poisons expel poisons? Can impurities deter impurities? Can nature throw off two or more burdens more easily than one? No! Poisoning a person because he is impure is like casting out devils through Beelzebub, the prince of devils. It is neither scriptural nor philosophical." – Dr. Russell T. Trall

ANTIBIOTICS FOR VIRAL INFECTIONS

It is said that over ninety-five percent of all acute sicknesses (cold, flu, etc) are caused by viruses. Given that our bodies only become prone to attack by these viruses from poor nutrition, it is interesting to me that, according to Dr. Joel Fuhrman, in his book *Super Immunity*, over ninety-percent of antibiotic prescriptions are prescribed for viral illnesses. Antibiotics are not made to kill *viruses*, they are created to kill *bacteria*, and they kill off our good intestinal bacteria too. Not only were antibiotics not created for killing viruses, they do not kill viruses, and they do not assist in any way in the recovery from viral illness.

When you go to the doctor for a cold, flu, sinusitis, or sore throat, which are all viral, and may also be linked to horrible food choices, most of these doctors will administer antibiotics for you to "get better." Not only does this make no sense, it is ridiculous and harmful. What we really need to do is start eating properly, avoid processed foods, and get some vegan "probiotics" rather than "antibiotics."

Many antibiotics come from the fungal kingdom. Certain species of fungi have defense mechanisms against bacteria and they produce antibiotics to fight off the bacteria. These natural antibiotics can destroy all harmful bacteria. What the pharmaceutical industry has done is extract the compounds that the defense mechanisms of these species of fungi consist of, and they have synthetically recreated, and chemically saturated them to destroy not only harmful bacteria, but all bacteria, including the good stuff that assists in digestion. If you want a good antibiotic, get some medicinal mushrooms. Chaga, reishi, maitake, lion's mane, and cordyceps are all powerful mushrooms with antibacterial properties.

VACCINES CAUSE DISEASE

The widespread myth that vaccination prevents disease is erroneous. While certain vaccines may assist in preventing particular diseases, they often create others. Over the years a number of toxins have been added to vaccines. According to the *Centers for Disease Control and Prevention*, they include formaldehyde, aluminum, thimerosal, polysorbate 80, MSG, streptomycin, neomycin, gentamicin, polymyxin B, soy, gelatin, egg, and yeast. Residual proteins from aborted fetal tissue, chick embryonic fluid, fetal bovine serum, guinea pig embryo cells, and monkey kidney cells have also been added to some vaccines.

Vaccines introduce toxins into the system. When they are not excreted, they inhibit enzymes from properly digesting nutrients. This begins the process of disease. If you look up the website, *vactruth.com*, you will read that *vaccines cause impaired blood flow (ischemia), chronic disease, illness, and death.*

"What vaccines have become is a multi-billion dollar annual industry that uses its money to manipulate laws, making it a requirement for more children to be vaccinated – not to protect the health of the children, but to protect the financial profits of the pharmaceutical industry." – John McCabe, Ignitingyourlife.com

Many common sicknesses and even horrendous degenerative diseases that children are plagued with today are a result of their being vaccinated. The most efficient way to prevent disease is to eat a clean diet, free from chemicals, and to make healthy lifestyle choices. This eliminates the need for vaccines.

"In many children, the introduction of attenuated germs or viruses, through vaccination, is sufficient to cause severe damage, brain dysfunction, diabetes, and rheumatoid arthritis." – Charlotte Gerson, The Gerson Therapy

If you are considering vaccinating your children, I strongly recommend that you research this topic thoroughly. You may save their lives by doing so. You may want to watch the documentary, *The Greater Good*, which features profiles of families impacted by life-altering vaccine reactions, and the perspective of vaccine experts. The website for the *National Vaccine Information Center* (nvic.org) provides us with more information on the topic of vaccines. Other great sites are *generationrescue.org*, and *thedoctorwithin.com*. Karen Ranzi wrote *Creating Healthy Children*, which includes a chapter on vaccinations. Andreas Moritz recently published *Vaccine-nation: Poisoning the population one shot at a time*. You may also want to read *The Sanctity of Human Blood: Vaccination is not Immunization,* 13th Edition, by Dr. Tim O'Shea. These resources will enlighten you about the truth behind vaccinations and help impact your decision on whether or not you will vaccinate yourself or your children.

CHEMICAL DRUG DENS AND SURGERY FACTORIES

A hospital, for many, is a place of security. It is the place to go for an *instant fix* of good health. The reality is, other than for emergency medicine, hospitals do very little, if anything, to help people improve from chronic diseases. They often make things worse. Many hospital patients are there because of malnutrition, due to ingesting processed foods, yet many leave more malnourished than when they arrive. In July 2008, an article was published in *Today's Dietitian*, titled *Malnutrition: A Serious Concern for Hospitalized Patients*. In the article, the author, Theresa A. Fessler, states that an estimated thirteen to sixty-nine percent of hospitalized patients are malnourished. This can be attributed to the basic four foods plan, which hospitals serve to all patients, and which was created by the meat, dairy, egg, and grain industries.

Around the globe, these hospitals contain hundreds of thousands of patients and are feeding them chemical-laden, processed foods that induce illness, while performing unnecessary and highly risky surgical experiments on them. These experiments include removing organs, such as the gall bladder, and even removing pieces of the intestines. It is time to put an end to this madness.

152

"One of the best-kept secrets in medicine is the brain damage caused during bypass surgery. During my forty years of medical practice I have never heard a doctor warn a patient before bypass surgery that an expected complication is memory loss. After surgery, when the family complains of dad's fits of anger, I have never heard a doctor admit that personality change is a common consequence of surgery. Yet these well-recognized side effects have been reported in medical journals since 1969." – Dr. John McDougall

Many of these surgical procedures result in post-surgical cognitive dysfunction, where the mind starts to deteriorate. More complications, like micro strokes, are arising from heart bypass surgery, when the plaque is disrupted during the surgery. Most internal problems that require surgery are brought on by poor eating choices, and they can also be reversed in many cases by changing the diet. This eliminates the need for bypass surgeries, or removal of other organs. Read *Preventing and Reversing Heart Disease* by Dr. Caldwell Esselstyn to learn more about the complications of surgery.

We are the most chemically contaminated species on the planet and hospitals are one reason for this. Have you been to the ER lately? Have you taken the time to look at all of the sick people who are dependent on chemical drugs and are only there waiting for another prescription? If you are one of these people who rely on chemical drugs to get through each day, I urge you to wake up and realize that you will never get better by continuing to be sedated by these drugs. You have to change your life. You have to change your diet.

WHY I CHOSE NOT TO BE A MEDICAL DOCTOR

"Young doctors who have just come out of college and are primed to the brim with vast stores of quite useless, and largely erroneous theoretical knowledge, are to be sure, confident that they know all about the nature of disease and its proper 'treatment,' under every conceivable condition. For have they not a drug for the treatment of nearly every disease? But with the older physicians, such is by no means the case." – Dr. Hereward Carrington

The difference between my education and a doctor's education is that I educated myself on the opposing sides of health – the medical side, and the nutritional side. Growing up, we see more than enough of what the medical side does. We see people continually relying on doctors, pills, and surgeries, but not getting better, and often becoming much worse.

I read books and taught myself about the human mechanism, and the way medicine works and dysfunctions. Although I grasped the concept of medicine, it did not make sense to me that we should poison the body when we are trying to relieve it of its poisoned condition. I have also eaten a diet cleaner than most Americans for the majority of my life. What I have noticed over the years is that the people who are sick are the ones who make poor eating decisions. As I began reading about raw nutrition and exploring the natural healing side of health, I realized this is the only way to erase sickness. After carefully examining both sides and making many observations, I decided I had to help bring out the truth behind sickness and disease. By continuing to educate myself, and spread my knowledge to others, I have found this is the only way to reveal the truth.

Where medical doctors go wrong is that they too often choose to become doctors for the money and social status, or to live up to the expectations their parents have placed on them, and too few times to help others. They are then forced to learn everything they know from the medical texts that have been formulated so that the only way to solve any health problem is to prescribe medicine and/or advise surgery. So the doctors waste several years of their lives, and space in their brain, with this mostly useless information about chemical drugs, which, outside of emergency situations, are usually not much of an answer to health problems – and may trigger illness. Chemical drugs are beneficial in situations involving emergency surgery, emergency pain care, and certain other conditions, such as infections or burn care, and when someone is experiencing extreme stress, or is in shock. As we learn more about nature's prescriptions, we may also discover remedies for these without chemicals.

"The older physicians grow, the more skeptical they become of the virtues of medicine and the more they are disposed to trust the powers of nature." – Dr. Alexander H. Stevens, NY College of Physicians and Surgeons

What I did differently is I stayed away from title and social status and absorbed all of the knowledge I could on both sides. Rather than being forced by some corrupt industry to abide by their false rules, I chose the option that works best for me, and for nature. I discovered that there is little need for chemical drugs used to maintain health. The medicine we need to experience vibrant health is in raw organic foods.

WHAT MANY DOCTORS DO NOT KNOW

"One thing that I think the public tends not to know is there's not a medical school in the United States that teaches nutrition." – Dr. T. Colin Campbell

As we make more and more money every year, we eat at fancier restaurants, and we drive nicer cars, we are falling further behind in terms of our health. We could acquire every material possession in the world, but a medical doctor could take them all away with one erroneous prescription.

"Almost every medical doctor will con you into eating poisonous medications that will actually make your conditions worse in the long run. Nearly all medical conditions are really lack of proper nutrition. How many times has a doctor told you to change your diet before they tried to sell you on toxic medicine?" – Dr. John McDougall

When you see a doctor for something as simple as curing hypertension, he will give you drugs and may expect you to take them forever. When you see a doctor because you have asthma, he will prescribe you an inhaler and may expect you to suck on it for the rest of your life without ever getting better. If you develop some type of ulcer, and see a doctor, he will most likely have you eating antacids. The same goes for allergies, diabetes, arthritis, and many other diseases. Every illness or condition for which you see a medical doctor, he will most likely prescribe you a pill.

The reason why these doctors prescribe harmful drugs is because they are not equipped with the knowledge they need to solve the problems we call diseases. The medical system fails to incorporate this into their education program. The answers are often fairly simple when you abide by nature; they become more complex when you go through years of medical schooling that teaches nothing but how to increase the profits of the pharmaceutical and surgical empires.

I read a medical study published in the *PLoS Journal* in 2011 titled, *Lack of awareness among future medical professionals about the risk of consuming hidden phosphate-containing processed food and drinks.* The study supports my claim that doctors do not know enough about nutrition to be treating chronic conditions by stating that, *"Because phosphate toxicity is an important determinant of mortality in patients with chronic kidney disease (CKD), CKD patients are advised to take a low phosphate-containing diet, and are additionally prescribed with phosphate-lowering drugs. Since these patients usually seek guidance from their physicians and nurses for their dietary options, the researchers conducted a survey to determine the levels of awareness regarding the high phosphate content in commercially processed food and drinks among medical and nursing students at the Hirosaki University School of Medicine in Japan. The researchers randomly selected 190 medical and nursing students, and provided them with a list of questions to evaluate their awareness of food and drinks which contain artificially added phosphate ingredients.*

While 98.9 percent of these students were aware of the presence of sugar in commercially available soda drinks, only 6.9 percent were aware of the presence of phosphate (phosphoric acid). Similarly, only 11.6 percent of these students were aware of the presence of phosphate in commercially processed food, such as hamburgers and pizza. Moreover, around two thirds of the surveyed students (67.7 percent) were unaware of the harmful effects of unrestricted consumption of phosphate-containing food and drinks. About twenty-eight percent of the surveyed students consume such 'fast food' once a week, while forty percent drink at least one, but no more than five cans of soda drinks/week. After realizing the potential long-term risks of consuming excessive phosphate-containing food and drinks, 40.5 percent of the survey participants considered reducing their phosphate intake by minimizing the consumption of commercially processed 'fast food' items and soda drinks. Moreover, another 48.4 percent of students showed interest in obtaining more information on the negative health effects of consuming excessive amounts of phosphate."

This study was conducted at a single school of medicine. I imagine the results would be similar at all other medical schools. While they were advising patients to eat a low phosphate diet, they were serving them high-phosphate foods. This should be enough evidence in itself that medical students should be required to learn more about optimal nutrition, and specifically the benefits of a plant-based diet. Instead, medical school cafeterias serve junk foods, and often have typical fast-food chain restaurants on campus. This paves the way for a generation of sickly medical doctors who will rely on prescription drugs for themselves, as well as for their patients.

THE PROBLEM WITH "SPECIALISTS"

"Many of the so-called health experts are people so personally addicted to a meat and dairy diet that they are in denial about the dangers that are posed to even their own health." — Dr. Brian Clement, Hippocrates Health Institute

I have a hard time understanding why any of us would continue to see a "specialist" when he does not offer a cure for our problems. A pulmonologist is considered to be a "lung specialist," yet never corrects a problem with the lungs. Pulmonologists only give you "treatments" and force you to breathe through a tube or to ingest chemical drugs. Those living with emphysema are often misled by these "specialists" into believing they have to breathe with oxygen tanks for the rest of their lives and that there is no cure for emphysema or that it cannot be improved. This is nonsense.

Most people with allergies see "allergy specialists" and these people offer no cure for their allergies. They prescribe them medicines that mask the problem and may create more adverse health conditions.

When the standard person has back problems they go see a "back specialist," and again, the problem persists. They offer no cures, just temporary relief — and often highly addictive drugs along with complicated and risky surgeries that may leave the patient in pain for life.

When an ordinary person has trouble with her vision, she sees an "eye specialist." Soon after, she is wearing glasses or contacts and her vision continues to get worse for the remainder of her life. Relying on these foreign lenses forever, her eye problems, however, never get better.

The truth, and what most fail to see, is that there is a reversal, relief, or cure and there may be permanent relief from many of these conditions. "Specialists" are nothing special at all. They may placate and mislead you into

156

believing you are some poor creature who has suffered a terrible fate, and must live with these unnatural conditions forever, while continuing to pay them for temporary relief while you experience gradual worsening of your conditions. It is time to empower yourself and discontinue your reliance on these not-so-specialists.

"The idea that even a single specialist treating cancer patients might have no idea about the impact of foods on cancer growth is appalling. Hundreds of scientific papers have been published, most in the last decade, on the affects of nutrients on cancer-cell growth. Yet, oncologists don't read them; instead, they read the articles about the latest chemotherapy agent or new combination therapy. After all, vegetable farmers are not going to take them out to lunch or invite them to exotic resorts in Hawaii." – Dr. Russell Blaylock, Health and Nutrition Secrets

When you change your diet and your lifestyle, you may find that you provide the cure for yourself. If you or anyone you know continues to see "specialists," you may want to consider the fact that you are being misled and explore other options.

"When numerous small injuries finally added up to being temporarily paralyzed, doctors mostly only offered highly addictive drugs and risky surgery. Luckily I refused their advice to undergo spinal fusion and have metal rods implanted along my spine. I now do everything they said I would never do: bike, run, and swim." – John McCabe, Igniting Your Life

THE ONLY THING GENETIC IS IGNORANCE

"Genetics loads the gun, lifestyle pulls the trigger." – Dr. Caldwell Esselstyn

I recently had a disagreement with a lady. She was attempting to strike up an argument with me claiming that genetics are responsible for every health condition. She claimed that heart disease is genetic and has nothing to do with diet or lifestyle choices. She also claimed that obesity is genetic and will occur even if someone eats healthfully, as long as their genes were predisposed to obesity. As I attempted to explain the truth to her, she insisted I was wrong because, "Her dad told her otherwise." Finally, after realizing she was a lost cause, I said, "The only thing genetic is ignorance."

"It is acidosis that causes degenerative disease, not genes. The genes dictate which of many degenerative diseases you will be prone to, but they do not cause the disease." – Dr. Robert Barefoot

If you are unfortunate enough to go to a medical doctor for a nutritional deficiency and bad diet that has resulted in diabetes, obesity, high cholesterol, cancer, heart disease, stroke, arthritis, or any other similar conditions, and that doctor tries to use his scare tactic of telling you that you are genetically predisposed and you cannot avoid the condition, do not believe him.

In the *China Study*, Dr. T. Colin Campbell lists eight principles of food and health. Principle number four states that, *"Genes do not determine disease on their own. Genes function only by being activated, or expressed, and nutrition plays a critical role in determining which genes, good and bad, are expressed."* When genes are not activated or expressed, they remain biochemically dormant. These genes then have no effect on our health. Nutrition is often the factor that determines the activity of genes.

Epigenetics is a term applied to the belief that gene cells can be turned on and off, and states that the environment of the cell determines which genes will be activated or inactivated. Diet and environmental conditions play the most important role in epigenetics. If you eat poorly and live an unhealthy lifestyle, chances are you will activate bad gene cells, which will also be passed down from generation to generation.

Genes do determine much; however, the only way many genes will lead to a degenerative condition is through diet and/or lifestyle choices. You eat what your parents eat and they eat what their parents ate and so on. If your parents were smokers or drinkers and you are also a smoker or drinker, then chances are you will develop a disease or health condition. If you eat processed foods, you are more likely to develop diabetes and/or cancer. If you eat meat and dairy, chances are increased that you will have high cholesterol and develop heart disease or cancer. If you feed your child fast food and/or processed foods, chances are increased that your child is going to have a lower IQ, weak bones, and be prone to serious disease. This is not genetic or hereditary, this is simply the fact that you are lacking an array of nutrients needed for vibrant health, and are consuming a variety of unhealthful substances.

It is outrageous for someone to see a medical doctor who misinforms them that their condition cannot be changed because of genes, that they must eat toxic medicine for the rest of their lives, and for them to accept this false diagnosis and prognosis. It is possible to reverse, or greatly relieve, many, or most, common health conditions. It is possible to turn gene cells off and deactivate them once they have become active. Most medical doctors simply lack the education needed to solve nutritional deficiencies and get their clients to clean up their diet to be free of toxins, which is the main way of overcoming many of the common degenerative and chronic conditions. If you are sick, even with a cold, fever, or flu, the last thing you need is chemical drugs. You need nutrients, you need internal cleansing, and you need to take measures to maintain vibrant health.

I observe people, things, places, and situations. What I have noticed is a common trend that takes place amongst girls and boys, men and women. They are all trapped in their ego so much that they trap themselves into being a part of the chain of sickness and disease. Their false sense of pride prevents them from going the other route.

No matter who you are, deciding to change your life to be at your best, taking action, allowing that change to occur, and making it happen, is the greatest thing you could ever do for yourself. When you are in a hospital bed dying from the worst diseases out there, you will wish you had made the changes earlier in life, so that you could have avoided the outcome of terrible food choices, lack of exercise, and other activities that brought you to be a pawn of the sickness industry.

Chapter 6: THE PROBLEMS CONTINUE

"Long surgical experience has proved to me conclusively that there is something radically and fundamentally wrong with the civilized mode of life, and I believe, that unless the present dietetic and health customs of the modern nations are reorganized, social decay and race deterioration are inevitable." – Sir Arbuthnot Lane, doctor and surgeon

Media does a great job shifting our attention away from the issues that are the most severe and most important, to the issues that are non-vital, such as celebrity gossip, entertainment, new products, and which politician is telling the most lies. The real issue we all need to be presented with daily is the war we are fighting for our own health, and our environmental health.

Right now, those of us who live in the United States are being robbed of our health and well-being by our food choices, the pharmaceutical industry, the GMO industry, the fossil fuels industries, the prison industry, the war industries – and by the government departments and corporations working in their interests. The marketing schemes of the drug companies have led us to believe that the simplest cures do not exist and that chemical drugs are beneficial to our health. The industrial, medical, and food industries have fooled us into believing calcium supplements, prescription drugs, dairy, eggs, and meat are necessary for our optimal survival. These industries have become so financially and politically powerful that they have scores of lobbyists and legal teams manipulating politicians and formulating legislation that gets passed into laws that protect the profits of the drug companies, hospitals, and industrial food companies. Concurrently, we are so worried about the celebrity scandal of the week, that we fail to see what is really going on.

The healthcare industry brings in more profits than oil, and costs our consumers much more than the price we pay for war. In a speech made by our First Lady, Michelle Obama, she mentioned that, *"Obesity, heart disease, cancer, and high blood pressure are all diet-related health issues that cost this country more than 120 billion dollars each year."* These numbers continue to rise annually, and our current healthcare system is not capable of reducing disease or improving health.

Although some types of cancer can be, have been, and continue to be cured through natural means, we are misled by medical doctors into believing there is no cure, and that chemotherapy and radiation are somehow helpful for "treating" advanced stages of cancer. Chemotherapy and radiation can trigger cancer to metastasize and spur the growth of other cancers. We have all been so misinformed that many doctors, as well as the medical staff, and employees of drug companies and medical technology companies, also choose to undergo radiation and chemo when they are stricken with cancer. In most cases, cognitive dysfunction is common after undergoing this treatment. While many doctors deny reported cognitive problems are in any way related to chemo, results from a study released in a November 2011 issue of the journal *Archives of Neurology* suggest otherwise. They found evidence that chemo can cause brain damage. Dr. Daniela Bota and Dr. Mark Linskey, co-directors of UC Irvine's Comprehensive Brain Tumor program, discovered that *certain chemotherapeutic agents destroy the stem cells in the brain that would have become neurons for creating and storing memories.*

Many conditions, such as high blood pressure, high cholesterol, an array of skin issues, common colds, influenza, ear infections, and headaches, have been taken out of context. Rather than eliminating the toxic foods and chemical additives that are triggering these symptoms, we are manipulated into believing we need chemical drugs to "treat" them. Most of these chemical drugs contain side-effect-warnings on the labels, and if you read them, you will notice that they cause more of these common symptoms to occur – and spur worse health events, such as ulcers, nerve issues, depression, suicidal thoughts, and cancers.

"This whole notion of deriving benefit or of becoming 'cured' through the taking of 'chemical drugs' in any form, or under any circumstances, is one of the most disastrous, as it is one of the most ludicrous fallacies; one of the most harmful beliefs existent, and one which the coming generations of free-thinking medical men will have to most vigorously combat." – Dr. Hereward Carrington, Vitality, Fasting & Nutrition

Much of the current medical profession provides erroneous treatment procedures, and the crimes which the pharmaceutical empire has committed over the past sixty plus years cannot be justified. Over 106,000 people die each year from adverse drug reactions. In addition to this staggering number, a study published in the *Journal of the American Medical Association* in 2006 reported 700,000 emergency department visits and 120,000 hospitalizations annually from adverse drug reactions. It is estimated that up to eight million children take one or more psychotropic drugs regularly. The *Centers for Disease Control and Prevention* reports that eighty-two percent of American adults take at least one medication and twenty-nine percent take five or more. The annual death toll from hospitalizations and outpatient care is over 400,000. Many of these deaths could be avoided.

"Our figures show approximately four and one half million hospital admissions annually due to the adverse reactions to drugs. Further, the average hospital patient has as much as thirty percent chance, depending how long he is in, of doubling his stay due to adverse drug reactions." – Milton Silverman, M.D., Professor of Pharmacology, University of California

In spite of the statistics, we continue to support the medical industry. We raise our children with the principles that growing up to be a medical doctor is a good thing. We allow laws to govern whether we can be cured of our conditions, and whether or not we can eat real food. Subsidy dollars are used to help pay for commercials, such as the *Got Milk* campaign – which lies to the public about the benefits of consuming dairy, and for assuring we can afford fast food dollar menu items and other health-degrading foods. In the meantime, our health care costs are steadily rising and currently have been reported at $2.6 trillion annually. Nearly seventy-five percent of these costs are associated with chronic diseases. A high percentage of chronic disease is linked to the consumption of animal products – meat, dairy, and eggs. What these dollars should pay for are more of the *Infect Truth* campaigns. The *Infect Truth* advertisements currently offer attention-getting scenes and hard-hitting facts about smoking, while encouraging teens to share the knowledge with their friends and family. These campaigns should also warn us about the dangers of eating meat, eggs, dairy, processed foods, and chemical drugs, rather than strictly warning against the use of so-called "illicit drugs."

Currently we battle with laws that are attempting to outlaw organic health care products. The corporate whore, Senator Dick Durbin, submitted the *Dietary Supplement Labeling Act of 2011* which would deny many Americans affordable access to the natural health products they rely on daily. His proposed plan would crack-down on the testing, labeling, and sales of supplements nationwide. Luckily this bill has not passed as a law just yet. We also battle with the GMO giant, Monsanto, and other GMO companies, such as Bayer CropScience and DuPont, over whether or not we can grow real crops.

We are in a war right now within our own country. We are battling big business, big pharma, and big agriculture against their attempt to drown our society inside of sickness and poverty. They continue to profit while many of us kill ourselves, each other, and our chances at being successful in life, with each drink of alcohol, each bite of fast food, and every pill swallowed.

They persuade us into believing we need vaccinations to "avoid" certain sicknesses and diseases. Well, the only way to avoid these sicknesses is to eat a clean, plant-based diet, live actively, and be aware of the link between sickness and our food and lifestyle choices. The "flu shot" and all of the vaccinations we have been poisoned with for all of these years may be causing more sickness and disease than they claim to prevent. On the *Centers for Disease Control and Prevention* website, it is stated that, *flu vaccines will NOT protect against infection and illness caused by other viruses that can also cause influenza-like symptoms. There are many other viruses besides influenza that can result in influenza-like illness.* That sounds like deception to me.

"*You assist an evil system most effectively by obeying its orders and decrees. An evil system never deserves such allegiance. Allegiance to it means partaking of the evil. A good person will resist an evil system with his or her whole soul.*" – *Mahatma Gandhi*

When we are sick, we most often do not need to see a medical doctor. We need to analyze our situation. We need to reflect on what foods and other substances we have been allowing to enter our bodies. We should consider our

162

lack of exercise, and the health of our environment and relationships. Sickness is not a medical issue. Being sick is a nutritional dilemma that can be solved by changing your diet and practices. A raw nutritionist or health coach could help you lay the groundwork for a new approach to food. Be sure that your nutritionist is not abiding by the food pyramid. Inform them that you wish to go the plant-based, organic, richly raw vegan route. If you cannot afford a nutritionist, join Facebook groups that are related. There are many free groups on Facebook that are full of good people who will happily reply to the questions you may have. A few examples of groups you can join are: *The Raw Cure, Living Tree Community, Naturally Healing, Inc, Rawgust, Raw Vegan Club, Vegan Super Fitness Group, and Raw and Delicious Lifestyles.*

Much of the sickness and many wrongs in this world are connected. The chemical saturation of foods, of the water, and of the medical industry often leads back to the same few corporations. Much of what we have been taught about nutrition since we were children has been false and misleading. We were fooled into being customers of the dairy, egg, and meat industries. They put synthetic food additives in packaged food items. They put chemicals in our water supply and added poisons to our infant formulas and children's "beverages."

In school, the children are taught to follow the deceptive food pyramid and eat from the four food groups of illness, which is leading to severe obesity and the development of diabetes, cancers, and heart disease at a young age. In increasing numbers, young children are having issues with high blood pressure. This is something many never imagined would happen fifty years ago. School lunches are toxic and put together using guidelines set by the animal farming industry and – what John McCabe calls its concierge service – the USDA. Medicine makes those who are sick even sicker and the worst part is that the laws and tax benefits hold all of it into place.

School lunch programs consist of a sad mess of toxic foods, laying the groundwork for a lifetime of illness we call chronic, autoimmune, and degenerative diseases. This profits the medical industry's trinity of pharmaceutical drug companies, hospitals, and doctors.

In July 2012, the *Physicians Committee for Responsible Medicine* (pcrm.org) petitioned the federal government to remove milk as a required food from the school lunch program. The committee labeled milk as an *ineffective placebo* and provided research showing that the consumption of milk does not improve bone health or prevent bone fractures. Elaborating on the petition to remove milk from school lunches, the committee's nutrition education director, Susan Levin, announced, *"Milk does not make children grow taller or stronger, but it will make them heavier. We are asking Congress and the USDA to place the interests of the children above the interests of the dairy industry. Focusing on milk as the single most important source of calcium in children's diets distracts schools and parents from foods that really can build bones, like leafy green vegetables and legumes."* The petition asks the *U.S Department of Agriculture* to recommend an amendment to the *National School Lunch Act,* excluding dairy milk as a required component of school lunches. Now we can hope the petition will create much needed change.

THE STANDARD AMERICAN GIRLS DILEMMA

As I was leaving a seminar in the city, I stopped in a 7-Eleven to purchase what I expected to be the winning lottery ticket. I was wrong, of course, about the outcome of the ticket, but as I was standing in the store, I could not help but notice they do not sell anything, aside from Clif Bars and maybe a few pieces of fruit, that has not been made synthetically with chemicals. There were no other items in the store that I consider to be food. The beverages seemed to be "gut- stretching" and organ straining, rather than thirst-quenching. Even the products they label as healthy were far from that. There were two young ladies in front of me. They had placed on the counter: a frozen pizza, a two liter bottle of a combination of chemicals known as Diet Cola, and a pack of chewing gum. They then had the man working behind the counter retrieve a large bottle of whiskey. After the purchase was made, one of the girls said, "Oh, I almost forgot. I need a pack of cigarettes."

I recently encountered a situation where a young lady could not find something in her purse, so she dumped out the entire contents onto the surface below her. Inside of her purse was: a pack of cigarettes, chemicals for her face (moisturizers and make-up), a pharmaceutical pill bottle for the relief of headaches, gift cards to a popular coffee shop, lip balm, and some chewing gum.

"We are prone to thinking of drug abuse in terms of the male population and illicit drugs such as heroin, cocaine, and marijuana. It may surprise you to learn that a greater problem exists with millions of women dependent on legal prescription drugs." – *Robert Mendelsohn, M.D*

Every day I see young ladies drinking blended coffee drinks, smoking cigarettes, polluting their beautiful faces with synthetic chemical make-up, walking around with orange skin from the toxic tanning lotions and bronzers they use, eating an array of medications they falsely believe assist them with their "bi-polar" or "anxiety" issues, drinking cocktails which are really alcohol mixed with high-fructose corn syrup and sodium benzoate, eating fast food, and chewing on gum. They seem unaware of how they are assaulting their systems with a continual flow of chemical stew. As I observe all of this, I am not only completely turned off by their lack of respect for their bodies and minds, but I am saddened because I begin to think of the rapidly growing percentage of young women who are developing cervical cancer, breast cancer, multiple sclerosis, cardiovascular disease, and an array of mental health issues.

In the past year I have known eight different women in their twenties who have developed some sort of cervical cancer or cancerous lump in their breasts. They are only a few of the hundreds of thousands who have poisoned their bodies with mass-marketed products containing the substances that trigger such cancers to grow. According to the World Health Organization, there are 132,082 women diagnosed with cervical cancer every year, and of those, 74,118 die. Globally it affects approximately 500,000 women. When they visit medical doctors or cancer "specialists," the procedure for them is to have the cancerous growths surgically removed. Not one thing is mentioned to them about diet, or clearing the onslaught of toxic foods and chemicals out of their lives – from soaps, deodorants, perfumes, and cosmetics, to fast foods and alcoholic beverages.

This cancer develops from many nutritional deficiencies, as well as the accumulation of toxins from the ingestion of so many chemicals in the products they have been considering food, and from what they have been putting on their skin and in their hair. As they continue to delve into these poor lifestyle and eating choices, the toxins continue to accumulate. Each time they get sick, they enervate, or halt, the natural elimination process with chemical medicine, and the toxins accumulate even more heavily. This build-up of toxins is known as toxemia. Toxemia is the root cause of much of the illness plaguing society. I discuss toxemia in a later chapter.

"The only disease is toxemia, and what we call diseases are the symptoms produced by a forced vicarious elimination of toxin through the mucus membrane." – Dr. John Tilden

The frozen pizza those girls purchased at 7-Eleven lacks natural ingredients. Instead, it contains a mixture of additives, preservatives, and other garbage, processed ingredients. Additionally, it contains dairy, salt, gluten grains, acrylamides, and glycotoxins. A small effort to improve the nutritional value is made by adding a few synthetic vitamins, which is known as "fortifying." Foods that have been fortified with synthetic vitamins are close to useless.

The bottle of Diet Cola they purchased is a stew of many toxic chemicals, and is highly acidic. Remember, for every eight ounce cup of Diet Cola (or any soda you drink), you need thirty-two eight ounce cups of water simply to dilute the acidity. I know quite a few people who drink can after can of this poison every single day. Soda consumption has been linked to many different cancers, osteoporosis, nerve disorders, oral health problems, and lupus. The high amounts of phosphates in soda from the phosphoric acid erode the myelin sheath that protects nerve cells and can trigger multiple sclerosis. The chemical additives, such as aspartame and sodium benzoate, have been linked to Parkinson's disease and Alzheimer's disease. The caramel coloring and refined sugars have been linked to cancer, and disorders of the liver and pancreas. An acidic blood pH is also directly linked to cancer and soda is highly acidic. The conclusion of a study published in *Cancer Epidemiology, Biomarkers & Prevention,* a journal of the *American Association for Cancer Research,* in February of 2010, revealed that, *"People who drank two or more soft drinks a week had an eighty-seven percent increased risk – or nearly twice the risk – of pancreatic cancer compared to individuals consuming no soft drinks."*

The chewing gum that a majority of people chew on daily are pieces of synthetic chemicals. Have you ever read the ingredients in chewing gum? I read the label of a popular brand and it consisted of maltitol, sorbitol, glycerol, aspartame, acesulfame K, and sodium bicarbonate. These sugars are not easy to digest and have been linked to irritable bowel syndrome. The aspartame in the gum has been linked several times to cancer, and is also known to trigger bi-polar disorder and anxiety. A study in the *Journal of Periodontology* in January of 2002, titled *Systemic Release of Endotoxins Induced by Gentle Mastication: Association with Periodontitis Severity*, showed a rise in harmful bacteria products in the blood after chewing gum. Researchers studied sixty-seven patients of whom forty-two were diagnosed with moderate to severe periodontitis and the remaining twenty-five patients were healthy individuals who had never received periodontal treatment. Blood samples were taken before and after patient's lightly chewed chewing gum fifty times on each side of their jaw. Researchers found *the number of patients with endotoxemia rose from six percent before chewing to twenty-four percent after chewing. Additionally, those with severe periodontal disease had approximately four times more harmful bacterial products in their blood than those with moderate or no periodontal disease.*

The alcohol that the young ladies purchased depletes B-vitamins, and damages intestinal flora by decreasing intestinal absorption of nutrients, sodium, and water. The mixers they use with the alcohol might also contain aspartame and refined sugars, and these combinations can play a role in irritable bowel syndrome, bi-polar disorder, and anxiety. The cigarettes steal vitality and reduce blood flow to the skin, accelerating aging. The coffee drinks, cigarettes, and sodas leach alkaline minerals from the body, creating acidosis in the blood. Acidosis, along with toxemia, can trigger breast cancer, cervical cancer, and many other degenerative or chronic conditions.

The *Journal of the National Cancer Institute* published a report in September 1974 that found excessive intake of alcohol raises one's risks for cancers of the breast, mouth, pharynx, and esophagus. When combined with smoking, these risks skyrocket. It also raises risks for stomach, liver, and colon cancers.

The amount of chemicals being added to cigarettes today is far greater in number than it was in decades past. Now that we have been warned of the dangers of cigarettes, the tobacco manufacturers are no longer held responsible for the damages their products cause. Those who smoke today develop disease by means of their own ignorance, defiance, and denial. The chemicals being added to cigarettes sold throughout the world is one reason why we are seeing more and more cancers developing at younger ages. Cigarettes, processed foods, and diets rich in fat and animal protein are major contributors to breast and cervical cancers. The *Centers for Disease Control and Prevention* reports that cigarettes are responsible for about one out of every five deaths per year.

The *Tobacco Atlas Report*, conducted by the *World Lung Foundation*, reported in March of 2012 that tobacco-related deaths have nearly tripled in the past decade and big tobacco firms are undermining public efforts that could save millions of lives. In the report, marking the tenth anniversary of its first *Tobacco Atlas*, the *World Lung Foundation* and the *American Cancer Society* stated, *"If current trends continue, a billion people will die from tobacco use and exposure this century – that is equivalent to one person every six seconds."* The report also includes that, *"Tobacco has killed fifty million people in the last ten years, and tobacco is responsible for more than fifteen percent of all male deaths and seven percent of female deaths. In China, tobacco is already the number one killer – causing 1.2 million deaths a year – and that number is expected to rise to 3.5 million a year by 2030."*

Meanwhile, have you noticed how we continue to be bombarded with cigarette advertising telling us that smoking is fun, cool, and sexy?

Today, many people are indirectly choosing to develop cancer, to have cardiovascular disease, to develop mental illness, and to gain weight by choosing to live low-quality lifestyles. By eating fast food, drinking alcoholic cocktails, sneaking lines of cocaine, sipping on sugary coffee drinks, and smoking cigarettes, they are creating acidosis and toxemia in their bodies. When acidosis or toxemia occurs, the breath often has an awful stench to it. The best way for them to cover up this odor is by chewing gum. Now the cycle continues.

The next time you crave a soda, my advice would be to grab a good fresh vegetable juice instead. Rather than indulging in sugary coffee drinks or cocktails, you could provide your body with enough alkalinity every day, by eating fresh leafy greens, so that you will no longer crave stimulants. Give up smoking while you are still cancer-free. If you continue to smoke much longer, you will be more prone to developing cancer, emphysema, and many other chronic conditions. Use virgin organic coconut oil on your skin when you are tanning rather than the chemical lotions they sell in stores, it will nourish your skin and provide some protection from the rays of the sun. Eat whole foods that do not come from a package or a fast food restaurant, but that are harvested from Mother Nature.

If you make these choices, you will gain more energy. You will notice that you no longer have bad breath so often, or maybe not ever. This will eliminate your dependency on chewing gum. You will develop a more positive outlook on life. This is your moment to wake up and experience nature's highs, rather than the synthetic chemical lows you have grown so accustomed to.

THE CONFUSION OF THE STANDARD AMERICAN GUY

These days, it seems that everywhere I go, I see the same cycle of defeat involving toxic ingestion. Many of my closest friends with whom I grew up are spiraling through this cycle. They drink alcohol daily, they use cocaine, they smoke cigarettes, and they regularly indulge in fast food. Their diets are meat – and dairy-heavy, fat-rich, fried, sugary, salty, gluten-thick, and sickness-inducing. As the years go by, and I continue to make things happen for myself, it saddens me to see them stuck in the same place each time I come back around to visit. I'll stop by in the afternoon and they will be just waking, feeling awful after a night of poisoning that they refer to as "partying." The first thing a majority of them do is smoke a cigarette. Then they follow that up by eating some other type of garbage food lacking true nutrition. How defeating is that?

I have friends who were amazing athletes and have let it go for alcoholism, gang violence, and drug abuse. I have friends who have huge hearts and have always been great people, who are in prison, struggling to live, or who are no longer living due to this dangerous cycle that confuses nature all the way down to the mitochondria and genes of the human cell. This pattern is becoming commonplace among young adults all around the world. Many people let their lives go while chasing "highs" and escaping from reality into a façade of replicating commercialism and the lie of celebrity culture. Then they wake up when they are fifty and realize they have nothing to show for all of the years they have been alive. They have become a waste product of a toxic culture.

I was convinced to go into a restaurant/bar in Chicago one evening, although I very much dislike any environment where alcohol is served. I do not eat the food or drink the water in most food establishments. There was live music playing, which was nice. The girl who was with me dragged me into going because her friend worked there. We sat down and she ordered a plate of fried chemicals in the form of some sort of cheese stick, to go along with an alcoholic cocktail. I sat and tried to enjoy the music, feeling satiated from the raw food I had eaten earlier that evening. There I sat, as she ate this cheese stick that is the product of the sickly dairy industry, which kills baby cows and sells their flesh as "veal," while taking the mother's milk and selling it as food for humans. Does she know? Would she care? Should I speak? Why was I there?

Sitting next to me was a sorry mistake for a man. He kept leaning towards us, while gluttonously drinking loads of mixed drinks. The old man was being entertained by the music and repeatedly shouting and applauding the musician. When the girl I was with left for the bathroom, he approached me and said, "What's wrong with you? Where is your drink? Where is your food?" I informed the man in a polite manner that I had already eaten. He then asked again, "Where is your drink?" I replied by telling him I choose not to poison my mind with chemicals and alcohol, and I like to enjoy life.

As the man stumbled off of his stool, almost fell over, and drooled on himself, while his eyes rolled into the back of his head, he grunted, "Be a man! You are a p---y! Be a man. You need to wake the 'f---' up and be a man." I kept my cool but I gave him a stern look and I said, "Well at least I will never be an ignorant old man who has no purpose in life. I would appreciate if you would not say another word to me." I then moved away from him and he shut his mouth.

Maybe something dawned on this man. Maybe he fell further into his drunken stupor. Maybe he forgot he had ever even spoken to me. The relevance of this situation is that he truly believes it is "manly" to drink alcohol. Many guys believe poor lifestyle choices are somehow masculine and this is why they continue to live their lives with poor health. I cannot count how many times I have listened to fat guys and degenerates insist that they eat meat or hunt animals for the reason, as they say: "Because I am a man."

"Of all the creatures, man is the most detestable. Of the entire brood, he is the only one that possesses malice. He is the only creature that inflicts pain for sport, knowing it to be pain. The fact that man knows right from wrong proves his intellectual superiority to the other creatures; but the fact that he can do wrong proves his moral inferiority to any creature that cannot." – Mark Twain

Guys fight because they believe it proves they are masculine and therefore boosts their "manliness." Guys become womanizers and believe they are "manly" when they break a girl's heart. In college, and at parties, and even in bars, many guys binge drink until they black out and wake up in places they never should have been, often times in jail. Data released by the *Substance Abuse and Mental Health Services Administration* in 2011, reported that nearly twenty-five percent of the 137,000 Americans surveyed, participate in binge drinking. What bothers me most about this is that the behavior is so widely accepted in our society. Even before the legal drinking age of twenty-one, it is common for parents and some police officers to be more lenient with kids, allowing them to drink alcohol as minors once they enter college. Then the kids fail out after their freshman year. College for many has become an entrance way to a lifetime of alcoholism, poor eating, and lousy values.

The whole cultural aspect of being a man has damaged the qualities of many men and taken away from the content of their characters in immoral and shameful ways. Guys today believe it is "manly" to eat meat. They believe it is not "manly" to cry or have feelings. They think "men" are the dominant gender and therefore, feel it is okay to control their women or to abuse them. They think "men" have to prove their "manliness" by belittling others, by insulting others, or by fighting and bullying others. This is their way of boosting their egos. In reality all it is doing is showcasing their insecurities and desperation for approval. They believe having money defines success and therefore makes them manlier. Two of the most insulting things I have ever heard are the comments, "Be a man, eat meat," or "Be a man, do a shot."

To me, the least masculine, least man-worthy thing anyone could do is hide behind a false and phony image of this "man" they dream of becoming, as they mask their pain with alcohol, and indulge in the dead flesh of poor innocent animals, all the while trying to act superior to anyone and everyone standing outside of their circle of friends, which most often consists of other lost, shadows of men.

"Every man is born an original, but sadly, most men die copies." – Abraham Lincoln

We have our values as "men" inverted. We think a nice car will drive us into manhood. We wallow in the idea that a nice home will comfort us as men. We think fancy dinners will nourish our manliness. We believe controlling women will gain us superiority as the "dominant" gender. What we do not realize is that we are driving these nice cars for the wrong reasons. We are letting our egos create our destinations, and so our journeys we take never find their ending points. We fail to see that while we have homes, they often consist of broken families, heartless holidays, negative energy, and no love. We are teaching our children all of the wrong ways to live because they learn from our actions not from our words. These fancy dinners we indulge in clog our arteries, rob our health, and diminish our spirits. We are served plates full of dead matter, and by consuming the remnants, we fill ourselves with dead energy, our cells become weak, and we fall into sluggishness and despair. These toxic foods cause impotence, which is then "cured" by use of erection pills, but is really a sign of cardiovascular disease. We do not realize that while we use the women in our lives to get us by, get us off, or show off as "trophy wives," we not only break their hearts, but we cast shadows of emptiness over their entire worlds while building our reputations at the expense of their happiness.

I have heard stories of guys who pick up old ATM teller receipts that show someone else's remaining, and impressive account balance, and keep them in their pockets until they meet a girl. Then they pretend that is the only paper they have in their pocket, using it to write their phone number on for the lady. When she sees the account balance, she calls thinking she has found this "successful" guy. What a great first impression. What ever happened to meeting someone and being drawn to them for their character, or for their personality, or for the way they make you feel? Many of my female clients in Miami have shared stories with me of the times they have had men hand them fake business cards as a way to flatter them and deceive them into believing they are successful. This is pathetic.

"Life begins at the end of your comfort zone, so get used to being uncomfortable. It won't kill you." – Bill Tikos

Some guys are very confused as to what being a man is. It is not manly to cheat on your wife. It does not make you anywhere close to a man to control or abuse a woman. It is not manly to hide behind a phony caricature. It is not masculine to kill animals; it is not even "feminine," that would be an insult to the female gender. It is not manly to eat steak dinners every night and fill your bellies until you can barely walk. It is not manly to be "the fat guy" who wakes up one day and cannot even see his sex organ, because he let his stomach get so big from allowing the food industry to rid him of his manhood with chemical additives and processed foods. It is not manly to develop degenerative diseases because your ignorance denies you a positive lifestyle change. It does not make you a man to drink alcohol. Alcohol defeats any man you may have in you and reveals ugliness, weakness, insecurities, poor health, and depression. All of those extra shots you took to "drink the other guy under the table," well, you pay for that as the "man" you believe yourself to be degenerates into a decrepit, weakened spirit, with deteriorated organs, weak bones, and disease. Alcohol robs you of your B vitamins, leaches alkaline minerals from your bones, destroys your intestinal flora, and warps your mind. In addition, it is not manly to smoke cigarettes. Cigarettes will kill you. Cancer is not fun. Heart disease is not a thrilling ride. Prostate cancer is not joyous. Eating junk food, rich in animal cholesterol and saturated fat, that clogs your penile blood flow to the extent that you have to take *Viagra*, is not manly. It is foolish.

A great start to becoming a real man is finding your purpose in life. Life is not a spectator sport. You can sit and watch others achieve their dreams. You can watch from a bar counter while you tell stories about who you "used to be," and how you "could have" done this, or "could have" done that, but you will never do any of these things; you will never be that person again, until you decide to wake up and make it happen.

There are not many things that upset me more than seeing wasted potential. There is nothing that irks me more than wasted dreams that are trapped inside of bottle after bottle of alcohol, exhaled as cigarette smoke, blown away in lines of cocaine, swallowed up with pill after pill of

171

pharmaceutical chemicals, and buried with diseased bodies that have become over-intoxicated and flaccid with the poisons of meat, dairy, eggs, sugars, fats, flours, and processed foods saturated with fried oils and synthetic chemicals.

"The better way to approach people is to put your ego under theirs. Be willing to lower your status. Don't flaunt your stuff, instead, show your weakness and ask for help." – Joe Vitale

I think it is time for us to shift our human consciousness and start winning. We have been losers for far too long. Be a man today; don't act like a spoiled child. Be compassionate; don't try to boost your ego by belittling others. The best way to boost your ego is by boosting the egos of others around you. Be a real lover to your woman, don't make her life miserable. Be a real father to your children, they need you, and they learn from your actions far more than your words. Be there to encourage them, to teach them, to love them. Have a heart for animals. Like you, they breathe air, drink water, have families and feelings, enjoy playing with their young, and are alive. Put that drink down, it is robbing you of your life. Stop worrying about what your friends, other family members, colleagues, coworkers, "boys", or "homies" think of you.

Maybe the old man in the restaurant was right about one thing, I did need to wake up. I needed to realize that there are many more misinformed people like him, and I need to spread a message to them so they will also wake up. What I have realized, and what I hope the rest of us will soon understand, is that when you follow a calling in life, rather than following the footsteps of others, and when you follow the shadows of your own calling, you will find that you receive more respect than you ever have. Our reputations as men have been shattered by gluttony, lust, greed, ignorance, weakness, ego, poor diets, poor lifestyle decisions, insecurities, and giving in to commercialism and celebrity culture. Let's take our reputation back and help make the world a better place.

What does it mean to be victorious in life? How do we decide whether or not we are winning? Should victory in life last forever? If we are winning and getting further ahead, why is it that we watch so many people falling further behind?

On a team we cannot win unless each one of our teammates is with us one-hundred percent. This means we should start treating life as a sport and including everyone around us on our team. If one of our teammates is down, sick, or losing, we are also losing. We cannot ignore their condition.

The very best way for us to help unite our team and rally everyone together is to start eating real food. We need to break away from the chemical addictions that are bringing us down. I like to win, and my mission in life is to help all of my teammates so we can be triumphant in victory.

What are you doing to help today?

Chapter 7: WE ARE NOT WINNING

"Those who are unaware they are walking in darkness will never see the light."
– Bruce Lee, legendary martial artist

We keep thinking we are winning and getting ahead, when in reality we are falling further behind in terms of our health and the fabric of who we are. We are conditioned to believe that the way our society is commercially structured resembles the patterns we should live by. We go to school, eat the lunches we are fed, follow the food pyramid, leave for college to pursue a degree, abide by the laws that govern our society, and fashion ourselves by common expectations. Those who break this pattern are rejected and frowned upon. Meanwhile, many of those following the pattern are developing common diseases and living miserable lives lacking in satisfaction.

Defying the best interests of the citizens, the *Food and Drug Administration* (FDA) continues to approve foods that result in the consumer eventually needing treatment for some kind of illness. The *FDA* is the concierge service for the pharma industry. They control the exact amounts of chemical additives that are allowed into food products. The approved amount will not kill the consumer in one serving; rather, it will gradually sicken them so they rely on expensive drugs, procedures, and surgeries. As the profits continue to rise, the pharmaceutical industry creates more labels of diagnosis to create a demand for more high-priced medications. On the *World Health Organization* website there are over twelve-thousand disease categories listed and the number continues to get larger every year. The companies that compose the pharmaceutical industry pay their employees to study and research ways these diseases are induced and they formulate chemical drugs to "treat" them. This adds to the amount of sickness already present in people by way of the side effects of the very same chemical drugs. In addition, they have created drugs for the animal farming industry, and these negatively impact human health. Some of the same companies making these chemical drugs also make synthetic vitamins and synthetic chemicals used in the food supply. These chemicals induce sickness in humans as well.

Many of the pharmaceutical companies invest in the companies making the synthetic chemicals added to common brand packaged foods. Whether they know it or not, by putting their money behind these toxic foods, the pharmaceutical companies are creating a demand for pharmaceutical drugs to provide "relief" from the sickness the food chemicals cause. This sickness you may experience is your body trying to eliminate the toxins that are contained within those particular foods. Then, the drugs provide you with temporary relief, so you eat the same poison again, and your symptoms worsen over time. By following this cycle, you are creating toxemia, candida overload, and acidosis in your body. When you have toxemia, your body becomes the terrain for disease.

When your body is in this toxic, altered state from the food and chemical drugs, and you introduce other poisons, such as illicit drugs, cigarettes, alcohol, dysfunctional and damaging relationships, and anonymous sexual encounters, you weaken your immune system further and then you become prone to diseases such as HIV, cancers, liver disease, hepatitis, cardiovascular disease, and many other disease labels.

It has become a tradition in medical schools to teach students chemistry so they can prescribe chemicals for diseases. They learn about medical technology and how to perform surgery. But, what about the cures? As the American Medical Association rules over those teachings, many medical doctors are realizing the systematic failures of it all, and concluding that what they were taught about treating the diseases was not the answer.

"There is no money in healthy people and no money in dead people. The money is in the middle. People who are alive, sort of, but with one or more chronic conditions." – *Bill Maher, Forks Over Knives*

When you cure something, it does not come back. There is no profit in a cure, so the pharmaceutically-managed medical school infrastructure instills into their student's minds the absurd idea that chemical drugs and risky procedures are the only way.

What you eat and the lifestyle you live controls whether or not you will contract or develop most medically declared "terminal" illness. If you are to contract a terminal illness, you will most likely panic and then be given many lethal and toxic drugs to "treat" your symptoms in ways that may temporarily relieve you from your pains. In addition to this, you might continue to eat junk food, dead animal bits, and dairy, while never ceasing to have meaningless sex in empty relationships, smoke cigarettes, ingest illicit drugs, and indulge in large amounts of alcohol daily.

The good news is that you do not have to die. Most "terminal" illnesses are not deadly unless you allow them to be. Gain a little faith and strengthen your spirit. Start eating a plant-based diet. Clean your colon with hydrotherapy. Detoxify your body with chlorophyll-rich plant substances. Keep in mind that the health and vitality of your immune system relies solely on the health and vitality of your colon and internal organs.

By eating an organic diet consisting of green leafy vegetables; delicious ripe fruits; superfoods, and sprouts, and by drinking green juices and blended fruit and vegetable drinks, you will crave poisons much less, and begin to feel wholesome again. You will gradually cut-out alcohol and you will stop smoking cigarettes. In exchange, you will begin exercising and educating yourself on ways to better who you are and strengthen your character.

When you regain your spirit and restore your health, these deadly viruses and diseases will lose their attraction to you and gradually disappear from your life.

THERE IS NO PROFIT IN HEALTHY SENIORS

Of all age groups, the senior citizens should be the most furious. After working for the majority of their lives, many of them sadly develop degenerative and chronic diseases that diminish their chances at living long enough to see their social security and other retirement benefits. They are misled into believing routine doctor visits, medications, and discounts on nutrient-deficient foods are of benefit to them. In reality, all of these things benefit the financial institutions, the food industry, the government, the pharmaceutical, surgery, and insurance industries.

When people become ill after they have lived long enough to receive their social security, the hospitals have teamed up with the banks, so now rather than paying for their hospital bills, the banks will pay for them in return for the mortgage on their houses. This is known as a *reverse mortgage*. I pulled this quotation from a popular website of a company that provides reverse mortgages, *"In fact, many of the seniors we help use the proceeds of their reverse mortgage to pay for mounting medical expenses."* Now they have nothing left to leave their children and grandchildren for inheritance. Everything they own becomes the bank's property and medical industry profits. The bank then gives their portion to the pharmaceutical companies to cover the medical expenses, and the house becomes bank property. These banks and hospitals get away with robbery and extortion. If you are a senior citizen and you have medical conditions, you may want to consider radically changing your diet. This will help you to avoid the medical dilemma and you will not be trapped or conned into the reverse mortgage program.

Many seniors are pitied and receive special favors to coax them to surrender into accepting that they are old. They give in by using excuses like, "Oh, I'm getting old." This is the worst attitude to carry with you later in life. There are plenty of people in this world who abide by a raw vegan diet, are in their sixties and seventies, and are looking quite youthful. I guarantee they would never accept senior discounts or go to meetings for seniors on "senior health." They are among some of the healthiest, happiest, and most loving people.

"The average life expectancy of a meat eater is sixty-three. I am on the verge of eighty-five and still work hard as ever. I have lived quite long enough and I am trying to die, but I simply cannot do it. A single beefsteak would finish me; but I cannot get myself to swallow it. I am oppressed with a dread of living forever. That is the only disadvantage of vegetarianism." – George Bernard Shaw

176

When I think of aging, I do not think of disease, sickness, walkers, wheelchairs, handicapped parking, and fifteen percent off at local diners that serve horrible food laced with chemicals. When I think of aging, I do not think of wrinkles on my body, developing Alzheimer's disease or arrangements for my funeral. When I think of aging, I think of maturing, of finding more ways to love myself, and of ways to share this love with the world. I think of Mimi Kirk's beautiful smile, Karyn Calabrese's dazzling appearance, Storm Talifero's extreme level of fitness, and Charlotte Gerson's brilliant mind. Aging makes me think of life in its most pure state.

If you want some inspiration, do a YouTube search for Annette Larkins. Annette is seventy years old, and could easily pass for forty. She eats an organic raw vegan diet, has her own garden, and exercises daily. Her DVD *Annette's Raw Kitchen* will motivate you to eat the way she does. I am confident she will not fall victim to any of the degenerative diseases and chronic conditions so many others her age are afflicted with.

By following a clean, plant-based diet, when we get old, we mature and solidify our character; we grow wiser, not become forgetful; we remain strong and active, not lay there helpless and sedentary. When we progress with age, we should do exactly that, progress. A majority of our civilization is doing it backwards. We are regressing with each year and watching helplessly from behind the scenes as our bodies degenerate, our skin sags, our vision blurs, our hearing fades, and our hearts falter. We have accepted this twisted fate that has been placed on our population by greed and the lust for profit.

If you are a senior, you must realize that this is your life. Each mammal in the animal kingdom is created to live to be seven times the age they are when they reach full maturity. As humans, we mature around twenty-four years of age. This reveals something that many of us fail to notice. We are created to live beyond one-hundred years. Much of the population settles for less than half of that. If you are a senior, you must take back the other half of your life. You cannot do this by lying around helplessly while you are sedated with medications, swindled by your medical doctors into believing you suddenly developed a genetically predisposed disease that you cannot do anything about, and yearning for pity everywhere you go while catering to the disease process that you believe has been set as your path.

It is time to take back your health and the only way to do this is by weaning yourself from chemical drugs and pills, while increasing your intake of raw organic fruits, vegetables, seeds, sprouts, and sea plants. These foods will add years to your life and give you vitality, causing your skin to glow, your eyes to brighten, and your energy levels to soar. You must eliminate all meat, dairy, eggs, flour, sugar, bottled oils, gluten grains, synthetic chemicals, acrylamides, glycotoxins, MSG, caffeine, alcohol, and nicotine from your diet. These deleterious foods, toxins, and lifestyle choices are a burden on your health, they are the cause of nearly all sickness and disease, and they are the reason why you have aged prematurely. You have to incorporate more live enzymes in your diet by eating raw fruits and raw vegetables. You must start drinking real water. You must taste life in its pure form and drink from the fountain of youth and wisdom.

I have a problem with the way we have been treated by the pharmaceutical industry. I have grown weary of watching people give in to misinformation, to not question authority, to ingest toxic foods and drugs, and to suffer unnecessary deaths. I have a problem with the way we treat those people who have nutritional deficiencies that have caused them to develop mental illness.

I have read hundreds of testimonials revealing that the vast majority of mental illnesses can be reversed. The ways of the past, where we lock the mentally ill in hospitals and asylums, obviously did not work. Today we need to change the way we mishandle these brilliant minds. We must reconceptualize our ideas about what mental illness is. We need to provide the mentally challenged who are institutionalized with real foods and take them off of these sickness pills we call sedatives.

We need to grant them their right to live and give them the elixir to their problems. That elixir is raw organic, plant-based foods, free of toxins, combined with intellectual stimulation, art therapy, physical activity, and fresh, lively, and engaging surroundings. Sedating them with chemical drugs while locking them in toxic rooms filled with artificial light should not be an option.

THE HOARDING OF THE MENTALLY CHALLENGED

The *National Alliance on Mental Illness* (NAMI) defines mental illness as any medical condition that disrupts a person's thinking, feeling, mood, ability to relate to others, and daily functioning. Serious mental illnesses include major depression, schizophrenia, bipolar disorder, obsessive compulsive disorder (OCD), panic disorder, post traumatic stress disorder (PTSD), and borderline personality disorder and other labels. The *National Institute of Mental Health* reports that one in four adults (around fifty-eight million Americans) experience a mental health disorder in a given year. According to the *US Agency for Healthcare Research and Quality*, treatment for mental disorders in children made up the bulk of the money spent on them for healthcare in 2006, equaling $8.9 billion. Psychiatric prescriptions for children have increased by fifty percent from 1996 to 2006, and adult use has risen seventy-three percent in the same stretch of years.

Often, when someone is labeled mentally ill, whether they have a mental illness, mental retardation, or autism, they are said to be disabled and require special attention for the remainder of their life. They frequently follow the same daily schedule and they do not get a chance to experience many of the joys of life. The *World Health Organization* has reported that four of the ten leading causes of disability in the US and other developed countries are mental disorders. What they are not reporting is that a big part of mental illness is not a disability, but rather, a nutritional deficiency combined with toxemia.

According to a review titled, *Nutritional Therapies for Mental Disorders*, published in Volume seven of the 2008 *Nutrition Journal*, "*The most common nutritional deficiencies seen in mental disorder patients are of omega-3 fatty acids, B vitamins, minerals, and amino acids that are precursors to neurotransmitters. For treating depression, the amino acids tryptophan, tyrosine, phenylalanine, and methionine are often helpful.*

Bi-polar patients tend to have excess acetylcholine receptors, which is a major cause of depression and mania. These patients also produce elevated levels of vanadium, which causes mania, depression, and melancholy. However, vitamin C has been shown to protect the body from the damage caused by excess vanadium. A double-blind, placebo controlled study that involved controlling elevated vanadium levels showed that a single 3 g dose of vitamin C decreases manic symptoms in comparison to placebo. Taurine is an amino acid made in the liver from cysteine that is known to play a role in the brain by eliciting a calming effect. A deficiency of this amino acid may increase a bipolar patient's manic episodes. In addition, eighty percent of bipolar sufferers have some vitamin B deficiencies (often accompanied by anemia).

In regards to schizophrenia, the most consistent correlation found in one study that involved the ecological analysis of schizophrenia and diet concluded that increased consumption of refined sugar results in an overall decreased state of mind for schizophrenic patients, as measured by both the number of days spent in the hospital and poor social functioning."

This report tells us that many of these mental illnesses are caused by insufficient amounts of several nutrients in our diet. By eating a well balanced plant-based diet, you easily provide your body with these nutrients, and as a result, the mental illness often decreases or fades away. This is most likely because many plants contain human neurotransmitters such as serotonin, dopamine, and melatonin, and a plant-based diet improves nutrient absorption.

In a September 2011 issue of the Journal *PLoS One, a study of 3,040 adolescents aged eleven to eighteen found that those who had poor diets filled with junk and processed foods were more likely to suffer mental health problems such as depression and anxiety.* The study suggests that eating plenty of fruits and vegetables could help protect teenagers from developing mental illness.

Intestinal toxemia, or bowel toxemia, has been linked to mental imbalances as well. Ammonia, phenol, and histamine, are each bowel toxins. When too many of these toxins accumulate in the body, symptoms of mental illness begin to occur and they gradually get worse, regressing into severe mental disorders. At an AMA conference held in 1917, two doctors, Dr. Satterlee and Dr. Eldridge, presented 518 cases of mental illness they had successfully cured by removing the intestinal toxemia from the patients. Many animal products and chemical drugs contain an abundance of these bowel toxins. Ammonia is produced by humans during animal protein metabolism. By fasting, refusing chemical drugs, shifting to a plant-based diet, and eliminating all animal products, the bowel toxins are flushed from the body and the mental symptoms are likely to vanish.

In his 1996 book, *Fasting as a Way of Life*, Dr. Allen Cott documents having success in curing a high percentage of schizophrenics by implementing water fasting. After the symptoms went away, when the patients again began to eat flesh foods and a high protein diet, they relapsed and the symptoms came back. He then had them remove animal products from the diet, and the schizophrenia again faded.

In the 1972 book, *Nutrition and Your Mind*, Dr. George Watson explains how it is possible to restore proper energy function to the brain by rebalancing cellular oxidation. In order to do this, he provides an adequate supply of nutrients to his patients. A diet of plant-based foods balances the body and therefore restores efficient brain metabolism. Once the energy function of the brain is restored, the mental illness fades away.

Dr. Gabriel Cousens more recently went into depth in his book, *Conscious Eating*, about the biochemistry of brain function. He states, *"Because our brain needs more glucose than any other body organ to function efficiently, our mental state is impacted when our glucose metabolism is thrown off. Our metabolic cycles create energy and they are driven by glucose, which is transformed by the action of enzymes and metabolites."*

In these energy production cycles, enzymes break down sugars, and niacin assists the break down of these sugars into glucose. When we are deficient in niacin, it throws off our glucose metabolism and slows down brain activity.

Mental illness is not a genetic predisposition. It is not an incurable condition. It is a nutritional issue that occurs when we lack a balance of vitamins, minerals, and other important nutrients in our body, and chances of it occurring increase on a junk food diet and substance abuse.

Niacin and tryptophan are essential nutrients for restoring brain function. The 2009 documentary, *Food Matters*, explains how niacin (vitamin B3) can diminish mental illnesses such as schizophrenia and depression. Dr. Andrew Saul explains this concept in the film.

Niacin is needed for the metabolism of tryptophan in the body. Depression and other mental disorders can result from a brain tryptophan imbalance. The role of tryptophan cannot be replaced. This is why Prozac does not always work. Prozac stops the enzymes that break down serotonin, and when more serotonin is present, all nerves function normally, but serotonin is only a by-product of tryptophan. By ingesting foods rich in tryptophan, one will no longer need to take Prozac pills, which have serious side effects.

Hemp seeds, raw nuts (almonds, pecans, brazil nuts, and pistachios), raw seeds (sunflower, poppy, pumpkin, and sesame), lentils, split peas, kelp, and beans (lima, navy, red kidney, pinto and black) are great sources for tryptophan.

Processed foods, refined foods, smoking, alcohol consumption, and synthetic chemical drugs can all contribute to a niacin deficiency. This inhibits the metabolism of tryptophan in the body.

For anyone with a mental illness who is looking to avoid psychotropic drugs that could lead to suicide and misery, I would suggest eating foods high in niacin and tryptophan to regulate the metabolic cycle which creates energy for optimal and efficient brain function. I also advise adhering to a low-fat, plant-based, raw vegan diet rich in raw fruits and vegetables.

To assure proper absorption of these nutrients, it is also important to cleanse internally. You will learn more about internal cleansing in Chapter 12.

ASPARTAME AND THE CREDIBILITY OF THE FDA

In his book, *Sweet Deception*, Dr. Joseph Mercola explains the story of how aspartame was approved for human consumption. The FDA was not always corrupt. The corruption began during the attempt for approval of aspartame back in 1981. After numerous attempts to get approval for the chemical in almost all diet sodas, they abused their power to make it happen.

Mercola explains that, *"The chemical manufacturer, GD Searle, hired Donald Rumsfeld, yes, the former Secretary of Defense under George W. Bush, to be their CEO. Rumsfeld had ties to Ronald Reagan and so the very first thing Reagan did was issue an executive order to limit the power of the FDA commissioner, so he could no longer unilaterally prevent aspartame from being approved. Following his limiting of power, they replaced him one month later with a man named Arthur Hull Hayes. Hayes became the President's and GD Searles' pawn and did anything they asked of him to get paid.*

Soon after, they had yet another vote for approval. With a panel of five, they still did not approve of aspartame because all of the testing revealed a direct link to epilepsy, brain seizures, brain tumors, and even death in monkeys. Because they still were unable to get approval, they hired a sixth panel member and informed him prior to his hiring that he would get the position only if he agreed to approve. With a three-three tie, the final say went to Hayes, who approved happily and became a very rich man."

Thereafter, the FDA protected the profits of the pharmaceutical industry rather than the safety of our society.

The FDA is seen by many as a big scam. Why food is even classified with drugs and why they are merged under one administration is a question I would love to receive an answer for. Could it be because they feed us poor quality foods to get us sick so we will buy their drugs that simply mask the problem? This is the cycle that our world revolves around.

FLUORIDE AND THE ULTERIOR MOTIVES OF THE ADA

There is a chapter in Dr. Russell Blaylock's book, *Nutrition Secrets That Will Save Your Life*, which explains in detail how the intentional poisoning of drinking water through fluoridation took place. I summarized Dr. Blaylock's explanation: *"It was Alcoa, the aluminum company that was spending millions of dollars a year to safely dispose of fluoride. Because of this, they convinced dentists – Dr. Gerald Cox in particular – to promote fluoride for the prevention of tooth decay. Dr. Cox worked for the Mellon institute, and Andrew Mellon happened to be the owner of both the Mellon Institute and Alcoa – as well as the US treasury Secretary. Shortly after, they hired an attorney by the name of Oscar Ewing and within a few months, Ewing became* the head of the Federal Security Administration (FSA). Both the Treasury and the FSA were in charge of the US Public Health Services and when they promoted fluoride this time, they hired Edward Bernays (the same guy who made cigarettes seem like a symbol of independence for women) to do their public relations.

After they found a way to channel their left over toxic waste into our water supply, they started discovering that the areas with less fluoride had less tooth decay. When dentists spoke out against this, they were quickly revoked of their ADA memberships. Their grant money was also taken away. This is how our country works. Everything revolves around profits. Alcoa saved millions a year for safe removal of fluoride, dentists made money on deadly fluoride treatments, and doctors and pharma continue to make money from the results of our exposure to the toxic chemical."

A reverse osmosis filter needs to be replaced every few months because of damage from fluoride. Imagine, then, what it is doing to the filters in our bodies (kidneys, liver, lymph system, etc). We cannot take those out and replace them every few months.

A story that had an impact on me, involving fluoride, was about the mayor of Sacramento, CA. Mayor Golding voted for the fluoridation of the city's water, and when she was asked why, she responded, *"I don't have to worry about fluoride toxicity because I have a reverse osmosis filter."* Well, how many other people in Sacramento are fortunate enough to afford the luxury of a reverse osmosis filtering system?

WHERE ARE THESE DONATIONS REALLY GOING?

According to a report in the *Scientific American* in 2011, *the US budget sets aside $29 billion for spending on Health and Human Services and another $28 billion on the National Institutes of Health.* It has also been determined that over $100 billion is spent annually on medical research.

A concern of mine is where all of the so-called research money is going from these different foundations that collect various donations. We have spent billions of dollars on this so called research; all the while the cures to these degenerative conditions have existed since long before the diseases developed. Fifty years into cancer research funding and billions of dollars later, the result is more and more food additives, more disease, and nearly four times the amount of deaths per year from cancer as there were before the funding began.

We can no longer trust these foundations. They have been hiding the cures from us for many years, while our donations continue to be spent on developing more harmful drugs. We are being manipulated by the crooks and crime syndicates that make executive decisions in the pharmaceutical industry and formulate legislation and government standards. I would never donate to one of these *causes*, however, I always welcome with open arms any person who comes to me to help them change their life for the better. I will never turn away any client, no matter what their financial situation, as long as they are serious about changing their life.

If anyone is looking for a charity to make a donation to, where you know the money will go to good use, contribute to **Kindness Trust** (kindnesstrust.com), **EarthSave** (earthsave.org), **Earth Island Institute** (earthisland.org), **Sea Shepherd** (seashepherd.org), **Earth First** (earthfirst.org), or the **Natural Resources Defense Council** (nrdc.org). The money will be of much better use than it would be if donated to medical research foundations. All of the time that has passed, all of the money that has gone to waste, and the millions of deaths yearly, have proven that these disease foundations are not putting that money to good use. By investing in preserving the trees and plants that produce the fruits which contain the natural medicines we need, we can help to erase sickness and infuse health.

John Robbins founded **EarthSave** in 1988. He also wrote **The Food Revolution, The New Good Life**, and several other books. Their mission is to educate and teach people how to make healthy food choices. They developed a thirty day **Meals for Health** intervention program which helps low-income participants reduce their health care costs, and puts them on a path of wellness and recovery, using a low-fat, plant-based diet. If we can spread this to everyone in the country, we can all contribute to saving this country from the dangers of the "healthcare" system. The philosophy for the **EarthSave** program is, *"May all be fed, may all be healed, may all be loved."*

THEY WANT OUR PETS TOO

Many of the largest toxic food manufacturers in the world also sell pet food. They take all of the left over by-products from the unhealthful foods they create and turn them into the food products marketed for our pets. This is why our pets are suddenly developing the same diseases as humans. This is not simply a part of evolution. Our pets are being poisoned just as we are, through toxic foods that induce illness.

There is no reason why a dog or a cat should have diabetes or heart disease. The reason why they are developing these diseases is because the chemicals we feed them for food are deficient in enzymes and lack quality nutrients. Dogs are omnivores (some can be vegan) and cats are true carnivores. They should be eating other animals and food from nature. They should not be eating human food. When these pets do not get their sufficient enzymes, just like humans, they develop disease and die.

If you really care about your pet, do not feed it the chemical foods they sell in most pet stores. Buy them organic raw food with its natural enzymes. Do not poison them with chemical foods. *Green Earth Pet Foods* (greenearthpetfood.com), *Paw Naturaw* (pawnaturaw.com), and *Pawgevity* (pawgevity.com) each offer frozen raw organic dog and cat food varieties, while Natural Balance, Newman's Own, and Organix offer organic options for pets.

OUR IGNORANCE IS DESTROYING US

Ignorance comes in the form of cigarettes being smoked, pharmaceutical drugs being ingested, drugs and alcohol being abused, vaccines being administered, processed and fast foods being eaten, toxic chemicals being added to our foods, and poisons being used to "clean" surfaces. Ninety percent of people still do not see what is happening, and nothing is being done about it.

The attitude we carry in life is reflective of the foods we eat. I observe people with poor attitudes who are angry in general, and when I see what they are eating, I realize why they express such negative attitudes. They stuff their faces with processed meats, all kinds of contaminated dairy products, poisonous eggs, and refined sugary sweets, then drink it down with sugary coffee drinks, contaminated with fluoride and harmful food additives. These are the ignorant people who choose to ignore what is happening right in front of their eyes.

"I'm gonna die anyways."

When I make decisions regarding my health, I think to myself, *"I still have at least another hundred years to live, do I really want to suffer through those years and possibly shorten them, or should I simply avoid eating and ingesting poor quality foods and beverages?"* What are the thoughts going through your head when you make decisions regarding your health?

THAT DEADLY DRINK OF ALCOHOL

Alcohol is one of the most dangerous substances to abuse. Alcoholism is a common societal problem. America alone has created nearly twenty million chronic alcoholics. This resembles the interconnection between mental and physical needs. In most situations, a shallow ego or low self esteem are characteristic of those who over-indulge in alcohol.

Alcohol destroys important nutrients, leading to vitamin deficiencies and mineral imbalances. The brain of an alcoholic becomes dehydrated and functionally impaired. Alcohol slows down reflex actions, perception, judgment and speech. The *Journal of the American Dietetic Association* published a study in February of 2011 which concluded that, *a dietary pattern with lower fruit and vegetable intakes in women, and a pattern characterized by higher consumption of red meat and alcohol in both sexes, were associated with an increased risk of acute myocardial infarction, and adverse cardiovascular risk profiles.* These findings highlight the importance of sustained recommendations for fruit and vegetable intake, and cautious guidance on consumption of alcoholic beverages.

Because alcohol alters blood sugar levels, most alcoholics crave sugars. The plain white sugar they sell in grocery stores is similar to the sugar found in alcohol. What happens after excessive alcohol consumption is that your blood sugar levels become dependent on your intake of alcohol.

When alcoholics abstain from alcohol, they tend to crave sweets and carbohydrates. They eat poor quality foods full of refined sugars because the grain and sugar ferment in the digestive tract after eating. This satisfies the craving. To relieve alcohol cravings and fulfill your craving for sweets, you can eat moderately sweet fruits, like berries. Grab a handful of organic blueberries, strawberries, or raspberries. Drinking Kombucha may also be helpful.

Dr. Charles Lieber, a professor of medicine and pathology at Mount Sinai School of Medicine in Bronx, NY, wrote an article published by the **National Institute of Alcohol Abuse and Alcoholism** in 2004. He writes that, *"Many alcoholics are malnourished, either because they ingest too little of essential nutrients (e.g., carbohydrates, proteins, minerals, and vitamins) or because alcohol and its metabolism prevent the body from properly absorbing, digesting, and using those nutrients. As a result, alcoholics frequently experience deficiencies in proteins and vitamins, particularly vitamin A, which may contribute to liver disease and other serious alcohol–related disorders. Furthermore, alcohol breakdown in the liver, both by the enzyme alcohol dehydrogenase, and by an enzyme system called the microsomal ethanol–oxidizing system (MEOS), generates toxic products such as acetaldehyde and highly reactive, and potentially damaging, oxygen–containing molecules. These products can interfere with the normal metabolism of other nutrients, particularly lipids, and contribute to liver cell damage. Nutritional approaches can help prevent or ameliorate alcoholic liver disease. For example, a complete balanced diet can compensate for general malnutrition. Administration of antioxidants (e.g., precursors of the endogenous antioxidant glutathione) can help the body eliminate reactive oxygen molecules and other reactive molecules generated from abnormal lipid breakdown. New agents currently are being studied as promising nutritional supplements for alcoholics with liver disease."*

In order to successfully stop drinking alcohol and overcome withdrawal symptoms, the body must be efficiently nourished and also cleansed of all stimulants. This includes caffeine, alcohol, nicotine, and sugars. This will shift the pH of the blood to a more alkaline state.

The alcoholic needs to be weaned from these sugars and other stimulants by eating a raw, plant-based diet. If you continue to add clarified sugars to your foods or eat foods containing these sugars, you will continue to damage your organs similar to how alcohol does damage.

The sugars and alcohols you are ingesting require some B vitamins to be metabolized. Because of this, foods containing B vitamins should be added to your diet. Fresh juices will provide you with the vitamins you need. A good juice blend would consist of: celery, cucumber, leafy greens, and algae. Hemp seeds and chia seeds are also helpful. Cantaloupe is excellent for hangovers, as it restores some B Vitamins. The more greens you consume, the better your recovery will be from the effects of alcohol.

"Addiction is not getting enough of what you never should have had." – Deepak Chopra

As for addiction in general, an addiction is a desire for a substance that has no connection with the needs of the mind and body. To overcome addiction, it can be helpful to eat wild foods, such as various seaweeds, plants, and roots. To learn more about wild edibles, visit Sergei Boutenko's *Wild Edibles blog* (sergeiboutenko.com).

Your main goal should be creating alkalinity in your system. When you are in an acidic state, the effects of alcohol can give you a false alkaline high and fool your system into believing you have reached an alkaline state. By eliminating meat, eggs, dairy, and other harmful foods from your diet, you can clear up the acidosis in your body and help create a real alkaline state. In doing so, you will no longer crave stimulants.

SMOKE YOUR LAST BREATH AWAY

"If you are smoking cigarettes, your body reacts by secreting excess mucus in the lungs to protect them from the vile smoke. This emergency measure reduces vital lung capacity and slowly undermines the body's oxygen transport system, so that the smoker dies slowly by degrees." – Ann Wigmore, The Hippocrates Diet

I'd like to share with you an excerpt from the *Hearing on the Regulation of Tobacco Products House Committee on Energy* and *Commerce Subcommittee on Health and the Environment.* Rep. Henry Waxman opened the hearing with a statement that included this quotation: *"The truth is that cigarettes are the single most dangerous consumer product ever sold. Nearly a half million Americans die every year as a result of tobacco. This is an astounding, almost incomprehensible statistic. Imagine our nation's outrage if two fully loaded jumbo jets crashed each day, killing all aboard. Yet, that is the same number of Americans that cigarettes kill every twenty-four hours. Sadly, this deadly habit begins with our kids. Each day, three-thousand children will begin smoking. In many cases they become hooked quickly, and develop a life long addiction that is nearly impossible to break. For the past thirty years a series of surgeons general have issued comprehensive reports outlining the dangers these children will eventually face. Lung cancer, heart disease, emphysema, bladder cancer, and stroke are only some of the diseases caused by tobacco use. And now we know that kids will face a serious health threat even if they don't smoke. Environmental tobacco smoke is a Class A carcinogen, and it sickens more than one million kids every year. In fact, five former surgeons general of the United States testified before this subcommittee this year, that the most important legislation in disease prevention that we could enact would be restrictions on smoking in public places."*

The purpose of cigarettes, as they are still distributed today, is to preserve the profits of the tobacco manufacturers. They profit from our sickness. The *Centers for Disease Control and Prevention* reports 443,000 deaths annually from cigarette smoking. Based on current cigarette smoking patterns, an estimated twenty-five million Americans who are alive today will die prematurely from smoking-related illnesses. This includes five million people currently younger than eighteen years of age. The average adult smoker will die fourteen years earlier than the non-smoker, yet, they will most likely suffer from painful diseased conditions for many of the final years or months of their life, and it will likely drain their finances as it steals their life.

If you are a smoker, today is the perfect day for you to quit. This moment is as great as any for you to take advantage of the opportunity you have to end your dependence on nicotine and refrain from supporting the sickness cartels that are the tobacco and cancer industries.

IS IT REALLY THAT HARD TO QUIT?

Nicotine is highly acidic. It is also very similar in molecular structure to niacin and nicotinic acid. By shifting to a more alkaline diet and establishing an alkaline pH in our blood, we greatly reduce, or completely lose our desire for this stimulant. Nicotine triggers the same cell receptor site as B3 (niacin), and whenever one smokes, they deceive their body into thinking it is receiving B3 by triggering this receptor site. This results in a B3 deficiency.

One reason why people crave nicotine is because their bodies are craving B3. If you overload with foods that are rich in B3 (see chapter three), your cravings might fade. The reason why many crave cigarettes more when they are drinking alcohol is because alcohol wipes out intestinal flora and that flora is needed to synthesize some B vitamins. Now their body craves B3 more, and they smoke to fulfill that craving with nicotine rather than eating foods that contain niacin.

Without healthy flora and good bacteria, some B vitamins cannot be synthesized, and as a result, you are more likely to remain addicted to cigarettes. The best remedy then would be to quit drinking, eat foods rich in B vitamins, and be sure to take in some vegan probiotics to maintain healthy flora.

While some may disagree with the 12-step program for alcoholics, it does help some people. However, many have found that they are greatly helped by improving their nutrition and following a clean, low-fat vegan diet rich in raw fruits and vegetables, and free of gluten, processed sugars, bottled oils, and junk. Reducing fat intake can help the system manage sugars and nutrients, while also improving the elimination of cellular waste.

BEAUTY PRODUCTS

I literally laughed out loud the last time I was in a retail store. There was a section in the store labeled "Health and Beauty." Being curious, I went over and checked out some of these "beauty" products. As I expected, there was no beauty involved. Everything they sold was full of toxic chemicals. Even the items they referred to as "natural" were far from being natural. There is nothing beautiful about synthetic poison. There is nothing beautiful about misleading shoppers into believing they are buying something that will make them "beautiful," when in reality it will degrade health.

Many shampoos, lotions, and cosmetics contain harmful parabens. These are chemicals that are added as preservatives and that are known to cause cancer. A comprehensive study published in the January 2012 issue of the *Journal of Applied Toxicology* provides evidence of a correlation between parabens and incidence of breast cancer. Researchers measured the concentrations of five esters of parabens using human breast tissue collected from forty mastectomies for primary breast cancer in England between the years 2005-2008. They were astonished to find that *one or more parabens were present in ninety-nine percent of the tissue samples and all five parabens were found in sixty percent of the samples.* These parabens are found in cosmetic cream, make-up, lotion, hand soap, lip balm, deodorant, and a majority of other hair, skin, and other body products. They are also added to some food items at fast food restaurant chains. Parabens are absorbed into the skin and likely bind to the fat cells in the breasts. This could be a reason for the high prevalence of breast cancer.

If you want some good advice, try to avoid shopping at typical commercial retail chains such as Wal-Mart, Target, or K-Mart. Always be sure that the products you put on your skin or hair are free of parabens and sulfates. If you really need something to put on your skin, use organic virgin unrefined coconut oil. You can use it for your hair as a gel, your skin as a moisturizer, and even use it as a tanning lotion to help protect your skin from oxidation. If you do not like the smell of coconut oil, shop for truly natural, and organic products sold in some health stores, or simply create your own.

To preserve the health of your teeth, get some organic toothpaste, do not use the chemical name brands you are so used to purchasing or that your dentists have recommended. For your deodorant, do not use the typical name brands. Use the "Crystal" fragrance-free deodorant. All it consists of are mineral salts. You could also use organic essential oils.

When choosing body wash and shampoo, make sure you use organic. Do not put chemicals on your skin. Anything we put on our skin we also absorb through our skin and ends up in the tissues, blood, and lymph. Some organic products still add sulfates and parabens, so be sure to check the labels, even when going organic. A good way to be sure your products are safe is by accessing the website of the non-profit *Environmental Working Group* (ewg.org), and searching for their review of the product you are using.

Brigitte Mars wrote an excellent book titled, *Beauty by Nature*, which has recipes for making soaps, shampoos, and all types of beauty products at home. The best way to be beautiful at all times is to fuel with living energy from eating raw, plant-based foods.

DID YOU SCARE THE SUN AWAY?

"The sun is good for you and does NOT cause cancer. Skin cancer comes from the wrong diet, chemicals, and stress." – Jeff Primack, Conquering Any Disease

The sun can play a role in skin cancer, but not all skin cancer is caused by the sun, and much of it may be a mix of sun overexposure and toxic chemicals, bad food, and horrible nutrition. Many of us have been fearful of the sun since childhood because certain people have gotten us to believe it is harmful. While overexposure to the sun does damage the skin, having no sun exposure is not good either. A study on ultraviolet radiation exposure and cancer risk published in April 2012 in the *U.S. International Journal of Cancer* found that, *"People who were exposed to more sunlight had a significantly lower risk of developing many types of cancer. The study followed more than 450,000 white, non-Hispanic subjects aged fifty to seventy-one over the course of nine years and calculated ultraviolet radiation exposure with the incidence of a variety of different cancers. A total of 75,000 participants in the study contracted cancer and many cancers were found to be reduced in those who were exposed to more sunlight."*

A similar study published in the *Cancer Journal* in March 2002 found that exposure to the sun decreases cancer rates. This was determined after analyzing 506 different regions in Western Europe and North America and finding that there was an inverse relationship between cancer deaths and sun exposure. The less sun exposure the participants had, the greater there chances were of dying from cancer.

Without sunlight we become deficient in vitamin D. The ultraviolet rays of the sun penetrate the skin to synthesize vitamin D from the solar energy. The liver and kidneys then create a hormone known as *calcitriol,* and this hormone plays a role in the development and maintenance of cells. When deficient in vitamin D, cellular growth can become abnormal and cancerous. Knowing this, we see that the sun can be helpful. If you want to know what is truly harmful, it is the chemicals in suntan lotion and sunscreen, not the sun.

Toxicology studies conducted at the *Missouri University of Science and Technology* found that zinc oxide, which is common in most sunscreens, may react with sunlight and cause a chemical reaction that releases free radicals. The study suggests that the longer the zinc oxide is exposed to the sun, the greater the damage it will cause to human cells. Dr. Yinfa Ma, a lead researcher conducting the study, believes that, *"When zinc oxide particles absorb UV rays, the ensuing reaction releases electrons that in turn create the unstable cancer-causing free radicals. Those free radicals then bond with other molecules and behave like parasites that damage the other molecules."* This study was published in the journal *Toxicology and Applied Pharmacology* in 2012.

The *National Institute for Occupational Safety and Health* labeled titanium dioxide as a potential occupational carcinogen. This is another common ingredient found in sun protection products. Octyl methoxycinnamate (OMC) is found in close to ninety percent of sunscreen brands, and researchers found that this chemical undergoes biochemical changes that cause mutation and cell death upon exposure to sunlight. When you apply these products that contain harmful chemicals to your skin, you are placing more of a burden on your health than you would by getting a little sun exposure.

Anything you put on your skin is absorbed into your system. Would you eat sunscreen? I know I would not. I also do not use sunscreen. I love the sun. I love being on the beach. I use the same stuff I apply to my skin after a shower.

Other than shade and clothing, protection from overexposure to the sun can be provided by virgin organic unrefined coconut oil. It was a primitive practice of the Islanders on the Fiji Islands to cover their bodies with this oil. If you ever wonder why many tanning lotions smell like coconut it is because the lotion companies first retrieve the protective compounds from the coconut oil and add it to the lotion before they taint it with the chemicals.

I have used coconut oil on my skin for years on the beaches in South Florida and never once have I been "burned" by the sun. I am also sure to moderate the amount of time I spend in direct sunlight. It is not wise to lay in direct sunlight for long periods of time.

In addition to zinc oxide, titanium dioxide, and OMC, benzophenones are more chemicals added to sun protection products. They are added because they can protect against UV rays and appear on sunscreen labels as oxybenzone. A study published in the May 2012 edition of *Environmental Science and Technology* measured concentrations of five different variations of these chemicals in the urine of more than six-hundred women who were evaluated for endometriosis. According to WebMD, *"Endometriosis is a painful condition that occurs when tissue from the inside of the uterus grows outside of the uterus. When this tissue grows in other parts of the body, typically spilling into the abdomen around the ovaries or fallopian tubes, it behaves as if it were still in the uterus, thickening and shedding each month in sync with a woman's menstrual cycle. Endometriosis can lead to scarring and infertility."* The study found these benzophenones present in ninety-seven percent of the women and concluded that women with the highest amounts of benzophenone-1 in their urine had a sixty-five percent greater chance of having endometriosis compared to women with the lowest levels.

As reported by Ross Horne, in his book, *Cancerproof Your Body*, *"Skin cancer develops when the blood supply to the skin is obstructed by unhealthful dietary fats and cholesterol."* A diet rich in animal protein, fried or highly heated oils, clarified sugars, sodas or colas, cholesterol, synthetic chemicals, gluten, acrylamides, glycotoxins, and heterocyclic amines, all play roles in cancer development. These toxins are excreted through the skin and some food components clog the oil glands. The blood flow is then blocked and adequate nutrients cannot reach the skin.

In the August 2000 *Cancer Research* journal, a study was published declaring that, *"Omega-6 fats are stimulators of development and progression of a range of human cancers, including melanoma."* This study also pointed out that, *"Long chain omega-3 fats inhibit the development and progression of cancers."* This study should raise awareness that if we simply add omega-3 rich foods such as raw fruits, raw vegetables, purslane, hemp seeds, ground flax, and chia seeds to our diet, while removing deleterious foods that contain cooked oils and free radicals, we could drastically reduce our chances of ever developing skin cancer.

When you make poor dietary choices, and you block your skin with carcinogenic chemicals that make up the majority of the ingredients in suntan lotions and sunscreens, you are helping to lay the groundwork for cancer. Please, avoid spending money on more chemicals. Get a bottle of coconut oil and moderate the time you spend in the sun. Even wild animals know to limit their sun exposure, and will seek shade to prevent overexposure. Be smart about the amount of time you spend in the sun, and always be cautious of what you are eating, and how it has an impact on your overall health.

WHAT TYPE OF PERSON ARE YOU?

There seems to be two main groups of people. The first consists of those who are more likely to become sick and fall into the medical system's trap of chemically induced temporary treatments that disable and drastically impair the body's natural defenses. They may eventually die from a variety of diseases. They give their lives to the profits of the pharmaceutical industry.

The other group consists of those who are more healthful, have pride in taking care of themselves, are more likely to preserve their youth, and will appreciate the nature of the world. They will avoid harmful foods that steal their immunity and weaken their health. They are more likely to avoid medication. They will enjoy the foods from the plants of Earth, and in exchange, they will increase their vitality. They are more likely to be positive in character, to radiate health, and to have healthier relationships.

You decide for yourself which type of person you will be. Different levels of energy are what carry us and attract us to different types of people, and in certain situations more than others, you will be guided into somebody else's life as a teacher to show them the right way.

Education is vital to whether or not you will survive the medical infrastructure that our society is enslaved by. You must be educated on all of the different foods you are eating, sicknesses you are being falsely diagnosed with, chemicals and additives that are in our cleaning products, hair supplies and hygiene products, and even in the water you are drinking.

My passion lies in educating you on these topics.

LESSON THREE:

THE CYCLE OF DISEASE

I NEVER TRUSTED THE DOCTOR

Growing up, I never trusted the family doctor. I always felt a distorted energy being emitted from him. He never looked into my eyes when he spoke. He told me I would grow up to be six feet, five inches tall and he insisted that I was genetically perfect. Well, I never did argue the genetic perfection, but I am only six feet tall. His false prediction led me to place a false expectation on nature and always wonder when I would hit that growth spurt and grow another five inches.

As a child, I felt worse after seeing him and therefore I rarely went to the doctor. It was also rare for me to get sick. My brother and I only went in for routine "check-ups," or to get the required shots that were mandated by public schools. To our parents, and to us, this seemed like the right thing to do and we knew no other way. We were always taught to trust the doctor as the Supreme Being who knows all and has a superior education.

I remember being congested with mucus at times as a kid, mostly after eating particular foods, and at times I wished there were some kind of a device that would clear all of it out of my throat. I forced myself to cough until it would come out. I had no idea it was the food I was eating that caused this and I continually searched for reasons why I was afflicted with this condition. Aside from that, I lived a good childhood, outside of the city limits, with nature and cornfields all around me.

As a boy, I had the idea instilled in my mind that one day I would find the cure for cancer or for AIDS. I did not, however, have any interest in becoming a doctor or a scientist. These jobs did not at all seem like what they were hyped up to be. To be a doctor or a lawyer seemed like every child's dream in their quest to live up to the expectations their parents had placed on them. How boring would it be to suggest pills and drugs all day to people who are dying or sick, and watch their conditions gradually worsen over time? I wondered why the people who were always visiting doctors seemed to degenerate more with each visit. In my mind, I held onto the idea that a cure existed for every problem. I also thought it would be a very simple cure, a lot less complicated than what this medical industry, and what science, had made it out to be. Maybe I was onto something...

Looking back, I feel fortunate that I did not have those high expectations placed on me. I feel like the expectations many parents place on their children change the way nature intends for them to evolve through life. I was taught to follow my own path and I did so very well. My family did not have much money. We were never given the materialistic luxuries in life that many people indulge in. We were, however, given the luxury of nature and unconditional love.

I rarely watched cartoons because I did not like sitting in front of the television. I spent my days journeying through the woods, climbing trees, eating fresh fruits from our fruit trees, berry bushes and grape vines, and most of all, playing sports. My mother told me I was born with a ball in my hand. I would throw the football to myself. Play baseball in the backyard with my brother, and I would shoot hoops on a basketball court my father had constructed to surprise me some time around my fifth or sixth birthday. Even in the cold Chicago winter, I would be out there shooting hoops, as if I were Michael Jordan, trying to make the winning shots.

Maybe it was my relationship with nature that made me the passionate person I am today. Maybe it was the love from my parents. Maybe it was the great opportunity I had to have a brother who was only seventeen months older than I, with whom I could share these experiences, and who I knew I could trust at all times. Maybe it was the good meals my father would cook for us when he got home. Perhaps it was a combination of all of these things. Whatever it was, I am grateful for it today.

HEALING MISSION

"Before the two-legged and the creature-beings arrived on the planet, the Earth Mother decreed that there would be no illness or disease among the ones with physical bodies that could not be healed. The power of healing any illnesses was given to the plant people.

The creatures were given instinct so that they would know which plants were going to heal them when they felt unfit. The human tribe was told to watch the creature-teachers in order to learn from them. The human beings learned for a while, and then, in arrogance, they adopted the idea that they were superior to the other creatures.

The Earth Mother frowned, because the further away from the natural world her human children strayed, the more illness they brought upon themselves. Finally, they had infected all their relations. The Earth Mother cleansed the natural world by freezing all of the sickness and started over.

Those who survived had heard the mothers' voice and were willing to respect their plant and creature relations. To this day, the human tribe is still looking for the pieces of the lost healing knowledge held by the plant tribe. The Earth Mother and the Great Mystery have promised that those cures are still there, awaiting rediscovery. They have also promised to freeze the Earth again if we fail in our missions to heal that which we have made sick or if we fail to clean the parts of our world we have harmed."

— Jamie Sams, Excerpt from her book Earth Medicine

Chapter 8: WHAT IS SICKNESS?

"When diet is wrong, medicine is of no use, when diet is correct, medicine is of no need." – Ayurvedic Proverb

Sickness is a sign that your body is working to detoxify and naturally eliminate toxins. When we overload our bodies with exogenous toxins (toxins from sources outside of the body) such as chemical food additives and synthetic medicines, these obstructions have to be eliminated. Sickness often starts with a cold, fever, or flu, and when enervated through synthetic medicine and bad nutrition, the toxins accumulate and the sickness becomes bronchitis, pneumonia, nerve dysfunction, compromised organs, cancer, and many other degenerative and chronic diseases – which are disorders.

The problem that arises in many of us is that we fear we are worse than we really are when a little sickness sets in. We should be thankful for the fevers, colds, and various attacks of influenza we may experience throughout the years. When we have these symptoms this means our body is still able to function properly and is naturally working to eliminate toxins. We should let the body do its work and refrain from eating chemical drugs. Pills and other drugs only force the sickness further into our system, leading to other illnesses. They postpone what we really need – to live more healthfully.

"The person who takes medicine must recover twice, once from the disease and once from the medicine." – William Osler, M.D.

The common cold develops most often when we are consuming dairy, eggs, heated flours, bleached foods, gluten grains, or too many sugars. Both dairy products and sugars are mucus forming. While mucus is necessary and normal, the overload of mucus is what we call illness – which is really an immune response. When we produce excess amounts of mucus, the toxins that come in with the dairy and garbage foods, and the toxins that are by-products of metabolism, accumulate in the mucus. Because we cannot properly eliminate mucus through the normal processes that take place when there is a healthful amount of mucus, and we have no way to remove the toxins, we are forced to excrete the mucus through the nose or throat. This results in a common cold or sinus infection. Someone who does not consume animal products, and eats a clean, plant-based diet, will rarely ever come down with a cold. They minimally, if ever, get sick.

Quite often people make the mistake of buying pills or cough syrup to alleviate their common cold or infection. They go see medical doctors who prescribe antibiotics for viral infections. This may worsen the problem as the drugs may enervate, or restrict the viruses and toxins from leaving the body. The antibiotics destroy the healthy bacteria of the alimentary tract that were once nourishing our bodies and synthesizing B vitamins. Once these bacteria are destroyed, we no longer synthesize much of these vitamins and candida yeast may grow out of control from the sugars and acids that are roaming free in our bodies.

"Why would a patient swallow a poison because he is ill, or take that which would make a well man sick." – L.F. Kebler, M.D.

After the sickness has been enervated several times and the problems start to spiral out of control, this is when the body has become a breeding ground for disease to settle in.

THE CYCLE OF DISEASE

Disease develops from any of the following:

1. A lack of something, whether it is water, activity, healthful digestive processes, or nutrients.

2. An excess of something, whether it be toxins, mucus, animal products in the diet, or cooked food.

3. The accumulation of poisons from inorganic nutrients, chemicals, and other foreign substances.

4. The enervation of the natural elimination process by means of chemical drugs.

5. A weakened immune system.

With the many thousands of names that doctors and those in the medical world have come up with to define the rapidly growing number of diseases that have been developing and continue to develop, I find that each of these is not necessarily a disease, but rather a symptom. A majority of these can be eliminated through true healing. The growing number of diseases is not a natural part of evolution, instead they are systematic reactions. What this tells us is that we are doing something unnatural, which is leading to disease.

"Meat-eating is the disease. Dairy consumption is the illness. Eggs being added to the diet are the sickness. Cancer, diabetes, heart disease, osteoporosis, hypertension, high cholesterol, macular degeneration, arthritis, gout, influenza, viral and bacterial infections, hatred, lack of compassion, and premature aging are the symptoms. Today you can go symptom free and remove much of this sickness, illness, and disease from your life by transitioning to a plant-based, cruelty-free, vegan way of living." – Jesse J. Jacoby

The human body has natural defense mechanisms that are activated to their full potential, with full strength, only upon receiving full nourishment in the form of real foods. By eating real food, we boost our immune system and our body becomes a shield that repels sickness, disease, and ailments.

When we are lacking nutrients, our normal processes in the body are altered. We tend to become too acidic and certain organs have to take on more work where others may be lacking. This extra burden, which often involves all organs, then triggers the development of a number of diseases, or disorders.

When we have excessive amounts of toxins in the body from cooked and processed food and animal products, our blood, liver, and lymph become compromised. This makes the role of filtering our blood much more difficult for the kidneys. Our lymph system, which is the filter for our cells, becomes slothful. Our liver, then, has to work extra hard to remove the toxins, and can become overwhelmed.

While all cells and systems are involved in detox, the liver is often mentioned as the center of detoxification. When it is clogged with mucus, foreign substances, toxins, and fat, it cannot perform at its peak. Many people who develop disease have a fatty liver. The liver creates bile, which emulsifies the fats and stores this bile in the gall bladder.

When we have excess amounts of inorganic substances, synthetic chemicals, and foreign animal hormones in our body, they can accumulate into gall stones which enter the gall bladder with the bile. They infiltrate our gall bladder and when the gall bladder is full of stones, there is a lack of space for excess bile to be stored. Now the fatty liver problem persists and the fats keep our blood sugar levels high, so the candida yeast, which feeds on the sugars, can grow out-of-control.

In the *European Prospective Investigation into Cancer and Nutrition* (EPIC) study, published in a 2009 issue of the *Archives of Internal Medicine*, it was reported that, "*Patients who adhered to healthy dietary principles (high intake of fruits, vegetables, and whole-grains), never smoked, had a body mass index of less than thirty, and had at least thirty minutes per day of physical activity had a seventy-eight percent lower overall risk of developing a chronic disease. This included a ninety-three percent reduced risk of diabetes, an eighty-one percent lower risk of myocardial infarction, a fifty percent reduction in risk of stroke, and a thirty-six percent overall reduction in risk of cancer, compared with participants without these healthy factors.*"

"Medical practice has neither philosophy nor common sense to recommend it. In sickness the body is already loaded with impurities. By taking drug – medicines, more impurities are added, thereby the case is further embarrassed and harder to cure." – Elmer Lee, M.D., Past Vice President, Academy of Medicine

It is the quality of the condition of the internal environment that is the real disease. When we abuse our bodies with poor nutrition and damaging lifestyle choices, we develop what is known as toxemia. Often, acidosis occurs, and frequently, candida yeast overgrowth takes place. The symptoms we get, such as colds, fevers, and influenza, are known as sickness. When we enervate this sickness with medicine and poor quality foods, we develop disease. The occurrence of disease is not necessarily that complex. There are three notable conditions we create in our bodies that become root causes for disease. The three conditions are: toxemia, acidosis, and candida overgrowth. Viruses also lead to a variety of cancers, and bacteria overload is problematic as well.

The solution is to keep the body nourished with real food that is free of toxins. By keeping our internal environment clean, we reduce the chances of developing the conditions that lead to most chronic diseases. We will be more likely to experience health and happiness.

"While keeping up the miserable delusion that diseases are all to be cured by drugging, homeopathy has been unintentionally showing that they would very generally get well without any drugging at all." – Dr. Wendell Oliver Holmes

TOXEMIA

As mentioned, when our diet is lacking in nutrients and we overload our bodies with chemicals in the form of synthetic food additives, acrylamides, glycotoxins, alcohol, cigarettes, and drugs, we compromise our systems. This results in toxemia. The blood becomes sticky, and then accumulates other toxins. The undigested foods ferment and decay into terrain for harmful bacteria. All of this shifts the blood pH from being alkaline to a more acidic level.

Dr. Thomas Lodi, founder of *An Oasis of Healing* in Mesa, AZ, established his own understanding of toxemia. His theoretic perspective is that, *"Because the colon is five feet long and reabsorbs water, when we do not defecate up to five feet of waste daily, we retain a substance that is toxic in our system, being the feces. Then when the water is continually reabsorbed, the toxins are absorbed into the blood. Once they reach the blood, this becomes what is known as toxemia."*

It is the state of the blood that makes all disease possible. Disease comes from this toxemia, as well as insufficient enzymes, acidosis, excessive growth of candida, and a clogged detoxification system. To avoid toxemia we have to cleanse our bodies of the toxic accumulation of synthetic medicines, drugs, cigarette residues, alcohol, processed foods, meats, eggs, dairy, and sugars. We have to cleanse the molecules of these substances, in addition to completely avoiding the substances.

"The greatest part of all chronic disease is created by the suppression of acute disease by drug poisoning." – Henry Lindlahr, M.D.

ACIDOSIS

When we eat animal proteins, the body produces uric acid as a toxic by-product from the protein metabolism. When we drink sodas, our bodies become overwhelmed with phosphoric acid. When we drink coffee we create excess chlorogenic acid. When we eat sugary food, the acids that are produced in the body can grow out of control. Consuming dairy creates excess mucus and is acid forming. All of this compounds into what is known as acidosis.

Disease starts to develop in the body when acidosis is present. In a sense, acidosis is equivalent to inflammation. We always want to avoid this condition. To reverse acidosis, we have to eat more alkaline forming foods such as leafy green vegetables and algae, and eliminate the acid forming substances. We have to break away from acid forming habits like eating meat, clarified sugars, eggs, dairy, gluten grains, bleached foods, synthetic chemicals and fried oils; drinking alcohol and coffee; and smoking cigarettes.

CANDIDA OVERGROWTH

"Many people are unknowingly infected with Candida albicans. This fungus deoxygenates our cells and the yeast grows until it eventually invades organ tissues, such as the lungs and liver." – Dr. Brian Clement, LifeForce

Candida is yeast that naturally occurs in the body. When we eat excessive amounts of sugars with fatty foods, the sugars cannot be properly metabolized and may linger in the system. When this happens, our blood sugar levels rise and the candida yeast feeds on the sugars, eventually growing out of control. If we eliminate the fats and allow our blood sugar levels to drop, we will metabolize the sugars, and the candida will no longer have a source of nourishment, eventually atrophying.

This candida yeast thrives on the sugars from dairy. Because we cannot properly digest dairy, candida yeast grows while feeding on its sugars. The best way to solve this problem is to eliminate dairy from your diet. If you have excess mucus and dairy in your system and you are overweight, chances are you have candida overgrowth. To help alleviate this condition, you will need a stronger bacterium that will eat the sugars before the candida. Just like a strong fungus kills another strong fungus, strong bacteria will kill a strong bacterium. This is where acidophilus and lactobacilli come into play. These two bacterial cultures thrive on the sugars in milk and they are not harmful to your body. To overcome candida overgrowth, after eliminating all dairy, it is helpful to take a vegan probiotic supplement to erase the food source for the candida. I recommend the supplement known as *Green Vibrance.*

The medicinal mushrooms known as chaga, reishi, and cordyceps can be brewed into a tea. By drinking this tea, you assist with the atrophy of the candida. The bark of Pau D' Arco is also known to be a powerful negator of candida.

During this time, raw organic fruits can and should be eaten frequently. As long as you are not eating fatty foods, these sugars will not bind to the candida. The nourishment from the fruits will help to improve your condition. You should get adequate exposure to sunlight and refrain from drinking alcohol, smoking cigarettes, and consuming animal products.

POOR HEALTH DELIVERS A POSITIVE MESSAGE

When we develop disease or sickness, or if something goes wrong in our body, this is a strong indicator that we are too toxic and we need to change our ways. Many times, rather than listening to our bodies, we take drugs, and/or undergo surgeries, which only cover up the issues while the toxins that are triggering them continue accumulating.

When our tonsils become inflamed, this is our body alerting us that we need to cleanse the toxins. Rather than solving the problem, a person might undergo a tonsilectomy. Now the problem gets worse without us having any signals from within.

When we have appendicitis, we might choose to undergo an appendectomy. While it is important to be sure the appendix does not burst, because it can infect the brain or kill us if it does, other steps can be taken to alleviate appendicitis without the requirement of immediate removal of the organ.

When we get wrinkles, rather than cutting out foods that contain flours and removing refined sugars from our diet, we may choose cosmetic surgery.

We should always keep our organs, as they do a good job of warning us when our body is in danger. Once we remove certain organs we become more prone to sickness and disease. If our organs act up, we know we must cleanse internally and choose a more healthful diet.

LEVELS OF SICKNESS

Each disease reflects diet and the lifestyle decisions we make. The lifestyle decisions we make lead directly to the development of different diseases, and these diseases gradually worsen, starting from a simple cold. A cold can only be enervated so many times and may lead to influenza. Then, when influenza is enervated with chemical drugs, toxemia develops. Once you develop toxemia, you are prone to a variety of diseases. When you develop toxemia and acidosis, as well as candida overgrowth, this is when you are likely to develop more serious diseases. With the lifestyle choices you make, you ultimately decide whether or not you will develop acidosis, toxemia, an overgrowth of candida, and common diseases. By eating clean and pure, you significantly decrease your chances of developing these conditions.

By living the lifestyle of abusing drugs, indulging in random sex, excessively drinking alcohol, and smoking cigarettes, you become more prone to contracting transmittable diseases, developing cancer, and laying the ground work for heart disease.

When you resort to the lifestyle of eating meats, refined sugars, and processed foods, you become prone to heart disease, cancers, hypertension, diabetes, obesity, and a weakening of your overall vigor. When you frequently dine out at restaurants or eat at fast food chains, you put yourself at high risk for developing common chronic ailments.

If you like to be sick, continue following these paths. If you would like to change your life, use a different approach. Adapt to a plant-based lifestyle. You will likely become a more enlightened and rejuvenated person.

PASTEURIZATION AND THE RELATION TO GERMS SAID TO CAUSE DISEASE

While some still cling to the belief that germs cause all disease and that we need to eliminate these germs by spraying them with toxic chemicals, this is far from the truth. When we keep our internal environment clean, these germs have a more difficult time setting up shop in our systems. The chemical poisons that we are using to clean our counters and spray everything we come into contact with are contributing to our sickness by weakening our immune systems. The poisons also poison us, and lead to stronger germs.

I will never understand how one could spray poisonous chemicals on counter tops, tables, and kitchen sinks, and somehow think they are "cleaning" the surface. I'd like to ask, "How clean is poison?" How can you justify using these toxins with the notion that you are "just cleaning it?"

I would much rather prepare food on a counter that has been wiped off with water, vinegar, peroxide, or some type of a plant-based cleaner, than a counter that has been treated or coated with poisons. All of this time we have been misguided into believing that we have to kill germs, so we are taught to spray chemicals on surfaces in order to do so. Yet, the entire time, these chemicals contain the compounds which are hazardous to our health. We have been cheated into poisoning ourselves, partially because of an incomplete piece of work put together by a man named Louis Pasteur.

By reading Ron Garner's book, *Conscious Health,* I learned more about pasteurization and the relation to germs which are said to cause disease.

206

Garner writes: *"We can blame Louis Pasteur, the man who started the pasteurization process, for the foolish belief that germs & viruses from the outside are what cause disease. He stole and plagiarized the work of a man named Antoine Bechamp who studied in France at the same time as Pasteur.*

While Bechamp was getting to the idea that small organisms are responsible for disease from within, meaning putrefaction and excess mucus and feces trapped in the body, Pasteur just stole a piece of the idea, not yet complete, and announced that the small organisms being referred to only came from the outside. He did not mention that these organisms all lose their virulence once exposed to air.

While on his deathbed, Pasteur admitted that a human's natural immunity is far more important than germs in the matter of disease and explained his logic for this after an experiment with germ cultures. He attempted to grow his germ cultures on fresh fruit, and they failed to grow. He instead had to grow them on rotting soup."

Even after his claims were debunked by his own admittance, we are still forced to pasteurize, and destroy, beneficial nutrients and enzymes in all packaged foods, and most juices that are sold to the consumer. This contributes to much of the sickness we are plagued with.

Additionally, we now know that some germs and viruses lose their virulence once exposed to air. This may reveal to us that disease starts inside the toxic body, not from "germs" outside. I think it is about time to give these "germs" a break from being our scapegoat, behind the disguise of the true cause of disease, which is largely poor nutrition, unhealthful foods, eating animals, lack of exercise, and poor lifestyle choices.

EVOLUTION WAS NOT MEANT TO BE THIS WAY

The thought that comes to mind the most for me is how we have come to accept sickness as a part of life. How is it that we decided that some of us are meant to suffer painful deaths from these agonizing diseases that are largely avoidable? None of it makes sense to me. Do you really believe we were created to evolve into this civilization of weak, sickly, and diseased creatures who destroy the planet any chance we get, and torture and murder billions of innocent creatures we call "farm animals" for the sake of profit and greed? This is not evolution.

We have decided this fate for ourselves. Now we can choose whether or not we want to reshape the way we are evolving.

The reason why so many who develop disease are never able to overcome that disease is largely because they think they know too much. They do everything they are told by doctors, or they read a single book, and think they have discovered all of the answers.

This limited thinking also limits these people from truly recovering, and in many cases, their own ignorance is what kills them. Either they know too much, or they listen to the doctors who may be misinformed, closed-minded, or simply not qualified to truly help the patient overcome their illness.

If you are sick and you want to get better, you have to open up your mind. You have to break away from tradition and go after the cure. You cannot settle for allowing yourself to be handicapped, wounded, or sidelined by some type of condition or disease for the rest of your life – especially when it may be so simple to rid yourself from it.

Do yourself a favor and admit that you do not know it all. Do some of your own research. Read books and medical studies, and clean up your diet while getting daily exercise.

Chapter 9: THE PROBLEM WITH KNOW IT ALLS

"When a man's science exceeds his strength, he perishes by his ignorance." –
Oriental Proverb

A lot of people have too much pride in what truly is their ignorance. They defeat themselves and feed their weight problems, their health issues, and their poverty by defending their state of denial. When they are approached or presented with ways to solve their problems, they refuse to open their minds and instead answer with, "Oh, I know."

If they really knew, they would not be sick today. They would not be overweight. They would not be bullied around by a doctor whose plight makes them sicker and adds to their health problems. If they really knew, chances are they would not read one book with poor quality content and allow it to mislead them into believing it is the only way, then declaring they know everything about the subject matter. The key is finding those books that have broken away from traditionalism and have no ulterior motives of selling products, or finding the ones that have not been funded by one of the deceptive industries that control our economy. The key is to open your mind. The key is to break away from tradition.

"Often, the less there is to justify a traditional custom, the harder it is to get rid of it." – Mark Twain

If you have a chronic health issue, chances are that it has a relation to diet and unhealthful choices, such as lack of exercise, substance abuse, and relying on bad medicine. Much of the medical literature has been influenced by the pharmaceutical industry. What may be the "common and acceptable" ways of treating your condition may simply be the result of drug company business interests. You may find that what is best for you is most likely unrelated to these common and widely accepted forms of "medicine."

WE ALREADY KNOW TOO MUCH

Dr. Weston Price tells a story of the native peoples living in Northern British Columbia in the Rocky Mountains. In winter, temperatures can drop to seventy degrees below zero. These people refused to eat any of the highly toxic processed foods that the white man had been giving to those in different areas. The result was that they rarely developed disease and never developed scurvy. Many of the other natives who were eating the modernized foods not only developed scurvy, but also tuberculosis, and many other degenerative diseases. Scurvy is a disease that comes from a vitamin C deficiency. If these people were not eating their fruits and vegetables, where in fact were they getting their vitamin C?

Dr. Price asked one of the natives for their secret. He asked why they had not told the white man. The response: *"The white man already knows too much to ever ask us."* This is a problem we face today. We all think we know too much. We learn things we should never have been taught, which are misleading and irrelevant to the natural processes of life. These natives had a remarkable remedy and preventative practice for their immunity to scurvy. After hunting for moose, they would cut the moose open near the back and pull out the adrenals, slice them up, and pass them around to other members of their tribe. After eating, they would develop immunity. Astonished, Dr. Price did research and found that the adrenals contain the highest amount of Vitamin C of all of the organs. The moose get their vitamin C from eating plants. These Indians had simply been drawn to it by nature. This does not mean we should start eating moose adrenals; that was a way of the past. This would be a terrible thing and would not work for us like it did for them.

We are fortunate enough today that we can obtain sufficient amounts of vitamin C from fruits of the Earth. We do not always need supplements and we definitely should not rely on animals. If we live in cold climates, we can gather food for the cold months, and grow our own sprouts, and other foods indoors. We need to avoid chemicals and eat fruits and berries. The indigenous did not need billions of dollars in research money to discover this. They did not need to create chemicals. They did not need to fry each others brains with radiation treatments, or perform unnecessary surgeries to "treat" symptoms. They simply abided by nature and realized there is a cause for every disease, as well as a way to heal the body from each disease. Because we failed to listen while gloating in our foolishness and so-called stellar education, we lost many thousands of lives until it was discovered that vitamin C and a diet rich in raw fruits and vegetables cures scurvy.

ALLERGIES

A perfect example of a "know-it-all" would be a woman I did a nutrition consultation with. She and her husband came in and we discussed nutrition. They were both significantly overweight and had numerous health conditions. She had allergies. When I mentioned to her that natural healers and holistic health practitioners cure most allergic conditions by having their clients simply cut dairy products, colas, gluten grains, artificial sweeteners, and synthetic food additives from their diet and increase their intake of water, she had a hard time accepting what I was saying. Her response humored me. Her response for me was, *"Oh no, I have studied the immune system for eight years. I know all about allergies. My allergist has been working with me for years and there is just nothing I can do about it. I have eight different allergies and they will not go away."*

210

So does that mean for every year she studied the immune system, she developed another allergy? With each new medical book she may have studied, she was misled into believing another prescription pill would help, and each new pill may have led to her developing another allergy. If she knew so much about the immune system, why was she not her own doctor? Why did she continue accepting advice from her "allergist" while not improving?

Allergies are triggered by the body's increased production of histamine. They are reactions to accumulated stores of toxins. Certain foods trigger and stimulate these toxins and we refer to these as "food allergies." At times, we may breathe in certain compounds that trigger the release of toxins and we refer to these as "environmental allergies." If you have an excess amount of potassium in your system and it is not balanced with organic sodium, this alone can trigger excess production of histamine. In some cases, allergies can be relieved by simply adding real water to your diet and introducing organic sodium. Many people with allergies drink sodas, or other soft drinks, regularly, and fail to incorporate pure water into their daily intake of fluids. They believe soda is water or can take its place as a hydrating fluid. This also leads to increased production of histamine. Keep in mind that fruit juice, and especially, bottled, jarred, reconstituted, or otherwise pasteurized fruit juice is also not a replacement for water, unless water is not available.

We can eliminate these allergies once and for all by cleansing the toxins from our system. The most efficient way to do this is by partaking in internal cleansing services, eating raw organic foods, being exposed to fresh air and sunlight, getting adequate exercise, and drinking plenty of good water.

All chemicals and foreign animal proteins should be removed from the diet. This means no processed foods, no meat, no dairy, no eggs, no sodas, no coffee, and no foods containing synthetic chemicals, including preservatives and artificial flavors, scents, sweeteners, and colors. This includes having to eliminate the use of unnecessary "beauty" products that we put on our skin and apply to our hair falsely believing they will enhance our beauty. If a skin moisturizer is needed, the use of virgin organic unrefined coconut oil will do the trick.

By following this advice, we begin to notice quality improvements in our health. Dr. Fereydoon Batmanghelidj provides a number of testimonials of patients who were cured of their allergies by drinking pure water and balancing their sodium and potassium levels in his book, *Your Body's Many Cries for Water.*

I do not know if the woman with the allergies followed my advice, but I know I at least motivated her to read other books on the immune system. What matters most to me is that I had the slightest bit of impact. Anything I can do to erase the health ignorance in this world is a win. I truly hope she did some real research after we spoke.

EMPHYSEMA

My grandmother is sixty-seven and has suffered from emphysema for several years from what she believes were her many years of cigarette smoking. Yes, the cigarettes were definitely a major contributor, but what she has failed to, and continues to refuse to accept, is the role her diet plays in the worsening of her condition. She quit smoking many years ago, but her diet consists of not an ounce of real food each day. Her cabinets are full of processed foods, packaged sweets, candy, and just about every "food" item that I listed on the unhealthy grocery list in chapter three. Her fridge is filled with processed sandwich meats, chemical-laden condiments, conventional pasteurized milk, cheese, and of course, sodas. Her freezer is full of meat and frozen microwave dinners. She follows the sickness-infusion diet.

A study conducted by the *College of Physicians and Surgeons at Columbia University* concludes that, "*The nitrites in cured meats significantly increase the risk of developing chronic obstructive pulmonary disorder (COPD) in women. The study consisted of 71,531 women who had no signs of COPD and were between the ages of thirty-eight and sixty-three. They were studied for sixteen years. The results of the study found that the women who did not eat meat and smoked were far less likely to develop COPD. A majority of the women who ate meat regularly and smoked, however, developed emphysema.*" There were 750 cases reported amongst the group of women. This study was published in a December 2008 issue of the *American Journal of Clinical Nutrition.*

A similar study was conducted by the *Department of Nutrition* at the *Harvard School of Public Health* where they studied the effects of cured meats on 42,915 men. The study concluded that, "*Men who eat cured meats regularly have a much higher risk of developing COPD.*" This study was published in the December 2007 issue of the *American Journal of Epidemiology.*

In, yet another study, published in the *Journal of Respiratory and Critical Care Medicine* in August of 2007, and that was conducted by the *Department of Medicine at Columbia University*, 7,352 participants over the age of forty-five were studied. The results found that, "*Frequent meat consumption was associated independently with an obstructive pattern of lung function and increased risk of COPD.*

Each meal my grandparents eat consists of unhealthful food choices. Most of their meals come from packages and are loaded with health-depleting ingredients. The lining of the cans in their cupboard contain harmful chemicals that have been linked to chronic diseases. My grandma adds MSG to her gravy. When I commented about it, she said, "*Oh Jesse, I wish I would have known you did not like it, I would not have put it in. I add MSG for the good flavor.*" For years she had been adding that poison to her food for the manipulation of

212

her taste buds, mistaking this for "good" flavor.

In addition to all of the hazards in their kitchen, my grandparents frequently dine out. They often order steak or prime rib, and they enjoy an occasional McDonald's Big Breakfast. She has been seeing doctors and so called "specialists" for many years, and not once have they inquired about her diet. Sadly, many of these overpriced doctors with overpriced degrees are eating similar foods. But, because they "know all," she will only listen to what they tell her.

When I mentioned to my grandma that emphysema can be improved, and the lungs also can be improved through a clean diet, she thought about it momentarily and said, *"Oh Jesse that just cannot be. If they did have a cure for my condition, my pulmonologist would have already cured me."* If her pulmonologist had a different education and one with a strong influence on optimal nutrition, her condition may get better. Judging by the foods she continues to consume, and her reliance on pills and more doctor appointments, these doctors are not doing her much good. And so, the illness keeps advancing, and she remains hooked to the oxygen tank, eating horrible foods.

A publication in the *Current Opinion in Clinical Nutrition and Metabolic Care* journal, titled, *Impact of nutritional status on body functioning in chronic obstructive pulmonary disease and how to intervene,* states that, *"Diet, as a modifiable risk factor, appears more as an option to prevent and modify the course of COPD."* The article mentions several important factors regarding nutrition and obstruction of the lungs. What I found most interesting is that one-third of all COPD patients have always been non-smokers. The article states that, *"Increased intake of dietary fiber has been independently associated with improved lung function and reduced prevalence of COPD* (meat and dairy products do not provide us with dietary fiber*)."* This strongly supports my claim that diet plays a role in the deterioration of the lungs. The article reveals that impaired glucose metabolism is associated with impaired lung function (refined sugars and chemical sweeteners cause impaired glucose metabolism). The article concludes that, *"Nutritional depletion has been widely reported in COPD patients. Diet may also play a role both in the development and the progression of the disease. Holistic management for these patients should include nutritional modulation."*

I showed my grandma testimonials of clients from the Gerson Institute who reversed their emphysema. I showed her literature declaring that her diet was worsening her condition. All of my efforts, and all of the evidence I have provided her with the hope for her to change her fate, have been ineffective because her "specialists" continue to reject my claims. They are worsening her condition each day with their negligence, and she with her reluctance to change her diet.

I asked my grandma if any of her "specialists" had ever taken a moment to speak with her about her diet, they had not. Because they have failed to inform her that diet plays a huge role in the worsening of her condition, my grandma continues to eat red meat with every meal. She continues to drink soda. She gobbles down "Jelly-Belly" candies. She drinks excessive amounts of milk for the "calcium." What she does not realize is that all of these poor decisions are robbing her of any chance she may have of recovering from her condition. Eating dairy alone is restricting her breathing capacity to a percentage of what it could be. Eating meat is diverting the energy in her body away from repairing and creating new cells and tissues, to the process of converting the meat into liquid for digestion.

In a prospective study of dietary patterns and chronic obstructive pulmonary disease among US women, published in the *American Journal of clinical Nutrition* in 2007, *a pattern was associated with a high intake of fruits, vegetables, and whole grains resulting in a decreased risk of COPD. Concurrently, a Western pattern was associated with high intake of refined grains, cured and red meats, desserts and French fries resulting in an increase of COPD.*

Eating clarified sugars and meat, consuming dairy products, and eating other processed foods is assuring her that she will never get better. She fails to implement the most necessary step for improvement, which is eliminating all of these toxic products from her diet. By ingesting easily digestible foods like sprouts, fruits, and fresh juices, her condition will begin to improve. Her body will divert the energy she has been wasting trying to digest these heavy, toxic "foods" back to repairing her lung tissues, repairing her damaged cells, and fueling her brain. In addition, there are certain herbs such as comfrey root, chickweed, marshmallow root, and yerba santa leaf which Dr. Robert Morse claims can rebuild lung tissue (Access *GodsHerbs.com* and search for his herbal products for the lungs).

My grandmother likely has plaque consisting of a variety of medicines and chemicals from over the years lodged in the walls of her intestines – when the famous actor, John Wayne, died, his autopsy revealed close to fifty pounds of plaque lodged in his system. Her lymphatic system likely has residues from all of the toxins she has been ingesting. She could benefit by drinking two ounces of lobelia extract each day. This would help her expel much of the excess mucus from her lungs. She does not accept the fact that doing simple procedures, like colon hydrotherapy with a chlorophyll implant, lymphatic drainages, and oxygen baths will help expel the toxins from her system and improve her condition. When I mention this to her, she gets sad and claims that her pulmonologist would have informed her if these would be of any benefit to her health. She needs help, but because her doctors and pulmonologists have repeatedly misinformed her over the years, and she believes them and limits herself to their advice, she cannot be saved.

If my grandmother were to cut all meat, dairy, eggs, cooked oils, processed salts, clarified sugars, gluten grains, and refined flours from her diet, I am certain her condition would improve. If she were to incorporate regular internal cleansing processes, she would breathe much easier. Once she began breathing on her own, she could add some light aerobic exercise to her routine.

I love my grandparents, and it saddens me seeing them so caught up in failing health, bad food, and bad medicine.

THE ACNE SOLUTION

Many dermatologists have resorted to internal poisoning for treatment of acne by prescribing antibiotics for what they refer to as a "solution" to the problem. A friend of mine recently informed me she has been taking an antibiotic every day for several years for her acne. She seems to be sick often. She had been unknowingly destroying her intestinal flora through the frequent use of antibiotics. Now in order for her to have a "clear" face, she must resort to having a disruptive bowel and she will frequently suffer from episodes of sickness.

The *Archives of Dermatology* published a study in March of 2012 that showed a positive association of pharyngitis with oral antibiotic use for the treatment of acne. The researchers from the *University of Pennsylvania* assessed 576 participants. *"Of the 306 with acne, thirty-six received oral antibiotics for its treatment and ninety-six used topical antibiotics. Of the total participants, 210 patients, or thirty-six percent, had a history of pharyngitis in the past month. Those taking oral antibiotics were 4.3 times more likely to have had an episode than those not on antibiotics."*

The skin is like a mirror of our internal organs and nutrition. If we have healthy skin, we most likely have a healthy internal environment. As a signal from nature, whenever we have a blemish or a problem with our skin, we are warned that our internal environment may need some cleansing and our diets may need to be altered. If we disrupt this natural signaling process, by taking antibiotics or chemical drugs, we will never know when our internal organs are unhealthy. Our skin will always appear to be healthy, when internally, there may be a problem. As a result, we have – as John McCabe refers to them – *toxemians* walking around, appearing to have healthy skin, while their internal organs could be deteriorating underneath.

Skin is our largest eliminative organ. When we consume low-quality foods containing substances that cause disorder, are difficult for our system to digest, and may damage the processes of the digestive tract, the toxins can end up accumulating in our system as residues, plaque, weight gain, and skin disorders, including acne and eczema.

One culprit behind pimples and acne is cooked oils. When we apply heat to "cooking" oils, these oils turn rancid. The fats that may have been healthy become equivalent to trans-fats. These trans-fats block the pores of the skin. In addition, they cause inflammation of the skin and clog arterial walls and cell membranes. Cooked fats are sticky, end up on cell membranes, and interfere with cell respiration, nutrient transfer and absorption, and cell waste disposal.

Cheese is a common food source for these harmful fats. The fats in the cheese, that have already turned rancid through the pasteurization process, are again heated at higher temperatures during cooking, thus creating more toxins. Fried foods are also high in trans-fats. Foods that are deep fried or pan fried in any type of oil (including olive oil) are detrimental to our health and the appearance of our skin.

Milk is another common source for trans-fats. Milk becomes enzyme-less and rancid once it is pasteurized. All milk purchased today, unless raw from an organic farm, contains the equivalent to trans-fats. Raw milk still contains casein, making it a poor choice of food for humans. Chocolate is also a food that is detrimental to our health. Although cacao in its raw state is a nutrient dense superfood, once it is heated and processed into chocolate, it loses its nutritional value and the fats turn rancid and become equivalent to trans-fats. It is okay to make your own raw chocolate using carob powder and to eat this sparingly.

Another ingredient that is added to food and does damage to our skin is flour. The starch molecule is known to clog the pores of our skin. In addition, there are hormones from meat, dairy, and eggs, as well as farming chemicals that lead to acne. Synthetic chemicals, free radicals, dietary cholesterol, acrylamides, glycotoxins, gluten grains, MSG, processed sugars, caffeine, lack of biophotons, and lack of true nutrients also play a role in the formation of pimples. Anything that clogs the lymph and stagnates the lymph fluid can cause acne.

A study conducted by the *Department of Nutrition*, at the *Harvard School of Public Health*, examined the role of dairy consumption in the occurrence of acne. *Researchers studied questionnaires submitted by more than 47,000 high-school-age girls, and found a positive association between acne and total milk and skim milk consumption. Further examination revealed that the association was due to the hormones and bioactive molecules found in the dairy products.* This study was published in a February 2005 journal of the *American Academy of Dermatology*.

By eliminating all acid foods, cutting out dairy, meat, and eggs, avoiding synthetic chemicals, coffee, and chocolate, refusing to eat foods that contain oils, especially cooked oils, refraining from drinking sodas and energy

216

drinks, avoiding all protein powders containing soy, whey, casein, egg, and artificial sweeteners, and by eliminating foods that contain flour and gluten grains, one can expect to have clear skin that truly reflects the cleanliness of their internal environment. Their energy levels will increase, they will end their dependency on chemical drugs to provide them with a synthetic skin appearance, and they will be closer to reaching an optimal level of health.

CROHN'S DISEASE

While speaking with a guy who works at a gym where I once provided personal training for a few of my clients, he mentioned that he has Crohn's disease. I informed him that many people have been cured of his ailment, to which he replied, "That is impossible." I asked him if he had ever considered fasting or doing a parasite flush. He insisted he had tried it all and none of it worked. I knew he had not tried anything outside of the medical world so I asked for details about his fast. His response was far worse than what I expected. He told me that he had done a three month liquid diet drinking only "Ensure." I am surprised he survived. I suggested that he try a real fast with something like wheatgrass juice. He knew better. He would rather eat chemical drugs all of his life while his condition gradually worsens and he ages prematurely.

He did not seem to care when I mentioned to him that Crohn's disease can successfully be reversed by eliminating cooked omega-6 oils from the diet and replacing them with raw omega-3-rich foods, while eating an abundance of raw organic fruits and cruciferous vegetables.

He could not seem to ponder the thought of possibly reversing his condition by avoiding all alcohol, cigarettes, meat, dairy, eggs, and processed foods, and internally cleansing until his condition went away. He already knew everything he needed to know because his doctor had already misinformed him into believing that he has to rely on toxic chemical drugs for the rest of his life.

Crohn's disease is a form of bowel disease that causes inflammation in the gastrointestinal (GI) tract. The most common age group to suffer from Crohn's is between eighteen to thirty-five years old. Those who take antibiotics at a young age (which are used for treating Crohn's disease) are known to be more prone to developing cardiovascular disease. When Crohn's disease occurs, the immune system attacks microbes in the intestines by sending white blood cells into the intestinal lining, and producing chronic inflammation. This is similar to the leucocytosis process where white blood cells attack cooked foods. All layers of the intestines may be involved and there could be healthy patches of bowel mixed in with diseased patches of bowel. While medical researchers claim they do not know where Crohn's comes from or how to cure the disease, many have identified the culprits as gluten, cooked oils, cooked corn, soy, bleached foods, and fiberless foods, such as meat, dairy, and eggs, along with other toxic foods. When these foods remain stagnant in the bowel, they decay and the body sends white blood cells after them in an attempt to remove them. This likely causes the inflammation.

Omega-3 fatty acids have powerful anti-inflammatory effects and can affect intercellular signaling. Raw fruits and vegetables contain omega-3 fatty acids, and by eating a plant-based organic diet, you can be assured you will receive these essential fatty acids in a proper abundance. Hemp seeds are rich in omega-3 fats, as are chia seeds and purslane. Omega-6 fats break down into arachidonic acid, and this acid converts into inflammatory eicosanoids, which interfere with immune function. Arachidonic acid is found in foods such as, egg yolks, liver, turkey, salmon, chicken, pork, beef, and all other meat sources. By eliminating these foods from his diet, a Crohn's patient can expect his condition to improve. A study published in the *World Journal of Gastroenterology* in 2005 suggests that *adding omega-3's to the diet is effective in maintaining remission of Crohn's disease. They studied thirty-eight patients and gave one group omega-3 fatty acid capsules and the other group received a placebo olive oil capsule. They found that the group who received the omega-3 capsules had a significantly lower rate of relapse and an increase of DHA and EPA. The patients most importantly had lower levels of arachidonic acid and eicosanoids.* Many Crohn's patients have an overabundance of arachidonic acid. Omega-3 fatty acids can inhibit the formation of this acid, altering eicosanoid production.

Many studies suggest that Crohn's disease develops from a bacterium in milk known as mycobacterium paratuberculosis. A study in the 1992 *Journal of Clinical Microbiology* states that these bacteria may be responsible for many cases of the disease. A separate study published in the same journal that same year found that *11.6 percent of cow's affected by Johne's disease (similar to Crohn's) produced milk that was positive for strands of these bacteria.* So-called health experts shrugged this information aside by claiming that the pasteurization process would not allow for these bacteria to survive and be passed on to humans. However, a study was conducted by the *Department of Pathobiological Sciences* at the *University of Wisconsin* that found *mycobacterium paratuberculosis is capable of surviving commercial pasteurization.* This study was published in the *Applied and Environmental Biology* journal in March of 1998. In 1996, the National Academy of Sciences documented that *mycobacterium paratuberculosis RNA was found in one-hundred percent of Crohn's disease patients, compared with zero percent of controls.*

Because humans cannot digest cow's milk very well, it lingers in the system long enough for the bacterium to settle in the bowel. This can be one reason for the development of Crohn's disease. By eliminating all dairy from the diet, the symptoms of Crohn's will begin to subside. As I mentioned in chapter two, good bacteria assist in breaking down milk proteins and sugars. For Crohn's disease, lactobacillus and bifidobacillus are needed in sufficient numbers to improve symptoms. For the colon to be healthy, this bacterium is a necessity. A study conducted by the **Department of Pediatrics at Tampere University Hospital** in Finland, found that *lactobacillus greatly improved the secretory immunoglobulin A (sIgA) in the intestine of patients with Crohn's disease.* The study was conducted on fourteen children with Crohn's and determined that lactobacillus could provide an adjunct nutritional therapy for the disease. This study was published in the **Annals of Nutrition and Metabolism** in 1996.

The best way to prevent this disease from reoccurring is to keep the bowel clean. Doing colon hydrotherapy with a chlorophyll implant and maintaining a healthful terrain for beneficial intestinal flora will help to prevent the inflammation process. To maintain this clean bowel, there cannot be any dairy, meat, eggs, cooked oils, gluten, synthetic chemicals, processed sugars, processed foods, alcohol, or cigarette smoke in the system. Someone suffering from Crohn's disease should give up all of these foods, go in for internal cleansing services, eat a raw, plant-based diet, consisting of many organic fruits and vegetables, and exercise regularly. By following this advice, you can expect significant improvements of your condition.

SHE ALREADY KNOWS

I met a girl who is a friend of my younger brother. She is a vegetarian. She is also a fun-spirited person. I think it is a beautiful thing to see children today standing up for their health and for the freedom of the animals trapped in the Animal Holocaust – which we refer to as "factory farming" and "animal agriculture." She began asking me a few questions and every time I would respond, she would say, "Oh, I know." She had recently added dairy back into her diet after her doctor informed her she was not getting enough calcium. He used scare tactics to make her believe she had some type of unknown medical condition that required her to drink milk. I heard a similar story from a client when they transitioned to a vegan diet. Their doctor alerted them they had an unknown medical condition that would get worse if they did not add dairy into their diet. When I suggested to her that she does not need to poison herself with a toxic substance like foreign milk, she already knew. When I told her she gets ten times more calcium from green leafy vegetables, she already knew. So, why is she listening to her doctor? Why did she ask me for advice? What is wrong with this world? The answer is we have too many mis-educated authorities stuck in the failing system. I have educated myself on a lot of things and I do claim to know a little, but I know there is much more knowledge out there for me to absorb and I keep my mind open. Many people do not, because they know already.

The most notorious of the mis-informed are the doctors, pulmonologists, allergists, dermatologists, and all of the "specialists" out there who claim their way is the only way based on their overpriced mis-education. They insist they know, but they know misinformation. They assume each patient they meet with knows nothing. The wording these medical professionals use can essentially scare a patient into believing that pills and surgery are the only ways to get relief. So, the patient ends up as a peg in the cluttered, dysfunctional medical system, taking pills and getting shots, and undergoing procedures. Each visit to them, while maintaining a toxic diet, accelerates the process of developing a degenerative disease. A sure way to eliminate ignorance from your life is to accept that you do not know, ask questions of the right people, do research using unbiased sources, and to open up your mind and break away from traditionalism.

The question still looms as to whether or not there is a cure for many of these diseases and conditions that have been labeled as "incurable." Can these so-called conditions, sicknesses, and diseases be cured?

Through all of my research, the testimonials I have seen and read, and after seeing these so-called "incurable" diseases be healed with my own eyes, I know there are natural ways in which people can greatly improve their health, even to the point of eliminating diseases and reforming their structures through true nutrition and daily exercise.

The first step towards reversing your condition lies in healing your body and mind. You must believe the body can be cured and you must know it deep within.

The first action to take is converting to a low-fat, organic vegan diet rich in raw fruits and raw vegetables. You must cleanse internally and you can never give up.

Please watch these documentaries: *Fat, Sick, and Nearly Dead*; *May I Be Frank*; *A Delicate balance*; and *Forks Over Knives*.

Chapter 10: CAN WE REVERSE DISEASE?

"There is no disease, whatever name it may bear, which cannot be cured; though there are patients whose physical strength is too far gone to complete the process of cure." – Dr. Louis Kuhne

Today many doctors are shifting towards the holistic approach of healing. Raw food healing retreats and institutes are becoming more popular. Many hospitals are starting to add holistic health programs as they notice the rise in demand for this natural method of healing and the insurance companies are realizing that many natural therapies cost less. As natural healers, we aim to understand the human body and how it works. We work to identify the root cause of disease, and in doing so, we seek ways of reversing positive risk factors. The easiest cure for disease is prevention, by means of eating raw, plant-based foods, and avoiding exogenous toxins (chemicals, alcohol, cigarettes, and drugs). Once disease develops, the best way to help reverse it is to internally cleanse, eliminate all toxins, and adapt to a raw, plant-based diet.

Cancer is one of the most feared diseases. According to *cancer.org*, 571,950 people died from cancer in the US in 2011. An additional 1,596,670 new cases are expected to be diagnosed in 2012. For every one person who dies from cancer, three more can expect to be diagnosed. If you wish to reduce your chances of experiencing cancer in your life, there are several ways you can go about doing this. One way of doing so is avoiding processed foods, with all of their health depleting components. Another is to restrict yourself from eating animal products. Give them up entirely. Studies conducted at institutions around the planet have concluded that certain substances are known to increase the risk of cancer, and those include meat, dairy, eggs, clarified sugars, processed foods, and cigarettes. Many chemicals found in common cosmetics and hair products have also been identified as carcinogenic.

CANCER- THE LOSING BATTLE OF CHOICE

"Don't give up. Don't ever give up." – Coach Jimmy Valvano

Jimmy V was one of the best, most well-known, and highly respected college basketball coaches to ever live. He was also a great family man and an overall terrific person. He is an idol of mine and his ESPY acceptance speech is one of my favorite speeches. Unfortunately, he was afflicted with cancer, and lost the battle.

If Jimmy V was eating the typical American diet heavy in animal protein, heated oils, bleached gluten grains, acrylamides, glycotoxins, heterocyclic amines, polycyclic aromatic hydrocarbons, processed sugars, and synthetic chemicals and farming residues, it should be no surprise that his body was overtaken by cancer. If he did not clean up his diet and follow one rich in raw fruits and vegetables, but kept eating the typical American foods while undergoing the "standard" cancer treatments involving cancer-causing chemicals and radiation, it should be no surprise that he died of his "disease." Unfortunately, the cancer research fund he started likely supports more of the same processes of toxic drugs and radiation, while overlooking what may be best.

Rather than prevent cancer and teach people about the proper ways to do so, the typical medical doctor advises toxic, cancer-causing therapies to "treat" cancer – which makes no sense at all. Rather than teach us the ways to heal our bodies, so our natural healing properties can cure and reverse these diseases, they expect us to spend money on their unnecessary drugs while they poison us with chemotherapy and radiation treatments that become the main cause of death in nearly every terminal case.

"Considered in its broadest terms, orthodox cancer treatment today is a failure and a disgrace. Contemporary cancer management, in a number of respects, constitutes professional malpractice." – Dr. Brian A. Richards, The Topic of Cancer

Counting on chemotherapy to cure cancer is like counting on winning the lottery to purchase your next meal. The odds are stacked so highly against you that the best option is to go another route. This is why we find jobs and we work to pay for our food. This is why some of us plant gardens and grow our own organic food. We cannot rely on luck to eat. What I have a hard time with is trying to understand why millions of people willingly throw their lives away to chemotherapy and radiation treatments. The survival rate of chemotherapy is in the single percentile range. Of the millions of people who undergo chemotherapy, only a small percentage survive and many of those who do survive often develop cancer again. This is partly because chemotherapy creates more acidity in the blood, and in some cases cancer develops because of acidity in the blood. So the chemo treatment may kill the cancer cells, however it also kills other cells that divide rapidly. Soon after, more cancer may develop and start to spread.

In a study that was published in *Nature Medicine* in August 2012, the lead researcher, Peter Nelson, from the *Fred Hutchinson Cancer Research Center* in Seattle, concluded that chemotherapy not only produces resistance to chemotherapy by cancerous tumors, but that it also stimulates the growth and metastasis of cancer cells. In his study he found that close to ninety percent of patients with cancer that had metastasized had also become resistant to chemotherapy. The study further concluded that chemotherapy may trigger the production of high concentrations of a protein named *WNT16B*, which is involved in the development of cancer cells. Exposure to excessive amounts of chemotherapy was found to stimulate the production of an abundance of these proteins.

As a result of chemo, the patient could also develop myelosuppression, mucositis, alopecia, and what is known as chemo brain. These conditions can also play roles in the patient being prescribed even more chemical "medications." Myelosuppression is suppression of the immune system. The patient may become so sick that they cannot walk. This may result in infections producing overwhelming amounts of bacteria in the blood. Mucositis is inflammation of the digestive tract, so this impairs the ability to eat, leading to severe malnourishment. Alopecia is an autoimmune disorder causing the loss of patches of hair. Chemo brain is a term applied to the damage done to the stem cells in the brain that store and create memories. The sad truth is that healing from cancer lies in the decision to change one's lifestyle, but many people are so lost in a system that fails them that they never heal.

"I am very much against chemotherapy generally. It simply makes the patients too ill. Remember, there are worse things than death. One of them is chemotherapy." – Dr. Charles Huggins, Nobel Prize Winner for Medicine in 1966

While the chances of surviving from chemotherapy are in the low percentile range, it is hard to determine the exact number, but I would bet a large wager that those who go to natural healing retreats, change their lifestyles, and incorporate raw, plant-based diets, have a survival rate much higher than those choosing the toxic medical "treatment." I have read testimonials of people "miraculously" healing their bodies from cancer by choosing to abide by nature rather than give in to the synthetic, chemically-induced disease-breeding choice. I have seen numerous video testimonials and pictures of massive tumors that gradually fade away by detoxifying the body and incorporating greens, grass juices, and sprouts into the diet. Rather than being forced to damage their brains with radiation (I have a friend whose father died after being burned by an overdose of radiation for a brain tumor), these people choose to break away from the trap, stand up for their rights, cleanse the toxins out of their system, and eat raw, organic foods from nature. Rather than agreeing to undergo surgery to remove tumors that are only symptoms of the disease, there are people who go the natural route and their tumors fade away. Look up Chris Wark and access his website (chrisbeatcancer.com). An inspiring story is of a woman who was given a death sentence by her cancer specialists. She decided to read *Sunfood Diet Infusion* by John McCabe, and the book motivated her to convert to a raw vegan diet. After only a year of following this diet, she is now cancer free.

"The failure of modern scientific medicine to solve the problem of cancer is due to the tenaciously held idea that cancer is a cellular aberration that can occur in an otherwise healthy body more due to bad luck than bad management, and that the cure for it is to cut it out or in some other way destroy it, a traumatic and expensive procedure that, as the statistics show, rarely succeeds." – Ross Horne, Cancerproof Your Body

I believe cancer is a chance for those diagnosed to wake up and realize they need a lifestyle change. Cancer is not a death sentence, instead, very often it is a manmade disease triggered by toxic foods, bad nutrition, and polluted water damaging immunity. It is fueled with toxic emotions. It stems from lack of movement and compacted energy. It is created by consuming slaughtered animal remains and by ingesting eggs, milk, and foods that contain them. By following standard medical cancer treatments, cancer can be more of a death sentence. Going the opposite route and converting to a raw, organic vegan lifestyle, not only can prevent cancer, but may also reverse it. It makes no sense that we are forced to poison and radiate our bodies to kill tumors when the procedure does not erase the root cause of the disease, which may often be food, nutrition, environment, and stress.

Misinformed doctors may use scare tactics to manipulate patients into undergoing chemotherapy and taking chemical drugs, but this is not wise. Lance Armstrong was one of a small fraction of the survivors of this pracice. His survival does not mean the next cancer patient will be so lucky. Lance changed his diet immensely, which boosted his immune system to a higher level. In 2012, he announced that he has been switching to a low-fat vegan diet, and has been experiencing many positive benefits from it. The doctors may do anything they can to get patients to follow standard treatments. They may even go to the extremes of getting the legal system involved and forcing parents by law to subject their children to chemo, radiation, and surgery.

A perfect example would be the case of Daniel Hauser, who was thirteen years old and suffered from Hodgkin's lymphoma. After his first term of chemotherapy, he felt so ill that he could not walk. He opted to not go back for a second term. The doctors took his parents to court and charged them with *medical neglect*. The judge then ruled that the boy must continue with chemotherapy and if the parents did not follow through, they would take the child away. The case was in Brown County, Minnesota. The ruling judge was John Rodenberg. What better defines *medical neglect*? Would it be the parents of this boy choosing not to force their son into frying and poisoning the cells and organs of his body with deadly chemotherapy and radiation? Or would *medical neglect* better be defined as the medical doctors who neglect the fact that their treatments may be deadly, that cancer could very well be reversed with optimal nutrition, and neglect to discuss the importance of a plant-based diet with their patients, instead forcing them to undergo harmful chemo and radiation treatments while ingesting an array of chemical drugs?

We have, to a degree, placed the same burden on ourselves that we have placed on the slaves, the animals in the Animal Holocaust, and the primitive cultures from all over the world throughout history. Could this be our karma coming back to us in the form of disease for the many years of abuse, torture, rape, and murder we have forced on the people and animals of this planet?

If Jimmy V had gone to a natural healing retreat such as the *Gerson Hospital and Healing Centre* (CHIPSA) in Tijuana, Mexico, or even the *Hippocrates Health Institute* in West Palm Beach, FL, he may still be alive today. This holds true for many of the people who have died from cancer. Many people have discovered that the natural way, free of toxic medicine and rich in true nutrition, is the answer. The problem we face, especially in the USA, is that natural solutions are not highly profitable so they are quickly shut down, rejected, and even covered up, or referred to as a scam or as fraudulent.

Max Gerson was a medical doctor who discovered natural ways of treating cancer. The medical industry would not accept his methods and did not allow him to practice in the USA. They paid his secretary to poison him and steal the manuscript of his first book, *A Cancer Therapy: Results of Fifty Cases and the Cure of Advanced Cancer*, which was eventually rewritten and published in 1958. He was able to escape the attempted poisoning and his work is now practiced in Tijuana, Mexico. His approach has successfully relieved thousands of people of their cancers, and each case has been documented. Although it was reported that the medical industry was able to successfully poison and murder Dr. Gerson years later, his daughter, Charlotte Gerson, has continued his legacy and continues to cure thousands to this day at her center in Tijuana, Mexico (Gerson.org).

Charlotte has written an excellent book titled, *The Gerson Therapy*. There are several DVDs which have documented the treatments Gerson uses. Three of these DVDs I recommend are: *The Beautiful Truth, The Gerson Miracle,* and *Dying to Have Known*. An additional DVD that everyone should watch is *Cancer Is Curable Now*.

At the Gerson Institute, they go about their treatment by internally cleansing the body with organic coffee enemas, eliminating all chemicals from the body, scrubbing the skin with skin brushes, providing exposure to sunlight, and giving their patients an intake of fresh organic vegetables, and juices. I strongly encourage anyone who has been diagnosed with cancer to seek their treatment. Start by watching these documentaries, and once you are inspired, seek out natural treatment, and avoid all toxic foods.

There are several natural healing centers in the USA as well, which abide by a similar healing protocol. Because of the strict medical laws, the staff may not tell you directly that they treat cancer, but they cleanse and detoxify the body so the cancer has a lower chance of surviving. There is the *Optimum Health Institute* located in San Diego, CA, and Austin, TX (optimumhealth.org/program/ohi-body.htm). In Mesa, AZ, you could check out *An Oasis of Healing*, operated by Dr. Thomas Lodi. In Wheaton, IL, there is the *Total Health Institute* (totalhealthinstitute.com/alternative-cancer-treatment). In West Palm Beach, FL, Dr. Brian Clement directs the

Hippocrates Health Institute (hippocratesinst.org). Hippocrates has a very good reputation for healing the body and mind and if I were diagnosed with cancer I would seek their treatment. An additional healing retreat where I would go for treatment is the *Tree of Life Rejuvenation Center* (treeoflife.nu) in Patagonia, AZ.

"There is no disease whose prime cause is better known, so that today ignorance is no longer an excuse that one cannot do more about prevention of cancer. But how long prevention will be avoided depends on how long the prophets of agnosticism (the belief that nothing is known) will succeed in inhibiting the application of scientific knowledge in the find of cancer. In the meantime, millions of men and women must die of cancer unnecessarily." – Dr. Otto Warburg, Max Planck Institute

To understand cancer, the root cause must first be determined. We know after years of successfully healing the body that poor nutrition is a main trigger of cancer. The *American Cancer Society* estimates that *nearly one-third of all cancer deaths in society are a result of poor nutrition.* In his book, *The China Study*, Dr. T. Colin Campbell states, *"There is enough evidence now that doctors should be discussing the option of pursuing dietary change as a potential path to cancer prevention and treatment. There is enough evidence now that the U.S. government should be discussing the idea that the toxicity of our diet is the single biggest cause of cancer. There is enough evidence now that local breast cancer alliances, and prostate and colon cancer institutions, should be discussing the possibility of providing information to Americans everywhere on how a whole foods, plant-based diet may be an incredibly effective anti-cancer medicine."* Dr. Campbell provides this evidence in the book.

Changing one's diet is imminent for any chance of survival. Cancer develops when, over its lifespan, the body is exposed to toxins. The main contributors to cancer are: meat, processed meats (such as sausages, bacon, bologna, lunch meats, etc), dairy, eggs, a high-fat diet, clarified sugars, free radicals, packaged, processed meals on shelves or frozen, microwaved foods, suntan lotions, beauty products, added chemicals in our food and water, pharmaceutical drugs, cigarette smoking, environmental toxins (farming chemicals, smog, industrial pollution), and alcohol abuse.

"Humans now carry dioxin levels in their bodies hundreds of times greater than the "acceptable" cancer risk as defined by the EPA, and ninety-five percent of this results from eating red meat, fish and dairy products. An EarthSave study of 11,000 people showed that those on a vegetarian diet have a forty percent lower risk of developing cancer than meat-eaters." – Jennifer Bogo, author of The Diet-Cancer Connection.

After nearly sixty years and many billions of dollars later, cancer research has helped spread cancer, hidden the real cures, and taken more lives per year than ever before. Where is this money going? Why are doctors not finding the root cause of cancer and then curing it rather than "treating" the symptoms while frying and poisoning the bodies of those with cancer through chemotherapy and radiation?

In his book, *The Cancer Survivor's Guide*, Dr. Neal Barnard states, *"For many years, researchers have been investigating how food choices can help prevent cancer, and when cancer has been diagnosed, how these choices can improve survival. While their work is by no means finished, what is already known is nothing short of dramatic. Certain diet patterns seem to have a major effect, helping people diagnosed with cancer to live longer, healthier lives. Other diet choices are risky propositions, increasing the toll cancer takes."*

As mentioned, ways of reducing the risk of cancer include, eating the right foods, and avoiding animal proteins, sugars, acrylamides, glycotoxins, heterocyclic amines, food chemicals, foreign hormones (from animal products), free radicals, and nitrates. By eliminating these from the diet, the cancer cells are less likely to take hold as our immune system is stronger.

"Dr. Davaasambuu cited a study comparing diet and cancer rates in forty-two countries that showed a strong correlation between milk and cheese consumption and the incidence of testicular cancer among men aged twenty to thirty-nine – rates were highest in high consuming countries such as Switzerland and Denmark and low in Algeria and other parts of the world where people eat less dairy. She also linked rising rates of dairy consumption to the increased death rates from prostate cancer (from near zero per 100,000 men five decades ago to seven per 100,000 men today) and noted that breast cancer also appears to be linked to milk and cheese consumption." – Andrew Weil, M.D.

To begin reversing cancer, it is important to immediately remove meat, sugar, eggs, sodas, and dairy from the diet. The most powerful cancer fighting foods are raw fruits, vegetables, and fresh organic juices. Asparagus and wheatgrass juice are especially effective. Asparagus contains an active compound known as *asparanin A,* which has shown to be a promising preventative and therapeutic agent against hepatoma. A study published in 2009 in the *Biochemical and Biophysical Research Communications* journal showed that *asparanin A induces G(2)/M phase arrest and apoptosis in human hepatocellular carcinoma HepG2 cells.*

In simpler terms, the compound, known as asparanin A, has anti-cancer effects and this could be the reason why asparagus has been effective in fighting cancers such as lymphoma and melanoma.

A study published in a 2011 edition of the *Turkish Journal of Medical Science* concluded that wheatgrass juice intake can kill cancer cells. There are several wheatgrass retreats offering wheatgrass therapy for treating cancer. They are the *Hippocrates Health Institute*: West Palm Beach, FL (hippocratesinstitute.com); the *Optimum Health Institute:* San Diego, CA, and Austin, TX (optimumhealth.org); the *UK Centre for Living Foods:* England (livingfoods.co.uk); the *Ann Wigmore Institute*: Puerto Rico (annwigmore.org); the *Creative Health Institute*: Union City, MI (creativehealthinstitute.us); the *Living Foods Institute*: Atlanta, GA (livingfoodsinstitute.com); and the *Hippocrates Health Centre of Australia* (Hippocrates.com.au). If you do not have the resources to visit one of these retreats, you can make your own wheatgrass at home. Organic red wheat berries are around three dollars per pound and all you need is a few pounds to go along with some wheatgrass trays and soil, and a juicer. Steve Meyerowitz wrote a book titled, *Wheatgrass: Nature's Finest Medicine*, and the book provides details on how to effectively grow your own wheatgrass. You can purchase readily available wheatgrass on his site at *sproutman.com*.

Those who have had success in reversing their cancer most often did so by simply removing meat, dairy, eggs, sodas, sugar, and all junk food from the diet and replacing them with green smoothies containing high amounts of raw asparagus and other greens, and drinking them daily. They also drink wheatgrass juice daily.

Another cancer fighting compound found in foods is saponins. They are a group of phytochemicals found in a variety of edible plants and they can prevent cancer cells from growing and mutating. In a study published in 2008 in the *Mini Reviews of Medicinal Chemistry* journal, it was found that *saponins have favorable anti-tumorigenic properties and can inhibit tumor cell growth by cell cycle arrest and apoptosis.* According to *livestrong.org*, their research has confirmed that saponins are found in the skin of grapes; legumes (especially chickpeas, red kidney beans, navy beans, and pinto beans); herbs and spices (alfalfa, ginseng, fenugreek, and paprika); and foods such as asparagus, beets, chives, garlic, leeks, oats, onions, peppers, spinach, and sprouts.

Mung bean sprouts have been used to treat cancer because they contain a high amount of vitamin B17. At the *Hippocrates Health Institute*, these sprouts are used with most meals. They can be grown in a sprouting jar using only distilled water and organic mung beans. I mentioned more on sprouting in chapter three. If you are seeking a book on sprouting that will take you through the sprouting process step-by-step, I recommend Ann Wigmore's, *The Sprouting Book*.

Prevention is the most important factor in beating cancer. If you have not been following a healthful diet, it is highly important to clean up your diet so that your system can begin to function on a better level and rid itself of toxins. Colon hydrotherapy, oxygen baths, infrared saunas and lymphatic drainage services can be beneficial for speeding up the removal of toxins.

WHY THE PINK RIBBONS?

The *American Cancer Society* reports that one in eight women risks developing invasive breast cancer at some point in her life. The most recent estimates for breast cancer in the United States in 2012 indicate that there are 226,870 new cases annually and around 39,510 of these cases will result in death. To promote the cancer industry and raise funding so they can continue to mislead us with chemotherapy drugs and radiation treatments, pink ribbons are distributed all over the country. These pink ribbons do nothing to stop the spread of breast cancer, or to find the cure. The truth is that the preventative steps are well known, yet not widely accepted or practiced. To efficiently advance forward with a cure, the cause must first be determined. We know the most common causes.

"While scientists are hard at work searching for specific breast cancer-fighting compounds, the safest approach is to apply what we already know: Diets that are highest in a variety of plant foods while avoiding heavy oils, meat, eggs, and dairy products, help prevent a great many diseases. The earlier in life we start, the better." – Dr. Neal M. Barnard

After assessing several international and migrant studies, Dr. T. Colin Campbell suggests in his book, *The China Study*, the possibility that we can lower our rate of breast cancer to almost zero if we make certain lifestyle choices. He learned from these studies that those people who migrated from one area to another, and then began eating the typical diet in their new residency, assumed the disease risk of the area to which they moved. This led to his belief that diet and lifestyle are the principle causes of these diseases. He points to a study conducted by Professor Ken Carroll from the *University of Western Ontario* in Canada, in which a relationship was shown between the intake of dietary fat and incidence of breast cancer. In this same study, Professor Carroll was able to show that breast cancer was associated with animal fat intake, but not with plant fat. When presented with this study, the cancer industry quickly overlooked his findings, and continued putting money towards developing new drugs that fail to prevent, reverse, or cure the disease. The study was published in *Cancer Journal* in 1986, and titled, *"Fat and Cancer."*

Those who were convinced that this increased intake of dietary fats is indeed linked to breast cancer began to lower their intake of fats, yet they did this by eating low-fat or nonfat animal products, rather than converting to plant-based diets. So, as the percentage of calories from fat began to decrease, the percentage of calories obtained from animal proteins increased. This could explain why we still have not largely eradicated this disease.

230

"Diet and disease factors such as animal protein consumption or breast cancer incidence lead to changes in the concentrations of certain chemicals in our blood. These chemicals are called biomarkers. As an example, blood cholesterol is a biomarker for heart disease. We measured six blood biomarkers that are associated with animal protein intake. Do they confirm the finding that animal protein intake is associated with cancer in families? Absolutely. Every single animal protein-related blood biomarker is significantly associated with the amount of cancer in a family." – Dr. T.Colin Campbell, The China Study

As I mentioned in chapter seven, the parabens that are added to beauty products trigger the development of breast cancer. The lifestyle choices we make also trigger breast cancer. The food choices we make play a role in the development of this disease as well. Prevention is the safest and most effective method for reducing your chances of being one in eight women who will be afflicted with this cancer. Prevention begins with abiding by a clean, plant-based diet. This means removing all animal products, processed foods, fast food, and food chemicals from the diet. Of all foods, dairy is the most detrimental. Several studies have concluded that the protein in milk, casein, is directly linked to breast cancer incidence. Of these studies, *The China Study* is the most comprehensive and up-to-date. If you have not done so already, I encourage you to read the book, and see the documentary, *Forks Over Knives*.

In addition to diet, it is important to avoid all chemicals in general. To do this one must refrain from using beauty products that are not organic, and that contain parabens or sulfates. Chemicals are absorbed through the skin and into the lymph fluid. If you enjoy cleaning, and use chemical cleaning supplies, it is also important that you replace your usual chemical cleaners with plant-based, chemical free cleaners, or simply use vinegar. Cigarette smoking, drinking alcohol, and using suntan lotions must also be eliminated.

What I find most appalling about the pink ribbon scam is that many of the retail stores, as well as fast food restaurants, that are accepting donations for pink ribbons, are selling the very same products containing substances known to increase the incidence of breast cancer, yet they still expect us to donate money to their cause. I find this to be backwards, disgraceful, immoral, and wrong.

"Some dairy products, such as whole milk and many types of cheese, have a relatively high saturated fat content, which may increase risk. Moreover, milk products may contain contaminants such as pesticides, which have carcinogenic potential, and growth factors such as insulin-like growth factor I, which have been shown to promote breast cancer cell growth." – The American Journal of Clinical Nutrition

A study published in *Mutagenesis Journal* in 2009, titled, *Dietary Intake of Meat and Meat-Derived Heterocyclic Aromatic Amines and Their Correlation with DNA Adducts in Female Breast Tissue*, showed that heterocyclic amines not only trigger cancer and promote tumor growth, but that they also increase its metastatic potential by increasing its invasiveness.

These cooked meat carcinogens are found mostly in bacon, fish, beef, and chicken, but are present in nearly all animal-based foods once heat is applied. Of the heterocyclic amines, PhIP is perhaps the most damaging to health. The study found that PhIP initiates tumor growth, promotes cancer due to its estrogenic activity, and promotes the invasiveness of breast cancer cells more than straight estrogen. This is alarming, especially knowing how common it is for women with breast cancer to continue eating animal products, and that the most frequent cause of death in patients with breast cancer is from the metastasis of cells from the primary tumor, to distant sites, such as the liver and lungs, where they can grow to form secondary tumors.

In a study conducted at *Harvard Medical School*, ninety thousand women were monitored from 1991 through 2003. The women completed regular questionnaires to record how often they consumed more than 130 different foods and drinks so researchers could determine a possible link between diet and cancer. The women were asked to report whether or not they had developed breast cancer bi-annually. Only women who were premenopausal with no previous cancers were included in the study. At the end of the study it was determined that women who ate a high-meat diet were found to be much more prone to developing hormonally reactive breast cancers. Women who ate more than one-and-a-half servings of red meat such as lamb, beef, or pork daily had almost double the risk of hormone receptor-positive breast cancer compared with those who ate three or fewer servings per week. The study was published in November 2006 in the *Archives of Internal Medicine*.

In the *Harvard Nurses' Health Study*, which included 120,000 women from all over the country and investigated the relationship between diet, lifestyle, and disease in women, it was determined after two decades that breast cancer risk increases by twenty-two percent with every 100g per day increment of egg consumption. This is equivalent to about two eggs per day. PhIP has also been traced in the urine of vegetarians who eat eggs, making eggs an even less desirable choice for those afflicted with this cancer.

In the same study, alcohol consumption was found to increase breast cancer incidence by forty-one percent for women consuming thirty to sixty grams of alcohol per day, when compared with women who choose not to drink.

"I performed multiple regression analysis on breast cancer incidence. The highest correlation with breast cancer incidence was from animal source calories as compared to plant source calories. The saturated fat in meat and milk products increases the risk of breast cancer." – **Dr. William Harris, author of *Cancer and Vegan Diet***

In his book, *Super Immunity*, Dr. Joel Fuhrman presents us with a list of foods he believes to have the most powerful immune-boosting and anti-cancer effects. He provides an acronym for these foods, being *G-BOMBS*. These are: Greens, Beans, Onions, Mushrooms, Berries, and Seeds. He claims these foods help to prevent the cancerous transformation of normal cells, and keep the body armed and ready to attack any pre-cancerous or cancerous cells that may arise. In one of his articles titled, *Fight Breast Cancer with G-BOMBS*, published October 8th, 2012, on *diseaseproof.com*, Dr. Fuhrman explains why he recommends these particular foods. He specifically mentions cruciferous vegetables as being associated with decreased risk of breast cancer, and increased chances of survival in women who have been diagnosed with breast cancer. He was inclined to include beans because they are high in fiber, and according to a study published in the *American Journal of Clinical Nutrition* in 2011, high fiber diets are found to reduce the risk of breast cancer. If you are going to include beans in your diet, learn to use a steamer basket or bamboo basket, or try a double boiler so the beans boil in the water but do not touch the hot bottom of the pan. Also be sure to add plenty of raw vegetables to your dish. Because onions contain organosulfur compounds, they can be effective in slowing tumor growth and killing cancer cells. Mushrooms contain compounds known as aromatase inhibitors, which can block the production of estrogen. In a Chinese study published in the *International Journal of Cancer* in 2009, it was determined that women who ate at least ten grams of mushrooms per day had a sixty-four percent decreased risk of developing breast cancer. This is equivalent to a button mushroom per day. Berries also contain aromatase inhibitors, as well as many antioxidants, which protect against DNA damage that could lead to cancer, and reduce inflammation. Some seeds, especially sesame and flaxseeds, are rich in lignans. These are plant estrogens that protect against breast cancer. A study published in the *Clinical Cancer Research Journal* in 2005 found that women who were diagnosed with breast cancer, and were given flaxseeds daily, had reduced growth and increased death of their tumor cells after only five weeks.

In June 2005, a study conducted by researchers in Italy was published in the *Journal of Nutrition*. The research team found that when they mixed raw cauliflower juice with breast cancer cells, not only did the cancerous cells stop growing, but when they were exposed to higher doses of the juice, the cells died. Normal cells however, were not impacted. The compounds in cauliflower juice that are responsible for killing these cancerous cells are known as isothiocyanates (ITC). ITCs are anti-cancer compounds formed when compounds called phytoalexins, or glucosinolates, which act as the defense system for the genus of plants known as brassica, are modified after being chewed, or blended. These brassica plants are also categorized as cruciferous vegetables. When we chew these plants, they produce an enzyme known as myrosinase, which converts the glucosinolates into ITCs. The ITC compounds then stimulate the liver to excrete the carcinogenic compounds that may be circulating in the body. This does not mean you can simply drink cauliflower juice and expect breast cancer to go away. This means that if you cleanse internally, avoid foods that nurture cancer cells, and incorporate the juices from cruciferous vegetables into your diet you will have a greater chance of reversing the condition – and preventing its recurrence.

Cruciferous Vegetables: Arugula, broccoli, broccoli greens, brussels sprouts, cabbage, cauliflower, collard greens, kale, mustard greens, radishes, turnip greens, watercress.

"The scientific evidence shows that women do have the power to protect themselves against breast cancer with powerful preventive lifestyle measures. Staying slim and active, focusing on healthful natural foods, and avoiding the disease-causing foods of the Standard American diet are strategies women can use to win the war on breast cancer." – Dr. Joel Fuhrman

If breast cancer has already developed and you happen to be living with this disease, this does not mean you will die. This also does not mean you will need to have a mastectomy. You will not need to go through unnecessary chemotherapy and radiation treatments. This means you must begin to cleanse internally, incorporate juicing into your daily routine, exercise, and change your diet and approach to life. Internal cleansing services such as the lymphatic drainage, oxygen bath, and colon hydrotherapy have all proven to be helpful in combating this disease. The lymphatic system operates by moving lymph fluids through connective tissues, and this can only be done through the movement of tissues. Because of this, as Ron Garner mentions in *Conscious Health*, "*Women should not always have their breasts bound tightly with bras. They should exercise daily wearing loose apparel that allows the breasts to move. The restriction of movement causes a constriction of fluids and obstructs lymphatic circulation. This long term restriction of the lymphatic drainage system in breasts blocks natural energy flow and can be a factor in the development of breast cancer.*" If you wear bras often, fail to incorporate exercise into your daily routine, and partake in activities that can cause the lymph fluid to stagnate, such as smoking, consuming dairy products, eating meat or eggs, and wearing cosmetics and anti-perspirants containing harmful chemicals, then going in for a lymphatic drainage would be a good idea. Beginning to exercise regularly, and remembering to wear loose clothing while doing so, will also get the lymph fluids moving again.

By eating the foods which Dr. Fuhrman recommends, eating cruciferous vegetables from the brassica family, drinking fresh organic juices, avoiding all animal-based foods, cleansing internally, getting exposure to sunlight, using plant-based cleaners, steering clear of cosmetics loaded with sulfates and parabens, exercising, and making healthy lifestyle choices, one diagnosed with breast cancer would be making wise choices in alignment with healing and prevention.

PROSTATE CANCER CAN BE BEATEN

On the website *cancer.org*, it is stated in their estimates for 2012 that 241,740 new cases of prostate cancer will be diagnosed, and 28,170 men will die from the disease. Prostate cancer is fatal, in many cases, and the reason behind this is a failure of medicinal and conventional treatments, and horrid dietary choices that trigger the disease into progression rather than remission. The most important factor in determining whether or not you will survive the prostate scare is education, mixed with action and preventive measures.

The proof is out there, through many different sources, and a number of studies, that there are positive correlations between the consumption of dairy, meat, eggs, and animal products, and a high fat diet in general, and the occurrence of prostate cancer.

Prostate cancer is so prevalent in wealthy countries because of the consumption of animal proteins, all dairy products, and high-fat diets. It does not matter whether dairy products are raw, organic, pasteurized, or homogenized. The truth is that all dairy products can trigger prostate cancer and make it more aggressive. Eggs, whether organic, raw, pasteurized, or cage-free also have the same negative effect on health. The countries which consume the most animal products have the highest incidence of prostate cancer. Lower rates of prostate cancer are found in Japan and China, where they formerly consumed mammal meat and dairy in far less amounts.

In 1997, the *American Institute for Cancer Research* concluded that *dairy products are contributors to prostate cancer.* The *European Urology Journal* published a study in 1999 that followed 384 men with prostate cancer over a five year period. *The men who consumed the most meats and dairy had three times the risk of dying from the disease than those with the lowest saturated fat intake.* Then, in April 2000, a study was published by the *American Association for Cancer Research*, again linking dairy consumption with prostate cancer. *The Harvard's Physicians' Health Study examined 20,885 men for 11 years, and found that having two and one-half dairy servings each day boosts prostate cancer risk by thirty-four percent, compared to having less than one-half serving daily.*

Robyn Chuter wrote an article published in a 2010 issue of *Natural Health and Vegetarian Life*, titled *Early Stage Prostate Cancer.* In the article she suggests, "A *healthy vegan diet based on vegetables, fruits, legumes, nuts, seeds, and whole grains; not vegan marshmallows and soy hot dogs. The diet should be rich in dietary factors like antioxidant vitamins, carotenoids, other phytochemicals, and fiber that help prevent many chronic diseases including cancer, and may assist in overcoming them. The diet is also low in saturated fat and cholesterol."*

In the publication, Chuter informs us that, *"Animal protein is a key factor in raising levels of a hormone called IGF-l, Insulin-like growth factor 1, which is a known risk factor for prostate cancer, and importantly that dairy products have no place in the diet of a man who wants to avoid dying of prostate cancer. Milk, yogurt, cheese, and other dairy products contain high levels of IGF-1 and also stimulate the body to make more of it. In addition, the steroid hormone 5alpha-pregnanedione [5alpha-P] present in milk, is converted to dihydrotesterone (CDHT), a hormone which drives the growth of prostate cells, and hence is involved in the development of both benign prostatic hypertrophy and prostate cancer."*

In his book, *Living Foods for Optimum Health,* Dr. Brian Clement explains the reasoning behind why animal products trigger prostate cancer. He states that, *"Animal products are turned into male hormones called androgens, which stimulate the prostate gland. After decades of running androgens through the prostate gland, it is not surprising that it becomes enlarged and cancerous."*

Luckily there are many natural foods that can help eliminate prostate cancer. Foods that contain high amounts of vitamin B17, zinc, and antioxidants (such as raw vegetables, raw fruit, and especially raw berries) should be eaten frequently. A good source of omega-3 fatty acids, like raw hemp seeds, chia seeds, and sprouts, should be added to the diet. It is also important to make sure levels of progesterone and testosterone in the body are in check.

The best food sources for zinc are raw organic pumpkin and poppy seeds, as well as raw organic pecans. Sprouts are an excellent source for zinc. Broccoli sprouts, brussels sprouts, cabbage sprouts, garlic sprouts, and onion sprouts are very high in zinc. In terms of dealing with the prostate, the best foods to consume would be different variations of sprouts and raw pumpkin seeds. The prostate gland contains the highest concentration of zinc of any organ in the body, but inflamed prostates have been found to contain around one-tenth of the amount that a healthy prostate carries. This makes it a must to add more whole food sources of zinc to the diet. The combination of pumpkin seeds with saw palmetto or with nettle root are known to be beneficial.

Vitamin B17 (laetrile) has anti-cancer properties and has been identified as working in favor of recovery from prostate cancer, as well as from breast cancer. In 1977, Dr Harold W. Manner released laetrile research he had conducted at Loyola University in Chicago. *In a study with eighty-four mice, seventy-five underwent complete regression of mammary tumors. The other nine showed partial regression.*

B17 was originally isolated from the seeds of the tree, *prunus dulcis* (bitter almond), but when the pharmaceutical and cancer industries discovered how powerful they were in fighting cancer, the seeds were banned from the US in 1995. Along with containing a good amount of zinc, pumpkin seeds also contain high amounts of B17. Also, apricot kernels are a must for anyone dealing with prostate issues. Some people who have naturally healed themselves of prostate cancer accredit the apricot kernels alone. B17 is also present in the seeds of the apple, cherry, nectarine, peach, and orange. Back in chapter three I listed foods that contain B17. If you have an enlarged prostate, I recommend you start eating those.

Raw organic, virgin unrefined coconut oil has been identified as a progesterone-stimulant. By producing progesterone in sufficient quantities, the body then balances out the effects of estrogen. After it was discovered that estrogens are implicated in prostate cancer progression, researchers from the *Institute of Pathology at University of the Saarland* in Germany conducted a study. The results were published in an issue of the 2001 *Prostate* journal and concluded that, "*Progesterone receptors can have an effect on the use of estrogens for prostate cancer progression.*"

If you know someone who has a high PSA level, he is most likely deficient in both zinc and omega-3 fatty acids, and having trouble with proper absorption of nutrients. These are essential to maintaining a healthy prostate. Find out if he eats enough zinc-rich foods. Determine whether or not he is getting sufficient omega-3 fatty acids. Raw fruits, vegetables, chia, hemp, and flaxseeds are excellent sources of omega-3's. A study from the *Division of Cancer Prevention and Population Sciences at the University of Texas*, published in the December 2008 issue of *Cancer Epidemiology, Biomarkers, and Prevention*, suggests that, "*Flaxseed is safe and may protect against the development of prostate cancer.*"

If I were told I had a high PSA level, or prostate cancer, the first thing I would do is declare that I am vegan, clear out my kitchen of all deleterious foods, including bottled oils and foods containing them, then go to the organic market and load up on foods that are rich in zinc, get a good source of omega-3 fatty acids, and incorporate those into my diet.

The second thing I would do is go in for a colon hydrotherapy session with a chlorophyll implant. Plaque in the colon may place pressure on the prostate and result in high PSA. The chlorophyll implant is inserted in the rectum, and will help detoxify the liver as well. A gallbladder flush may also be helpful, as gallstones may have accumulated there.

I have read studies showing that lycopene found in watermelons and organic tomatoes can lower PSA levels by up to twenty percent in only three weeks by ingesting it three times a day for three weeks. Start incorporating more watermelon into the diet. Lycopene is found in higher concentrations in cooked tomatoes, but cooked tomatoes may be acid forming. A better way to release the lycopene is to blend the tomatoes raw. Eggplant and peppers are also fairly rich in lycopene.

Another beneficial phytochemical is curcumin, which is found in the turmeric root. Curcumin is excellent for detoxifying the blood and liver. Throw some fresh organic turmeric root in a blended drink or in the juicer as a blend and start drinking that. The other two food sources that help to shrink the prostate are saw palmetto and red maca. Make sure it is the red maca.

By changing your diet, eliminating acidosis in the body, cleansing internally, and most importantly, removing animal products and alcohol from your life, you will see your condition improve.

THE DISEASED HEART

In the 1800's many of the people who developed heart disease were the rich. Why do you think that is? Because the staple food for the rich was meat, and the poor could not afford to eat meat as often or as abundantly. As a result, the poor were richer in terms of health and the well-off were dying from over-indulging in animal flesh.

In April 2006, Lewis Kuller, M.D. from *University of Pittsburgh* made the announcement that, *"All males over the age of 65, who have been exposed to the traditional Western diet, have cardiovascular disease and should be treated as such."*

Heart disease is known as the silent killer. The *World Health Organization* (WHO) reports that cardiovascular disease is the number one cause of death globally. They estimate that 17.3 million people died from the disease in 2008 and predict that 23.6 million will die annually by 2030. The *Harvard Stem Cell Institute* documents in the background section of their *Cardiovascular Disease Program* that one American dies from cardiovascular disease every thirty-eight seconds. If we want to reduce that number, we must start by changing our food choices.

In the U.S., cardiovascular disease starts to form in children as young as preschool. After the Second World War, a scientific study published in the *Journal of the American Medical Association* revealed evidence of the disease in soldiers with an average age of twenty-two. The study states that, *"Military medical investigators examined the hearts of three-hundred male soldiers and upon dissecting their hearts found 77.3 percent of the hearts examined had evidence of heart disease."* The staple of the military soldiers' diet was meat. This study should enlighten us on how dangerous meat consumption is and how much of an impact it can have on the health of our heart, even at a young age.

In chapter two, I included information from a study that was published in March of 2012 about the association between eating meat and developing heart disease. Regularly eating red meat was found to significantly increase the risk of death from heart disease and cancer. The study was conducted on over 120,000 people over the course of twenty-eight years. The findings were published in the journal, *Archives of Internal Medicine*. *Scientists documented 23,926 deaths, including 5,910 from heart disease, and 9,364 from cancer, and found a striking association between consumption of red meat and premature death. Each additional daily serving of unprocessed red meat, equivalent to a helping of beef, lamb, or pork about the size of a deck of cards, raised the mortality rate by thirteen percent, while processed meat increased it by twenty percent. When deaths were broken down into specific causes, eating any kind of red meat increased the chances of dying from heart disease by sixteen percent, and from cancer by ten percent. Processed red meat raised the risk of heart disease death by twenty-one percent and cancer death by sixteen percent.*

A 2011 study published in *Nutrition and Metabolism* concluded that *vegetarian men weigh less and have lower cardiovascular disease risk, compared with non-vegetarian men. Researchers compared 171 vegetarians with 129 non-vegetarians of the same age and found that the vegetarian men all weighed less, had much healthier arterial walls, and lower levels of blood pressure, triglycerides, and total cholesterol.*

Heart disease is far less common in nations and among cultures where meat, dairy, and eggs are also less common. Meat, dairy, and eggs all contain cholesterol and saturated fat that are problematic for the people eating them. When these people are also deficient in nutrients found in raw edible plants, such as fiber, vitamins, enzymes, omega-3 fatty acids, and antioxidants, the health problems are compounded. The saturated fat in meat, dairy, and eggs triggers our system to produce unhealthful amounts of cholesterol. The cholesterol in animal products also is not good for human health. This all leads to plaque in the veins, arteries, and capillaries, narrowing blood passageways, which is cardiovascular disease – the terrain of heart attacks and strokes.

Dr. Matthias Rath explains one cause of heart disease in his book; *Why Animals Don't Get Heart Attacks but People Do.* He mentions the bear, which has the highest known cholesterol rate of any animal. Bears never suffer from heart disorders. One reason for this, he discovered, is that bears, like other carnivorous creatures, can produce vitamin C in their liver. Humans cannot do this. The reason why humans do not produce vitamin C is most likely because vitamin C is synthesized in plants. Since we are created to eat plant-based diets, we should never worry about vitamin C deficiencies.

When humans eat the flesh of dead animals and consume animal products, they are nurturing heart disease. When we are exposed to too much foreign cholesterol, we naturally use up our vitamin C to attempt to buffer the levels and eliminate this foreign substance. When our vitamin C is gone, our endothelial cells are damaged by free radicals. These cells line our arterial walls and when they are damaged, blood passageways narrow as nitric oxide production is reduced, and disease forms. We then develop heart disease, according to Rath, and Dr. Caldwell Esselstyn, from a lack of vitamin C, as a result of eating meat, dairy, eggs, and cooked oils.

What we need to realize is that it is virtually impossible for most of us to develop heart disease if we do not eat animal products, follow a low-fat vegan diet, and refrain from smoking. This means no meat, no dairy, no eggs, and nothing that has ever been a part of an animal in any way. It is also important to carefully monitor your intake of oils if you have heart disease. Your diet should consist of no more than eleven percent plant-based fats.

Simply adding kale, or kale juice to your diet, could benefit the health of your heart. In the April 2008 issue of *Biomedical and Environmental Sciences*, a study was conducted on participants who all had cholesterol levels above 200mg/dl. They were each given 150mL of kale juice daily for a period of twelve weeks. At the end of the study blood tests showed a twenty-seven percent increase in HDL cholesterol levels (good cholesterol), and a ten percent decrease in arterial plaque formation, as well as levels of LDL cholesterol.

If you would like to know more about how to reverse heart disease, I suggest you watch the documentary, *Forks over Knives,* and read the books, *Prevent and Reverse Heart Disease,* by Dr. Esselstyn; *The China Study*, by Dr. Campbell, and *Sunfood Diet Infusion* by McCabe.

WHY IS MY CHOLESTEROL HIGH?

Healthful blood levels are considered to be:

Total Cholesterol: < 150 (3.85 mm/L)
HDL Cholesterol: < 65 (1.7 mm/L)
Triglycerides: < 75 (0.82 mm/L)
Glucose: < 85 (4.7 mm/L)
Uric Acid Men: < 4 (0.24 mm/ L)
        Women: < 5 (0.30 mm/ L)

Not a lot of us know that there is a better correlation between excess consumption of refined sugar and heart disease, than there is with cholesterol consumption and heart disease, yet it is true. Sugar greatly increases the oxidation of LDL molecules. High sugar intake interferes with vitamin C absorption, thus lowering antioxidant defenses, and increasing the likelihood that LDL and triglycerides will oxidize.

In April of 2010, the *Journal of the American Medical Association* published a study concluding that, *"People who get at least twenty-five percent of their daily calories from added sugars of any kind were significantly more likely to have lower levels of the 'good' HDL cholesterol than those who* consumed five percent or less of their daily calories from added sugars. The study also found that those who consumed more than 17.5 percent of their calories from these sugars were twenty to thirty percent more likely to have high levels of the blood fats known as triglycerides." 6,113 American adults participated in the survey from 1999-2006 and this was conducted by the *Centers for Disease Control and Prevention.*

Taking all of this into consideration, think about what is added to some of the "filler" in cholesterol lowering drugs. Do clarified sugars cross your mind? Some presription drugs have sugars added as "filler." This is another reason why chemical drugs do not work.

According to Dr. Russell Blaylock in **Health and Nutrition Secrets,** "There is no statistical evidence linking reduced cholesterol levels to fewer heart attack deaths. These cholesterol lowering drugs are actually increasing mortality rates caused by other conditions. They damage nerves in the brain stem, causing cancer in many test animals. What many people do not realize is that there are two types of LDL, smaller LDL and larger LDL. The smaller molecules are harmful and the larger are actually protective like HDL. These cholesterol drugs actually break down the larger LDL molecules into the more harmful, smaller molecules and this actually worsens the heart condition. The only way any of these LDL molecules can be harmful is when they are oxidized. To protect these LDL molecules from becoming oxidized, it is important to have high levels of Magnesium, Vitamins E and C, carotenoids, and flavonoids."

Something simple, like exposing yourself to the sun, can help lower your cholesterol levels. Cholesterol that we produce naturally on a vegan diet gets converted into vitamin D by sunlight. Sunlight can help lower cholesterol levels. However, this does not make it okay for you to eat dietary cholesterol from animals, then lay out in the sun believing you will be okay. Most likely, your doctors have never told you this. There is a lot they will not tell you, mostly because they do not know. As I stated previously, there are not many medical doctors out there who really study true nutrition and how the body works. Most of them only know how to prescribe chemical drugs that will mask symptoms and make your condition worse.

The *Cleveland Clinic* physician, Dr. Caldwell Esselstyn, tells of a study in his book, **Prevent and Reverse Heart Disease**, where he *placed seventeen patients with severe coronary artery disease on a low fat, plant-based diet. Group members had previously experienced forty-nine cardiac events, and five patients had been given less than a year to live. Twenty-three years later, all were still alive and free of heart disease symptoms.*

During his *"Uprooting the Leading Causes of Death"* presentation, Dr. Michael Greger mentions a 2012 study published in the **American Journal of Cardiology**. The study was based on 65,396 hospitalizations from 344 hospitals and it was found that *nearly seventy-five percent of heart attack patients fell* *within recommended targets for LDL cholesterol, demonstrating that the current guidelines may not be low enough to cut heart attack risk in most that could benefit.* The **American Journal of Cardiology** provides a statement as well that explains, *"For plaque progression to cease, it appears that the serum total cholesterol needs to be lowered to the 150 mg/dl area. In other words, the serum total cholesterol must be lowered to that of the average pure vegetarian. Because relatively few persons are willing to abide by the vegetarian lifestyle, lipid-lowering drugs are required in most to reach the 150 mg/dl level."*

I think the real issue is that the doctors fail to present the option of following a vegan diet, and rather, they offer drugs as the only method of treatment. When someone has high cholesterol levels, the best option for her is to cut out all meat, dairy, eggs, and sugars from her diet, adapt a low-fat, plant-based diet, and get daily exercise. A low-fat, plant-based diet, and a shift away from a sedentary lifestyle, have proven in cases of high cholesterol to lower levels.

If you want to reduce your chances of ever having a high level of cholesterol, the very best preventative measure you can take is eliminating all meat, dairy, and eggs from your diet. You should also be sure to consume foods rich in carotenoids, phytosterols, and flavonoids, that is: raw fruits, vegetables, and certain sprouts, nuts, and seeds. Phytosterols are plant-based compounds that are chemically similar to cholesterol and found in excess in raw nuts and seeds. They can partially block the absorption of dietary cholesterol, therefore having the capacity to lower cholesterol levels. A November 2005 issue of the *Journal of Agricultural and Food Chemistry* suggests that raw pistachios and sunflower seeds have the highest percentage of these compounds, with almonds and macadamia nuts trailing close behind.

> ***Good sources for carotenoids:*** apricots, bell peppers, cantaloupe, carrots, collard greens, kale, leafy green veggies, mangoes, pink grapefruits, spinach, sweet potatoes, swiss chard, and tomatoes.

> ***Good sources for flavonoids:*** apples, apricots, artichokes, bananas, berries, broccoli, buckwheat, celery, flaxseeds, grapefruits, lemons, limes, millet, mung bean sprouts, onions, oranges, peaches, pears, pecans, pistachios, plums, tomatoes, and walnuts.

242

BONE STRENGTH

"The most important dietary change we can make, if we want to create a positive calcium balance that will keep our bones solid, is to decrease the amount of proteins that we eat each day." – **Dr. John McDougall, author of *The Starch Solution***

The *National Osteoporosis Foundation* reports that over ten million Americans have osteoporosis and thirty-four million more have low bone mass. Through it all, these "specialists" still claim they have not discovered the cure. But, we sure do know the cause. We are weakening our bones from eating meat, drinking sodas, drinking coffee, eating clarified sugars, drinking alcohol, and consuming dairy (including milk, cheese, butter, yogurt, cream, whey Kefir, and casein). All of these are acid forming habits and they leach calcium from our bones.

In a study of 460 high school students, conducted in 2000, at the *Harvard School of Public Health*, it was found that, *"Girls who drank carbonated soft drinks were three times as likely to break their arms and legs as those who consumed other drinks. Dark drinks such as Coca-Cola, Pepsi, and Dr Pepper seemed to be even more dangerous than fruit-flavored sodas like Sprite: Girls who downed colas were five times as likely to break arms and legs in their teen years as girls who abstained from carbonated beverages."*

According to a 1988 study published in the journal of *Clinical Endocrinology*, *"Animal protein tends to leach calcium from the bones, leading to its excretion in the urine. Animal proteins are high in sulfur-containing amino acids, especially cystine and methionine. Sulfur is converted to sulfate, which tends to acidify the blood. During the process of neutralizing this acid, bone dissolves into the bloodstream and filters through the kidneys into the urine. Meats and eggs contain two to five times more of these sulfur-containing amino acids than are found in plant foods."* This condition where calcium is excreted in the urine is known as hypercalcuria.

In his book, *Diet for a New America*, John Robbins mentions a study in which *female meat eaters at age sixty-five were studied and found to have an average bone loss of thirty-five percent compared to vegetarians at the age of sixty-five who had only an eighteen percent loss.* Additionally, a 1994 report in the *American Journal of Clinical Nutrition* found *that eliminating animal proteins from the diet results in calcium losses being cut in half.*

When dairy is consumed, the phosphorus in the dairy combines with the calcium in the digestive tract and prevents absorption of the calcium. Dr. Amy Lanou, nutrition director for the *Physicians Committee for Responsible Medicine* in Washington, D.C., states that: *"The countries with the highest rates of osteoporosis are the ones where people drink the most milk and have the most calcium in their diets. The connection between calcium consumption and bone health is actually very weak, and the connection between dairy consumption and bone health is almost nonexistent."*

The common treatment for osteoporosis is a calcium supplement. Doctors and specialists encourage their patients to drink more milk for the calcium. This again reveals that they know very little about nutrition or the way the body works. A twelve year *Harvard Nurses Health Study* conducted on 77,761 women between the ages of thirty-four to fifty-nine, found that *those who consumed the most calcium from dairy foods broke more bones than those who did not drink milk.* This data did not support the hypothesis that higher consumption of milk or dairy foods, said to be rich in calcium, would protect against bone fractures. If you look on the *Harvard University Medical School* website, you will see they no longer promote dairy as being a healthful food. All of the misleading propaganda that we grew up being exposed to, telling us we need milk for strong bones, has resulted in us having the weakest bones of any country in the world.

In 1994, the *American Journal of Epidemiology* published results of a case-controlled study of risk factors for hip fractures in the elderly. The study concluded that *consumption of dairy products, particularly at age twenty years, was associated with an increased risk of hip fracture in old age.*

Bok choy, broccoli, cabbage, chard, collards, dried figs, kale, oranges, and spinach all contain utilizable forms of calcium. Dairy products do not contain a highly utilizable form of calcium, and are devoid of magnesium. You must take in your calcium with magnesium and manganese to form hard tooth enamel and prevent calcium from accumulating in your kidneys. Essential fatty acids also aid in the absorption of calcium and in depositing it into the bones. Raw nuts, seeds, and avocados are good foods to combine with calcium-rich foods.

The key to preventing and reversing osteoporosis is removing acidic foods and beverages from the diet, and replacing them with more alkaline foods. The best way to start is converting to a plant-based, vegan diet rich in greens.

DIABETES – THE MAGICAL DISAPPEARING ACT

At the 2012 *TEDx Conference* in Fremont, Dr. Neal Barnard declared in his speech on reversing the diabetes epidemic, that there are currently one-hundred million Americans that are prediabetic or diabetic. The *Centers for Disease Control and Prevention* estimates that one of every three children born after the year 2000 will develop the disease. What we eat, and what we feed to our children, has more of an impact than we may have previously thought. We did not evolve as humans for our children to develop diabetes, live sickly, depend on pharmaceutical drugs, and die young. In order to stop this trend, we have to begin by educating ourselves on what is causing this disease.

According to a study published in the February 2012 edition of the *American Journal of Clinical Nutrition, processed meat consumption significantly increases the risk of developing diabetes.* Researchers conducted a study on more than two thousand Native Americans living in the Southwestern United States. When the study began, they were all free of diabetes. Those who ate processed meats, such as bacon and sausage, were more likely to develop diabetes after five years.

In 2011, the *Journal of Nutrition* published a study conducted on 15,200 men and 26,187 women throughout the United States and Canada. The participants were grouped as vegans, lacto-ovo vegetarians, pesco-vegetarians, semi-vegetarians, or non-vegetarians. *Incidence of diabetes was almost four times higher in the non-vegetarian group. The other groups were twice as likely to develop diabetes compared to the vegan group. The study makes it obvious that eating fewer animal products greatly reduces your risk for developing diabetes.*

By simply cutting out all animal products, white potato products, fried foods, refined sugars, and high fat foods in general, it is possible to reverse Type II diabetic conditions within a few days to a few weeks. It is also important to eliminate alcohol from the diet. All of these foods enlarge the pancreas and lead to its failure to produce adequate amounts of insulin. Fat also interferes with cellular/insulin interaction. So, it is important to lower fat intake to about ten percent, with those sources being plant-based foods.

All clarified sugars, including agave nectar, brown sugar, cane sugar, corn syrup, honey, powdered sugar, sugar in the raw, and white sugar should be avoided by diabetics. Contrary to what many believe, eating raw, unheated fruits is helpful when reversing diabetes. As long as diabetics eat a low-fat diet, free of animal products, they should not have any reason to worry about the sugars in fruit. The sugars we eat start out in the digestive tract, and then pass through the intestinal wall and into the bloodstream. From the bloodstream, these sugars move into our cells easily. By eating a high-fat diet, the sugars can get trapped in the bloodstream, and the organs are then overworked trying to move them out. Many of these dietary fats can stay in the blood for an entire day before clearing up. This elevates blood sugar levels and leads to diabetes, candida, fatigue, etc.

Although fruits may be high on the glycemic index, the glycemic index only demonstrates how fast carbohydrates turn into blood sugar, failing to inform us how much of these carbohydrates are in a serving of each food. The glycemic load is more accurate for determining how a food elevates blood glucose levels than the glycemic index. All fruits (aside from watermelon) are in the low or medium categories on the glycemic index and glycemic load. Those that are in the medium range (aside from bananas) on the glycemic index are in the low range on the glycemic load. Because fruits consist of mostly water, they have a low glycemic load, even if they are a little higher on the glycemic index. To be sure, we are speaking of raw fruits.

The fibers in fruits tend to slow sugar absorption, so it is better to eat fruits whole, ripe, and raw. While they enter the bloodstream quickly, they also leave the bloodstream and enter the cells quickly. Once in the cells, these sugars provide us with fuel that allows for us to function, as they provide energy. Essentially, we need these sugars for energy, and to sustain life.

Fructose (fruit sugar) enters the cells through diffusion from the bloodstream, rather than via active transport. Glucose enters the cells by active transport. What this reveals to us is that glucose requires insulin to be transported across the cell membrane walls or else uses its stored energy (ATP) for active transport. Fructose requires no adenosine triphosphate (ATP) or insulin because it is absorbed through the cell wall by the diffusion process. This makes fructose (from fresh ripe whole fruits) the perfect sugar for diabetics because it does not create excessive glucose levels in the blood like complex (refined) sugars do.

In a study published in 2004, researchers from **Brigham and Women's Hospital** in Boston and **Harvard Medical School** analyzed data from the **Nurses' Health Study II**, an ongoing trial tracking the health of more than 51,000 women. None of the participants had diabetes at the onset of the study in 1991. Over the following eight years, 741 women were diagnosed with the disease. Researchers found that, *"Women who drank one or more sugary drinks a day gained more weight and were eighty-three percent more likely to develop type 2 diabetes than those who imbibed less than once a month."*

In two separate studies, both published in the *New* England Journal of Medicine, the combination of a reduction of dietary fat and energy, and increased physical activity, was shown to reduce the incidence of diabetes by fifty-eight percent. The reduction in dietary fat (energy density) and increase in fiber were the strongest predictors of weight loss and diabetes protective effects. A sure way to lower fat intake is to avoid bottled oils and remove animal products.

A study was published in the July/August 1982 issue of **Diabetes Care**, which was conducted by the **Department of Surgery** at the **UCLA Medical Center**, and found that, *"Twenty-one of twenty-three patients on oral medications and thirteen of seventeen patients on insulin were able to get off of their medications after twenty-six days on a near-vegetarian diet and exercise program."*

Another contributor to diabetes is the consumption of fried foods, especially foods containing white potatoes. Fried white potato products (potato chips, French fries, etc) are loaded with trans-fats. When these foods break down into sugars, they spike blood sugar levels, causing the pancreas to produce insulin to bring the level back down. When there is fat on the inside of the muscle cells – known as intramyocellular lipids – this interferes with the ability of insulin to let glucose into the cell, so these sugars cannot enter the cells. The fats basically trap the sugars, keeping blood sugar levels high, while the pancreas is doing extra work to bring levels down, and this constant battle for the pancreas eventually leads to it shutting down, resulting in the condition named diabetes.

A February 2006 issue of the *American Journal of Clinical Nutrition* published a study that examined the relation between potato consumption and the risk of developing Type II diabetes. The *Nurses' Health Study* was conducted on 84,555 women and the results found *that the intakes of potatoes and French fries were positively associated with the incidence of type 2 diabetes.* It is not only potato products that induce diabetes. Eating a diet that is high in fat, sugars, and animal protein, especially dairy, is a major cause.

By cutting out high fat foods, such as dairy, eggs, meat, fried foods, and bottled and cooked oils; and eliminating alcohol and clarified sugars from your diet, chances are greater that there will be little, if any, fat inside of the muscle cells, and you can expect your condition to improve. A low-fat, raw vegan diet has proven without failure to reverse this condition. I suggest you read Dr. Gabriel Cousens' book, *There is a Cure for Diabetes*, to find out more about reversing this condition. Dr. Neal Barnard also has a program for reversing diabetes. His book, *Tackling Diabetes*, will walk you through the reversal process. If you have not done so already, I strongly encourage you to read T. Colin Campbell's *The China Study*. Additionally, there is a documentary titled, *Simply Raw: Reversing Diabetes in 30 Days*, which is very insightful and will help you get on the right track to recovery. Type II diabetes is easily curable as long as you are properly educated on the cause of the disease, and maintain good dietary discipline throughout the recovery process.

TOOTH DECAY

"If the teeth are properly treated, they would never decay. There is no more reason, except abuse, why the teeth should ulcerate or become loose, than there is for the fingers or toes, or the ears or the nose, to rot and fall off. The teeth are the densest, firmest of all organic structures and should be the very last, instead of the first, to decay." – Dr. Hereward Carrington

Dental decay is primarily caused by nutritional deficiencies and low-quality food choices. Having unhealthy teeth contributes to poor health. In some cases, poor oral health is an indicator of heart disease, or other underlying disorders. The introduction of white sugars, white flours, canned foods, pasteurized milk, cooked and hydrogenated oils, coffee, cigarettes, and baked foods greatly increased the rates of tooth decay. They are also

247

contributors to heart disease, weakened immune function, obesity, and other maladies. Of these, sodas and baked sweets are considered to be the most damaging.

In a series of studies conducted by Poonam Jain, *Director of Community Dentistry at Southern Illinois University School of Dental Medicine*, Jain stated that, *"Sipping on cola is like bathing your mouth in corrosive acid. Soda eats up and dissolves the tooth enamel."* Jain tested various sodas by measuring their pH – an indication of acidity. Battery acid has a pH of 1, while water is a neutral 7. Jain found that sugary sodas came in at about 2.5, while diet sodas scored 3.2. *"The acidity can dissolve the mineral content of the enamel, making the teeth weaker, more sensitive, and more susceptible to decay,"* Jain said. By eroding the enamel, soda speeds up the decay process, making it easier for bacteria to enter the teeth.

A receding gum line may be the result of calcium deficiency or phosphorus overdose. Individuals who experience tooth decay may not be getting enough calcium, phosphorus, magnesium, or iron, and they may also lack other essential vitamins. They may have an acidic chemistry and would benefit by alkalizing their diet.

If you are experiencing tooth decay, another factor you may want to consider is that you may be lacking vitamin K2. While it is widely recognized that eggs are the best source for K2, this is not the complete truth. If you are looking for a good food source of K2, go for Natto over eggs. Natto is a fermented soy product. I do not eat soy myself, but it is a much better alternative than eggs. Natto has the highest amount of K2 of any food source. It is also not acid forming or detrimental to your health, as are eggs.

We synthesize K2 from our intestinal microflora. As long as we are eating enough foods rich in vitamin K, we will use our healthy bacteria to synthesize K2. There is no reason to worry that you need animal products. You don't.

Foods rich in vitamin K include: kale, kelp, spinach, broccoli, broccoli sprouts, cabbage, asparagus, tomatoes, alfalfa sprouts, turnip greens, wheatgrass juice.

You also need to be sure your intestinal microflora is healthy. If you are in the beginning phases of your diet, a good vegan probiotic supplement could be helpful. Once you have cleansed your system, these will not be as useful, as long as you continue to eat clean, low-fat, and rich in raw fruits and veggies.

To prevent and reverse tooth decay, it is important to eliminate all clarified sugars, refined flours, processed foods, coffee, cigarettes, dairy, and meat from the diet. Eating all plant-based foods will provide your body with the nutrients needed to strengthen tooth enamel and synthesize vitamin K2, resulting in healthy teeth.

HELP ME WITH MY ANXIETY

The *Anxiety Disorders Association of America* reports that anxiety disorders are the most common mental illness in the US, affecting nearly forty million Americans aged eighteen and older. Anxiety disorders cost the US more than forty-two billion dollars annually. With the profits that the medical industry rakes in from the drugs associated with "treating" anxiety, there is a slim chance they will ever bring forth a cure.

What strikes me most about this disorder is that it occurs most commonly among those aged eighteen and older. This is the age when adolescents reach adulthood and begin to smoke cigarettes, drink alcohol, and get out on their own and make unwise food choices. A similar number of adults aged eighteen and older regularly drink alcohol and/or smoke cigarettes. When they drink alcohol and consume refined sugars, they become dehydrated. Dehydration decreases the level of energy generation in the brain. This is one cause of anxiety. Those who like to drink alcohol, smoke cigarettes, drink sodas, coffee, or tea, and eat processed foods containing MSG and other additives, will most likely develop what they call anxiety. Nicotine increases physiological arousal (vasoconstriction) and makes the heart work harder, triggering symptoms of anxiety. Caffeine stimulates an adrenal response, provoking anxiety. Many prescription drugs contain caffeine and amphetamines, thus leading to anxiety. Recreational drugs, like cocaine, have the same effect.

Therefore if you would like this condition to go away, you must refrain from the things that trigger the symptoms of anxiety. This means avoiding gluten grains, sugars, coffee, tea, cola, cigarettes, energy drinks, excitotoxins, MSG, and all food chemicals. Casein, which is the protein in milk and dairy products, should also be avoided because it can cause many symptoms of bi-polar disorder and depression. The main goal for beating anxiety is to alkalize the diet. This can be done by eating plenty of green leafy vegetables and sea vegetables. Incorporating yoga into your life can also help to relax the mind, rejuvenate the spirit, and overcome some symptoms of anxiety.

Studies are revealing that alcohol and anxiety are linked and that those who suffer from anxiety tend to drink more often. A study published in the January 2011 journal *Alcohol and Alcoholism,* states that, *"Those who have anxiety and drink alcohol tend to drink more alcohol over a span of time. Researchers found that sixty-five percent of teens with anxiety who reported drinking at the start of the study continued to drink weekly two years later."*

Clarified sugars and chemical sweeteners, known as excitotoxins, are another anxiety trigger. In the *Anxiety and Phobia Workbook*, E.J. Bourne suggests for those suffering from anxiety to, *"Reduce intake of sweet refined foods, as these affect the blood sugar, and can lead to anxiety and mood swings while also affecting how the brain functions."*

Try replacing your alcoholic drinks with fresh organic green juices containing pinches of dulse and kelp, for the alkalizing minerals. Eat raw organic fruits and vegetables rather than processed foods.

A study recently showed that *nutritional and herbal supplements are an effective method for treating anxiety without side effects.* This study was published in the October 2010 *Nutrition Journal* and suggests *herbal supplements containing passionflower or kava as a remedy for treating anxiety as well as nutritional supplements containing L-lysine and L-arginine.* By eating an array of fruits, vegetables, nuts, seeds, sprouts, seaweeds like kelp and dulse, algae like spirulina and chlorella, and drinking fresh green juices, you will provide your body with these amino acids and other nutrients without the need for nutritional supplements.

An additional report I found to be interesting was published in a 2010 issue of the *Nutrition Journal. Researchers looked at sixty vegetarians and seventy-eight meat-eaters in the Southwestern United States and found that vegetarians scored significantly better on standardized mood tests that measured depression, anxiety, and stress.* This suggests that we should not only cut out alcohol and sugars from the diet to alleviate symptoms of anxiety, but also all animal products. As animals are being slaughtered, stress hormones and adrenaline rush through their system, and this triggers symptoms of anxiety in humans when they eat the contaminated flesh.

GETTING PAST ANEMIA

Centers for Disease Control and Prevention reports that there are roughly 5.3 million annual visits to ambulatory care, with anemia as the primary diagnosis; this number rises each year, and iron deficiency is thought to be the most common cause globally. When we are low in iron, we need magnesium. We store magnesium in our tissues and because of this, blood tests may show we have a sufficient amount, yet we may still be lacking magnesium in our tissues. This helps to explain the high occurrence of anemia. We may not be getting enough magnesium. Therefore, a good way to improve conditions of anemia is by including chlorophyll in our diets. Chlorophyll is centered on the magnesium atom. We can do this by drinking shots of wheatgrass juice three to four times a day and implanting chlorophyll rectally using enema therapy.

A 2008 article published in Nutrition Journal noted that inflammation and iron deficiency are two important causes of anemia. However, little was known about whether magnesium had an impact. After they conducted their study on 2,849 men and women, they found that *the lowest risk of developing anemia was observed among participants with the highest intake of magnesium.* This study supports the claim made by C.L. Kervran in his book, *Biological Transmutations*, that magnesium is biologically transmuted into iron as it is needed in the body. By maintaining a sufficient amount of magnesium in the tissues, the chances of developing an iron deficiency are low.

Wheatgrass juice is rich in chlorophyll and chlorophyll can detox and purify hemoglobin. *A study was conducted between the years 2003-2006 on two-hundred sickle-cell patients who required blood transfusions to determine whether they could reduce the need for transfusions if they were to drink wheatgrass juice. They found the wheatgrass juice had a unique iron-chelating property. After six months of wheatgrass juice therapy, only twenty-four of the study subjects required transfusion. The researchers concluded from the study that wheatgrass juice is an effective alternative to blood transfusion and its use should be encouraged for anemia patients.* The study was published in **Blood**, the **Journal of the American Society of Hematology**, in 2007.

Often, a B12 deficiency may show as symptoms of anemia. If you have low levels of B12 and are experiencing symptoms of anemia, please go back to lesson one and read about B12 deficiency. While many carry the false belief that anemia can be cured by eating red meat or drinking milk, it is important to note that a larger percentage of meat-eaters have anemia than do vegetarians. Green leafy vegetables, which are rich in chlorophyll, arc far superior to meat in iron content. Kale contains nearly fourteen times the amount of iron as red meat.

The *Vegetarian Resource Group* reported that per 100 calories, cooked spinach has 15.7 mg of iron, while sirloin steak has 0.9 mg, and chicken breast has 0.6 mg. Steak, chicken, and animal products provide heme iron, while spinach contains non-heme iron. To absorb this non-heme iron properly, it is important to combine vitamin-C rich foods with foods containing non-heme iron. Heme iron, which is found in animal products, is said to be more easily absorbable, however, it also plays a role in iron-loading related to heart attacks, and the development of cardiovascular disease.

By cutting meat out of the diet, and incorporating wheatgrass juice, raw fruits, and raw green leafy vegetables, you will provide your body with plenty of non-heme iron, as well as vitamin C, and the symptoms of anemia can be expected to subside.

WAIT, I FORGOT MY ALZHEIMER'S

"There is no cure. Doctors don't have a clue how to stop or even prevent this destructive disease. They aren't even sure what causes it. Fortunately, however, there is a way to both prevent and reverse Alzheimer's. It doesn't require drugs, surgeries, radiation, or high tech medical devices. The solution involves coconut ketones – a high energy brain food." – Bruce Fife, coconutresearchcenter.org

Centers for Disease Control and Prevention estimates that as many as five million Americans have Alzheimer's disease. About five percent of men and women between the ages of sixty-five to seventy-four suffer from this disease, while it affects nearly half of all men and women eighty-five and older.

Dr. Bruce Fife states that, *"The fundamental problem associated with Alzheimer's disease is the inability of the brain to effectively utilize glucose, or blood sugar, to produce energy. This defect in energy conversion starves the brain cells and weakens their ability to withstand stress. The brain rapidly ages and degenerates into dementia."*

The solution to the problem, he claims, *"Is to restore the brain's ability to produce the energy it needs to resist stresses that harm the brain, enable it to repair damage, and stimulate growth of new cells."* He suggests eating raw coconut oil to alleviate symptoms. To learn more about his treatment, I suggest reading his book, *Stop Alzheimer's Now*.

In *Sunfood Diet Infusion*, John McCabe states, *"Heterocyclic amines, which form in cooked meat, have been identified as playing a role in the development of neurological disorders, and specifically tremors, or the shaking that people often associate with old age, a condition called kinetic tremor or essential tremor. People experiencing this are also more likely to develop dementia. Other diseases of dementia include Alzheimer's and Creutzfeldt-Jakob disease. In cows, the related disease is Bovine Spongiform Encephalopathy (BSE), also known as mad cow disease. Mad cow disease can be transferred to humans through the consumption of meat. How many cases of Alzheimer's may actually be a misdiagnosis of Creutzfeldt-Jakob disease? We don't know, because the U.S. does not test for CJD in autopsies. We wouldn't want to damage the meat and dairy industries, would we?"*

Even one of the leading experts on Alzheimer's disease, Dr. Rudolph Tanzi, states that there is a clear connection between Alzheimer's disease and meat consumption.

A study published in *Neuroepidemiology* in 1993 found that *heavy meat-eaters have an increased incidence in dementia as do those who are vegetarian.* The *People for the Ethical Treatment of Animals'* (PETA-peta.org) website states: *"Recent research suggests that Alzheimer's disease, like heart disease and strokes, is linked to the saturated fat, cholesterol, and toxins found in meat and dairy products. Studies have shown that people who eat meat and dairy products have a greater risk of developing Alzheimer's disease than do vegetarians. Research also shows that diets high in animal fats have the highest correlation with Alzheimer's disease prevalence. In fact, people who eat large quantities of saturated fats, like those found in meat and dairy products, have twice the* risk of developing Alzheimer's. Meanwhile, people who eat very small amounts of saturated fat in favor of more polyunsaturated fats (found in vegetables and nuts) have a seventy percent reduction in Alzheimer's risk."

It is important to note that plants provide phytochemicals and nutrients such as antioxidants, vitamins, and minerals, which substantially lower the risk of developing Alzheimer's disease. *Harvard researchers discussed the role that fruits and vegetables may play in Alzheimer's disease and evaluated nearly 13,000 participants in a study. They calculated the intake of fruits and vegetables amongst women between 1984 and 1995 and correlated these values with performance on tests of cognitive function conducted between 1995 and 2003, when the women were in their seventies. Those who consumed the most green leafy vegetables and cruciferous vegetables, which are high in folate and antioxidants such as carotenoids and vitamin C, declined less than the women who ate little of these vegetables.* This was discussed at the ***Ninth Annual Conference on Alzheimer's Disease and Related Disorders*** in Philadelphia in July of 2004.

Aluminum toxicity and the food additives known as excitotoxins, such as MSG and other chemical sweeteners, are also contributors to this disease. According to a study published in February 2003 in the ***Archives of Neurology***, "*Those who eat meat, dairy, and eggs as a part of their diets high in fat, cholesterol, and total calories, while being low in fiber, fruits, and vegetables, have a far greater risk of developing Alzheimer's disease.*"

"*In Alzheimer's disease, abnormal accumulations of beta-amyloid are present in the brain. These deposits increase the neurotoxicity of glutamate in the brain. When MSG is consumed, these beta-amyloid proteins then make it more harmful.*"

A study was reported in the ***Journal of Neuroscience*** in 1992 concluding this to be true. Two separate studies published in 1983 in the ***Neuropharmacology*** journal and 1989 in the ***Neurotoxicology and Teratology*** journal reported that MSG demonstrates significant alteration in brain neurochemistry. Despite these reports, the pharmaceutical industry adds MSG and aluminum to medications that are ingested by elderly patients. The foods which elderly patients, and those who suffer from Alzheimer's, are served in hospitals and nursing homes, also contain MSG. The IV's which are administered to Alzheimer's and elderly patients often contain mannitol, an alcohol sugar, which leads to cellular dehydration. This could help explain why no cure is yet to be discovered by the medical industry.

By drinking at least two quarts of pure water every day, cutting meat, dairy, and eggs out of the diet, avoiding all foods and medications containing aluminum and excitotoxins, like MSG and other chemical/artificial sweeteners, and increasing intake of fresh, raw organic fruits and vegetables, and organic unrefined coconut oil, Alzheimer's may be prevented and perhaps somewhat reversed. Fresh vegetable juices and blended green drinks will also do wonders for improving memory.

WHERE HAS MY VISION GONE?

The *Vision Council of America* reports that approximately seventy-five percent of adults use some sort of vision correction, with sixty-four percent wearing glasses and eleven percent wearing contact lenses, either exclusively, or with glasses. The most well documented reason for why we lose our vision is macular degeneration, which is associated with eating meat, dairy, and eggs, which are all rich in free radicals. Free radicals are also produced by the play between light and tissues in the eyes, especially the macula region. A diet high in free radicals, including meat, dairy, eggs, and high temperature cooked foods, overwhelm our system with free radicals, which also damage veins and arteries, and age tissues. Over ninety percent of our population eats meat, dairy, eggs, and high temperature cooked foods. This, in part, explains why we suffer from vision loss. We need antioxidants from plants to clean up the free radicals, and to maintain eye health.

A link was found that positively associates eating red meat with loss of vision. Researchers from the *Royal Victorian Eye and Ear Hospital* found that, *"People who eat red meat more than ten times a week experience increased macular degeneration, leading to vision loss. They found that excessive meat intake – more than ten servings of red meat per week – was associated with a forty-seven percent increased association of early and late macular degeneration. The results come from a study involving 6,734 people from Melbourne, Australia that began in 1990-1994. A follow up study from 2003-2006 determined that higher red meat intake was positively associated with early age-related macular degeneration."* The study also found that a diet high in trans-unsaturated fats is associated with prevalence of late macular degeneration, while a diet low in trans-unsaturated fats and rich in omega-3 fatty acids reduces the risk of this macular degeneration. Trans-fats can be avoided by removing cooked oils from your diet and avoiding dairy, meat, eggs, chocolate, and processed foods. Eating a diet rich in fruits, vegetables, nuts, seeds, and sprouts, especially hemp and chia seeds, will provide omega-3 fatty acids. This was reported in the *American Journal of Epidemiology* in 2009.

In the *Age-Related Eye Disease Study*, it was concluded that *the use of vitamin A as beta-carotene, vitamins C and E, antioxidants, zinc, and copper, can each be beneficial for improving conditions from macular degeneration.* The eye is one of the more susceptible tissues to develop injury from the

254

absence of vitamin A, which we store in our eye tissue. It is far better to eat whole foods containing vitamin A than to take supplements. If you have bad vision, it is important to eat colorful fruits and vegetables, which are naturally rich in antioxidants. We see in colors, therefore it is important to eat colorful foods to help us see more clearly. Free radicals in the body can be damaging to the macula, and especially retina, and providing the body with antioxidants can be very helpful for improving vision and preventing vision loss. Lutein and zeaxanthin are both antioxidants that inhibit damage to the retina from free radicals. These two antioxidants are abundant in foods such as, corn, grapes, kale, kiwi, spinach, and squash. Zeaxanthin is most concentrated in orange bell peppers and yellow corn. Lutein is rich in avocados. By eating avocados with orange bell peppers, this will help to protect, and may improve eyesight. The two carotenoids are absorbed much more efficiently when ingested with good fats. This makes avocado an excellent choice.

The *American Journal of Clinical Nutrition* published a study in March 2011 showing a link between eating meat and developing cataracts. *27,670 participants were divided up into six groups. Those that followed a vegan diet were forty percent less likely to develop cataracts, while the vegetarian group was thirty percent less likely, each being compared to the group that ate meat regularly.* These cataracts are also partially the result of an over-abundance of free radicals and a lack of antioxidants.

Over the years we have discovered that visits to the eye doctor, and wearing glasses, will make your vision far worse over a span of time. When you realize your vision is starting to blur, you should take note that you may be lacking vitamins A, C, or E, antioxidants, and other nutrients. You may want to start eating foods rich in these nutrients before seeing an eye doctor. All cooked oils, meat, heated chocolate, gluten grains, baked foods, dairy, and eggs should be removed from the diet – including both sauteed and fried foods.

If you develop bags under your eyes, this could be a result of eating too much salt. Try balancing your sodium with potassium by eating a few dates, and a banana or two. Dates are richer in potassium than bananas. If you have dark areas under your eyes, this can indicate that you are getting too much potassium and not enough organic sodium. Try balancing these levels by eating organic celery stalks. Dark patches around the eyes can indicate liver toxicity from bad diet, substance abuse, and lack of raw greens.

LIBIDO FUNK

According to the *Minnesota Men's Health Center*, one in every ten men in the world experience erectile dysfunction. Thirty million men in the United States suffer from this condition. Jeff Primack, author of *Conquering Any Disease*, states that, "*Sexual health requires good blood circulation, a healthy nervous system, a functional prostate gland, adequate testosterone levels, healthy adrenal glands, freedom from chemical drugs, and abstinence from smoking and excessive alcohol intake."*

If you are lacking a sex drive, chances are you are doing something you should not be doing. Low libido can be linked to cigarette smoking. Smoking restricts blood vessels, altering the delivery of nutrients to the tissues and damaging the tissues in your body. One who smokes a pack of cigarettes a day is said to increase their chances of developing this condition by more than fifty percent. Alcohol is also linked to low libido.

In the April 2011 issue of the *Journal of Urology*, it was reported that daily use of Aspirin, and other nonsteroidal anti-inflammatory drugs (NSAIDS), is associated with a twenty-two percent increase in the risk of developing erectile dysfunction. 80,966 men aged forty-five to sixty-nine were studied over the course of nine years at the *Kaiser Permanente Los Angeles Medical Center*. The research team, led by Dr. Joseph M. Gleason, assessed the men's use of NSAIDS based on Kaiser's pharmacy records of filled prescriptions and the men's answers to questionnaires about over-the-counter drugs. Roughly forty-percent of the men studied were considered regular NSAIDS users, and nearly thirty percent of them reported moderate or severe erectile dysfunction. The team screened for a variety of other confounding factors, including age, smoking status, diabetes, and other conditions. One factor they did not screen for was consumption of animal products.

In other cases, lack of libido is linked to excess animal proteins, gluten, saturated fat, cholesterol, fried and sautéed oils, bleached foods, lack of exercise, stress, glycotoxins, acrylamides, heterocyclic amines, MSG and other excitotoxins, soy products, and cooked fats in the diet. By removing animal products, soy, and all of these other substances from the diet, while adhering to a raw, plant-based diet, and increasing frequency and duration of exercise, the sex drive will more than likely improve. There is no reason to take chemical pills like Viagra or Cialis, which do temporarily boost libido, when you follow these tidbits of advice. The documentary, *May I Be Frank*, features a man, *Frank Ferrante*, who had no libido prior to his transition to a plant-based diet, and once he began eating plant-based foods, his libido returned.

In September of 2011, a study was published in the *Journal of the American College of Cardiology* that involved 36,744 participants and evaluated the association between erectile dysfunction and the risk of developing cardiovascular disease. The study found that the incidence of *erectile dysfunction is a significant indicator of cardiovascular disease, coronary heart disease, stroke, and all-cause mortality.* Dr. Robert Kloner, a cardiologist at USC's Keck School of Medicine, described the reasoning for this, stating, *"Because arteries in the penis are smaller, atherosclerosis shows up there sooner, perhaps three to four years before the onset of cardiovascular disease."* The results of this study show that the penile arteries can be clogged with plaque sooner than the coronary artery. Eating foods high in cholesterol and fats, such as meat, eggs, dairy, and fried and sauteed foods are leading contributors to a build-up of plaque in the arteries.

An analysis of studies published in the May 2010 issue of the *Journal of Sexual Medicine* reported that, *"Men who eat a diet high in red meats, processed meats, and refined carbohydrates have higher incidence of erectile dysfunction than men who eat more nuts, fruits, and vegetables."*

A study published in the July/August 2011 issue of *Nutrition* journal showed how *ingestion of large quantities of soy-based products in a vegan-style diet results in a sudden onset of loss of libido and of erectile dysfunction. In the study, blood levels of free and total testosterone decreased after the soy was consumed.* This is another reason why soy is not a favorable food to consume on a vegan diet, especially for men.

Because celery stimulates the body to release the sex hormone, androsterone, through sweat, eating a few stalks of celery can enhance libido. The high sodium content also boosts the volume of extracellular fluid, increasing blood volume. Walnuts and watermelon are also excellent foods for reviving libido. Walnuts contain L-Arginine, the amino acid responsible for nitric oxide production and blood vessel dilation. A low-fat diet also improves nitric oxide production. Watermelon is high in L-Arginine, as well rich in lycopene, which is good for the prostate and improves sexual function. Zinc is also a precursor to testosterone and eating foods rich in zinc can boost the libido. Try eating raw pecans, pumpkin seeds, poppy seeds, and ground coriander seeds.

PLEASE MAKE THIS MIGRAINE GO AWAY

The *World Health Organization* indicates that two-thirds of males and eighty-percent of females in developed countries suffer from headaches. They report that migraine alone is nineteenth among all causes of years lived with disability.

I have had several people seek advice from me regarding migraines. This condition can often be easily reversed and alleviated by, first, cleansing internally, and then, maintaining a clean, low-fat, raw organic vegan diet free of gluten. Other foods that should be eliminated include meat, dairy, eggs, caffeine, clarified sugars, and alcohol. On the website for the *Physicians Committee for Responsible Medicine,* they state that, *"Meats, dairy products, and eggs, are best left off your plate permanently. Aside from being among the worst migraine triggers, they also tend to disturb your natural hormone balance, which contributes to migraines."* These foods also break down into bowel toxins, which trigger headaches.

Dr. Robert Cohen, organizer of *notmilk.com*, lists alcohol, cheese, and chocolate as the three most common triggers for migraines. He references a study published in the *Pediatric* journal in 1989 suggesting that, *"Dairy products may play a major role in the development of migraine headaches."*

As explained by Dr. Henry Bieler in *Food Is Your Best Medicine*, *"A migraine headache originates in the colon or stomach. It is a sign of indigestion due to excessive eating, allergic reactions, and fermentation of starch and/or putrefaction of protein, which produces a wide range of toxins in the stomach. The resulting detoxification activities overwork the liver and kidneys; the endocrine glands attempt to direct the toxins to other eliminative organs. This hyper function can cause them to swell. As the pituitary gland enlarges, it presses against its bony enclosure, causing the severe pain of a migraine headache."*

Because of relation between headaches and digestion, I suggest colon hydrotherapy to detoxify the colon. A neurologist or medical doctor will rarely suggest this; they are more likely to prescribe medicine, and little else, leaving patients relying on the false and defeating hope in drugs.

Dr. Norman Walker used colonic irrigation to erase migraine headaches in patients. He lived to be one-hundred and sixteen years old. He states in *Become Younger*, *"A headache may usually be an indication that waste matter in the colon is either clogging up that organ excessively or that it has been allowed to overstay its welcome and as a result is causing poisons to be absorbed from the colon into the system. In my study of thousands of cases of migraines, the colon has been the greatest headache of all, because people will not stop to think, and realize the relation between it and the pain."*

He also goes on to say, *"When we are bothered with a migraine, it is the nerves that are sounding the alarm to do something constructive to help remedy whatever has gone wrong in our system. To take aspirin or medicine for example, merely deadens the nerve to stop the warning. It is exactly like cutting the wires of your front doorbell because your neighbors have come to warn you that your house is on fire. Whatever we take to 'kill' or deaden pain, numbs or drugs the nerves. It may be alright to give us temporary relief, provided that we do something to remedy the cause and thereafter promptly take steps to get the painkiller out of the system."*

"By far, the larger share of headache has its origin in that foul state of the system, particularly the stomach and the bowels, caused either by bad dietetic habits or by an insufficient elimination of morbid matter through the bowels, skin, lungs or kidneys." – Dr. Martin Luther Holbrook

My best advice for relieving symptoms of migraine headaches is to go in for a colon hydrotherapy session. This will assist in the elimination of plaque that is coating intestinal walls, and the walls of the bowels. Then, follow this by adhering to a clean and alkaline diet, rich in raw greens, with additional chlorella and spirulina. Avoid all meat, dairy, eggs, alcohol, clarified sugars, caffeine, MSG, gluten, excitotoxins, fried oils, and chocolate, and replace them with more raw fruits, vegetables, and plant-based foods. Sometimes simply drinking water and eating juicy fruits can relieve headache symptoms.

ADHD AND NUTRITION

According to the *Centers for Disease Control and Prevention*, 4.5 million children in the United States are afflicted with *Attention-Deficit Hyperactivity Disorder* (ADHD). The *U.S. National Library of Medicine* states that this is the most commonly diagnosed behavioral disorder of childhood, affecting anywhere from three to five percent of school-aged children. As with all diagnosed conditions in their profession, medical doctors do not hesitate to write up prescriptions and pass out drugs to these children. If children stopped eating toxic foods, but got true nutrition, there would be no reason to prescribe drugs, and we could resort to much less poisoning of our children by means of dangerous prescription drugs.

In a July 2012 study published in the *Pediatric Journal*, it was determined that the amount of prescriptions handed out for ADHD drugs increased forty-six percent from 2002 to 2012. In an attempt to explain the increase, Dr. Scott Benson, a child and adolescent psychiatrist and spokesperson for the *American Psychiatric Association*, stated, *"For the most part, I think the overall increase reflects a reduction in the stigma. It used to be believed that, 'You are a bad parent if you cannot get your child to behave, and you are a doubly bad parent if you put them on medicine.'"*

According to a March 2011 study published in the *Lancet Journal*, the lead author, Dr. Lidy Pelsser, of the ADHD Research Centre in the Netherlands, announced that sixty-four percent of children diagnosed with ADHD are, in fact, experiencing a hypersensitivity to food. Researchers determined this by placing children on a very elaborate diet. After a few weeks, the diet was restricted. According to Pelsser, *"After being on the diet, the children simply behaved the way normal children do. No longer were they easily distracted, or forgetful, and their temper tantrums subsided."*

In a May 2011 study published in *Pediatrics Journal*, it was found that the organophosphate pesticides found in conventional fruits and vegetables also play a role in the development of ADHD. In this study, the levels of pesticide residues found in the urine of 1,100 children aged eight to fifteen were measured. Researchers recognized that the children with the highest levels of pesticides also had the highest incidence of ADHD. A 2008 *Emory University* study found that children who converted to eating only organically grown fruits and vegetables had their urine levels of pesticide compounds drop to undetectable, or close to undetectable levels.

Often, children are experiencing sensitivity to casein, which is the protein in cow's milk, or gluten, the protein in wheat – found in many grains, cereals, and other common food items. This may cause the hypersensitivity relating to ADHD. By removing gluten grains, replacing cow's milk with almond, coconut, or hemp milk, cutting out refined sugars, and being sure our children consume nourishing organic fruits and vegetables, their mental health would improve. Resorting to nature and real food is always the best option for overcoming any health condition.

EPILEPSY

The *Centers for Disease Control and Prevention* reports that epilepsy results in an estimated annual cost of $15.5 billion in medical costs and lost or reduced earnings. They claim that epilepsy affects nearly two million Americans. Epilepsy is defined as a chronic neurological condition, characterized by recurrent seizures. Medical science still fails to provide a reason for the development of this condition, nor do they provide a cure – but still relies on drugs as a solution.

In 1987, the U.S. senate held a hearing which was titled, *NutraSweet: Health and Safety Concerns*. During this hearing, several people from all walks of life testified about their aspartame-induced grand mal seizures. Each one reported that their seizures went away after abstaining from aspartame.

Aspartame consists of phenylalanine and aspartic acid, which bypass the blood-brain barrier, and directly alter neurological function. Aspartic acid triggers aspartate receptors, contributing to epilepsy. Sufficient levels of magnesium have been shown in studies to block the activation of these aspartate receptors.

Magnesium deficiency is often common amongst those who suffer from epilepsy. Many who experience epileptic seizures have improper mineral assimilation, most commonly with calcium and magnesium. A deficiency of vitamin B6 has also been linked to epilepsy.

The journal of *Neuroscience and Medicine* reported a study in 2010 showing that low cerebrospinal fluid magnesium is associated with epilepsy. The study included seventy-two patients and seventy-five healthy subjects with ages ranging from nineteen to ninety-three years. In the group of patients with convulsive seizures, low levels of magnesium were revealed. The study found that, *"Magnesium regulates the binding, or function, of opiate and N-methyl-D-aspartate (NMDA) receptors. Magnesium, at physiological concentrations, blocks NMDA receptors in neurons. Many NMDA receptor antagonists have a potent antiepileptic properties and activation of NMDA receptors may also contribute to epileptogenesis."* This study tells us that magnesium in the tissues will block the aspartate receptors, while low levels of magnesium will activate these receptors and make the subject more susceptible to epileptic seizures. The results of the study indicated that *magnesium deficiency may play a role in seizure manifestation.*

My best advice for freeing yourself from epileptic conditions would be to include rich sources of chlorophyll in your diet. Chlorophyll is centered on the magnesium atom. If possible, drink wheatgrass shots daily. Drink plenty of vegetable juices containing the juice of green leafy vegetables. Eat foods rich in magnesium (spinach, kale, chard, pine nuts, sprouted pumpkin seeds, sunflower green sprouts, wheatgrass juice), foods rich in B6 (brussels sprouts, cabbage sprouts, sprouted mango seed, sprouted sweet potatoes, wheatgrass juice), and foods rich in organic calcium (dried figs, freshwater algae, green leafy vegetables, green beans, sea algae, sprouted sesame seeds, sprouted sunflower seeds). Drink raw organic apple cider vinegar daily. Avoid all refined foods. Avoid all refined sugars, including corn syrup and agave. Stay away from excitotoxins, such as MSG and chemical sweeteners. Get plenty of exercise, mentally and physically. Practice yoga regularly. Sleep in a dark room, avoid blinking lights, and refrain from using fluorescent bulbs. It is also important to get fresh air, some sun, and even moonlight.

LYME DISEASE

If noticed immediately, Lyme disease can be successfully treated within weeks, but after Lyme disease (borrelia burgdorferi) enters the body, it leaves the bloodstream and travels into the lymph and tissues. Once this has happened, it is difficult to treat. A study published in the May 2011 issue of *PLoS Pathogens* journal provides a reasonable explanation for this process. The author summarizes that, "*Once infected with live* Borrelia burgdorferi *spirochetes (the bacteria that cause Lyme disease), live spirochetes collect in the lymph nodes. These lymph nodes then swell up and start producing large numbers of antibody-producing cells. Although many of these antibodies can recognize the bacteria, they apparently lack the quality to clear the infection. We hypothesize that by moving into the lymph node, usually a site in which strong immune responses are induced, Borrelia evades the immune response: it goes to the lymph nodes and tricks the immune system into making a very strong but inadequate response.* "There is an internal cleansing process known as a lymphatic drainage, which stimulates the lymph fluid and draws out toxins. This procedure may help draw the bacteria out of the lymph system.

Dr. Russell Blaylock theorizes in *Health and Nutrition Secrets* that, "*The neurological damage associated with Lyme disease is most likely produced by an immune-triggered excitotoxic reaction.* "What he means is that the body secretes glutamate and quinolinic acid when inflicted with this

261

disease. This tells us it is important to avoid all excitotoxins, especially MSG, aspartame, and artificial sweeteners if one hopes to heal from this disease.

If I were diagnosed with Lyme disease, I would go in for internal cleansing, combining lymphatic drainage with wheatgrass juice enemas. I would also be sure to drink wheatgrass juice daily and refrain from eating foods that clog the lymph system, such as dairy, meat, eggs, fried oils, bleached foods, and gluten. In addition, I would exercise daily, especially including cardiovascular exercises.

THE COLD REMEDY

The body creates mucus to protect the tissues and to help contain and rid the body of foreign substances. The onslaught of bad foods, foreign cholesterol, and a plunge in fresh food consumption during cold months backs up and confuses the system. Taking drugs to try to alleviate the symptoms can add to the toxicity, backing up the system even more. It is best to do a juice cleanse when you are feeling a cold begin to creep up on you.

Prior to him transitioning from a vegetarian to vegan diet, my younger brother would ask me to make him remedies if he ever felt a cold or sinus infection coming on, and this is what I always had him do:

I first informed him that he was feeling this way because he had been eating dairy. I instructed him to avoid all dairy and animal products. Then, I had him eat slices of organic black radish (black radish ihelps rid excess mucus). I also had him eat organic figs (another highly mucus dissolving food). He then inserted slices of fresh organic garlic into each nostril. Be sure that you do not snort the garlic slices into the sinus cavity, only breathe in the vapors. The allicin in garlic is what they add to the antibiotics being prescribed for treating sinusitis and other common cold symptoms. Rather than poison the body with synthetically created antibiotics, the garlic provides the anti-bacterial compound in its more powerful and natural state. He finished by drinking a mixture of organic wheatgrass juice with raw organic apple cider vinegar, diluted with a little water.

In a 2001 study published in the *Advances in Therapy* journal, one-hundred forty-six volunteers were randomized to receive a placebo or an allicin-containing garlic supplement over a twelve week period and any common cold infections were reported. *The group ingesting garlic had significantly fewer colds, while the placebo group reported significantly more days challenged virally.*

One can also gargle with apple cider vinegar several times throughout the day. Fresh citrus, not citrus juice that has been canned, bottled, jarred, reconstituted, or otherwise pasteurized, can also be helpful for alleviating symptoms of colds. Pasteurization kills nutrients and also separates the methane from the pectin, and that is not good for the nerves. It becomes almost like a very gentle neurotoxin, weaker than chocolate, which does contain a stronger neurotoxin.

SKIN IS A MIRROR OF THE INTERNAL ORGANS

Our skin is the largest eliminative organ of the body and the condition of our skin is a direct reflection of our internal organs. If we have a condition on the skin such as eczema, dermatitis, acne, or psoriasis, this reveals that our internal environment is overloaded with toxins and we must cleanse internally.

In cases of eczema, sensitivity to gluten could be causing the reaction. Most patients with eczema have elevated levels of anti-gliadin antibodies. Gliadin is one of the two proteins in gluten. Those with celiac disease and gluten sensitivity are unable to digest gliadin. This results in the body attempting to eliminate the gliadin through the skin, causing formation of eczema.

It is best for everyone to avoid gluten in general. In 2000, the *British Journal of Dermatology* published an article finding that *sixteen percent of psoriasis patients also had elevated levels of anti-gliadin antibodies.*

In the case of psoriasis, it may be a sign of an unhealthy condition in the liver. The results of a prospective study were published in a 2010 issue of the *Archives of Dermatology* linking an association between alcohol consumption and psoriasis. 116,671 US women between the ages of twenty-seven to forty-four were studied over the course of fifteen years. Overall, *women drinking more than 2.3 alcoholic beverages per week were at greater risk for psoriasis. The risk was 180 percent higher for those who drank five or more beers per week than for those refraining from alcohol.*

Cigarette smoking has also been linked with psoriasis. In January of 2012, the *American Journal of Epidemiology* published an article where *investigators examined research projects that followed more than 185,000 medical professionals in the United States for as long as two decades. They looked specifically at 2,410 people who had been diagnosed with psoriasis. The researchers found that current smokers were 190 percent more likely to develop psoriasis.* Dr. Joel Gelfand, who is the medical director of the *University of Pennsylvania's Department Of Dermatology Clinical Studies Unit,* explained the possible reasoning for this by stating, *"Since psoriasis is an inflammatory disease, it is plausible that smoking lights the fire that leads to chronic inflammation of psoriasis in people who are susceptible."*

The use of cocaine has been linked to psoriasis. I have read reports of cocaine addicts entering treatment facilities and in a large percentage of them, the skin condition was documented. I know several people who have psoriasis and use cocaine. This drug is a hazard to your health and longevity.

A study published in the ***Archives of Dermatology***, titled, ***Low-Protein Diet and Psoriasis***, determined after a hospital study that, *"Limiting the intake of animal proteins will lessen the severity of psoriasis and conditions will begin to fade."* The ammonia and uric acid that is created from the metabolism of these proteins is most likely the reason for this occurrence.

Furthermore, experimental data and clinical evidence obtained by the ***Institute of Food Science at the University of Hannover*** in Germany showed that *diet plays a role in the etiology and pathogenesis of psoriasis.* The data, which was published in a 2005 issue of the ***British Journal of Dermatology***, suggested that *fasting periods and vegetarian diets improved psoriasis symptoms.*

Atopic dermatitis is a common condition in children today. In May of 1998, the ***European Review of Medical and Pharmacological Science*** reported that *cow's milk is the most common food linked to this condition.* It was estimated that fourteen percent of children suffer from atopic dermatitis and nearly twenty-five percent from adverse reactions to cow's milk. *In a separate study, researchers excluded milk and eggs from the diet of fifty-nine children aged two to eight with severe atopic dermatitis and recorded the effects it had on the condition. Clinical improvement was observed in eighty percent of the cases.* The results were published in the ***Journal of Allergologia et Immunopathologia*** in Spain. By removing cow's milk, and eggs, from the diet, the condition subsides in children.

These studies reveal that it is highly important to eliminate all gluten, dairy, and refined foods from our diet to alleviate skin conditions. Because animal protein has been linked to many cases of psoriasis, it is wise to avoid all meat, dairy, eggs, and foods containing them. By drinking fresh juices, eating raw organic fruits and vegetables, and eliminating prescription drugs, cocaine, gluten grains, cigarette smoke, and alcohol from your life, you can expect your skin conditions to improve.

NO MORE PAIN

Centers for Disease Control and Prevention reports that an *estimated fifty million adults have claimed that they have been told by a doctor that they have some form of arthritis. One in five adults reports having doctor diagnosed arthritis. From 2007-2009, fifty percent of adults over sixty-five reported having an arthritis diagnosis.*

The most common form of arthritis is osteoarthritis. Gout, fibromyalgia, and rheumatoid arthritis are other related conditions. The ***Arthritis Rheum*** journal reports the following: *an estimated twenty-seven million adults had* osteoarthritis in 2005; an estimated 1.5 million adults had rheumatoid arthritis in 2007; an estimated three million adults had gout in 2005 and 6.1 million reported ever having gout; an estimated five million adults had fibromyalgia in 2005.

In 2006, *Arthritis and Rheumatism* journal estimated that, by the year 2030, sixty-seven million Americans aged eighteen and older are projected to have doctor-diagnosed arthritis. In 2007, the *Arthritis Care and Research* journal estimated that 294,000 children under the age of eighteen have some form of arthritis or rheumatic condition. This is approximately one in every two-hundred fifty children. Nowhere in human evolution were we meant to be predisposed to having such extreme pain as those who suffer from arthritis experience.

What these statistics tell me is that there is something unnatural that we are doing that is causing the prevalence of arthritic conditions to be so high. Eating animal products is unnatural for the human system. Eating meat acidifies the body and produces uric acid, which is a waste product of protein metabolism. When the blood is too acidic, arthritic conditions often begin to develop. Uric acid is also a by-product of the metabolism of clarified sugars. The liver and the kidneys can only excrete about eight grams of uric acid in a twenty-four hour period of time. One pound of meat contains around sixteen grams, so you are taking in double the amount your body can handle with each pound of meat eaten. This uric acid then lays the groundwork for gout and arthritis to develop. Therefore, it is important to alkalize the blood with plant-based foods and sea vegetables.

In his book, *Foods that Fight Pain*, Dr. Neal Barnard presents a four-week anti-arthritis diet. In this diet, he lists several foods that are arthritis triggers. These foods are: all dairy products, all meats, eggs, corn, wheat, oats, rye, potatoes, tomatoes, and coffee. The majority of these are acid-forming foods. The reason why dairy is a burden is not the fat content, but the protein it contains. Therefore, skim milk is also harmful. To free yourself from arthritis, you must make an obligation that you give up all animal products.

Dr. John McDougall conducted a study that was published in a 2002 issue of the *Journal of Alternative Complementary Medicine*. He studied the effects of a low-fat vegan diet on subjects with rheumatoid arthritis and found that *after only four weeks on the diet, almost all rheumatoid arthritis symptoms decreased significantly.*

In a November 2000 issue of *Toxicology,* a study was published which was conducted by the *Department of Physiology* at the *University of Kuopio* in Finland, and concluded, *"A raw vegan diet, rich in antioxidants and fiber, decreases joint stiffness and pain in patients with rheumatoid arthritis."*

If you have an arthritic condition, it is important to filter your water. Tap water is high in total dissolved solvents, which may accumulate in the body, causing calcification of the joints. Drinking distilled water may help pull out the inorganic deposits that have accumulated and are causing your arthritic pains.

"I have found distilled water is a sovereign remedy for my rheumatism. I attribute my almost perfect health largely to distilled water." – Dr. Alexander Graham Bell

If you want your arthritic conditions to subside, you must refrain from eating meat, dairy, eggs, nightshade plants, and all other arthritis triggers from Dr. Barnard's list. Nightshades consist of tomatoes, tomatilloes, potatoes, peppers of all types, eggplants, and chilies. Try cutting all of these foods from your diet, drink distilled water, take a daily shot of Bragg's raw organic apple cider vinegar, and be sure to get enough vegan probiotics. Maintaining healthy intestinal flora has been shown to improve conditions.

In his book *Conquering Any Disease,* Jeff Primack provides a recipe for *Ginger Firewater.* The recipe requires chopping a large piece of organic ginger root and boiling it with five to six cups of distilled water and a small handful of goji berries. You can also add some turmeric root. Boil the mixture until there are only about two cups of water remaining. This should take about an hour (depending on where you live, sea level or mountains). Then, after cooling, drink the entire serving in one sitting. Ingesting this is said to naturally reduce pain and inflammation.

HOW COULD I BE ALLERGIC TO FOOD?

If you have sensitivity to fresh fruit, the disturbance from the fruit enzymes may be due to the over-acidic nature of your blood and body. As I mentioned in a previous chapter, I met a girl who thought she had allergies to fruits. I observed her situation very closely and realized all of the fruits to which she reacted were the ones that contain the highest amounts of pesticides. When she switched from conventional strawberries to organic strawberries she was fine.

Dr. Stuart Berger wrote the book, *The Immune Power Diet,* as he attempted to help his mother beat cancer using optimal nutrition. He worked with several clients to help rid them of their allergies. He found that there are seven foods that cause a reaction over all others in the majority of his client base. These seven foods are: *cow's milk products, wheat, yeast, eggs, corn, soy products, and cane sugar or refined sugars.* By eliminating these seven foods from your diet, your food allergies may subside.

The reason why we have food allergies and digestive problems may simply be because we do not know how to properly combine foods. A typical plate from the Standard American Diet has a meat, mixed with a cheese, mixed with a starch (gluten grains, bread, pasta, potato), and in some cases, an overcooked vegetable. That platter is also filled with a variety of heat-created chemicals.

The starch molecule and meat both require different mediums of digestive juices for digestion and when they are eaten together, the juices neutralize each other, to a degree, and the food does not break down efficiently. Rather, the meat putrefies into harmful bacteria, and the starches ferment. The cheese and dairy being eaten create excess mucus.

In *Guide to Diet and Detoxification,* Dr. Bernard Jensen writes, *"An amazing number of food allergies clear up completely when supposedly allergic individuals learn to eat their foods in digestible combinations. What they suffer from is not allergy, but indigestion. Allergy is a term applied to animal protein poisoning. Indigestion results in putrefactive poisoning, which is a form of animal protein poisoning. Normal digestion delivers nutrients, not poisons!"*

SAY GOODBYE TO THAT INHALER

In 2009, the *American Academy of Allergy, Asthma, and Immunology* reported that approximately 24.6 million people in the United States have asthma. They estimate that three-hundred million people suffer from asthma worldwide. Many believe asthma is a condition they were born with that cannot be reversed; I'd like to present a different perspective.

Asthma is often linked to the consumption of cow's milk, all dairy, dietary fat from meat and eggs, alcohol, and caffeine and excitotoxins, including MSG, and artificial sugar. Therefore, if you want to reverse asthma, start by eliminating these from your diet. Childhood use of antibiotics also increases asthma, as does gluten, and certain other food chemicals. The use of antibiotics in pregnant women has also been shown to increase asthma in the child.

In his *Encyclopedia of Natural Healing,* Professor Gary Null writes, *"In all respiratory conditions, mucus-forming dairy foods, such as milk and cheese, can exacerbate clogging of the lungs and should be avoided."* When more of this mucus accumulates in the lungs than can be expelled, asthma attacks are most likely to develop. Dairy is linked to asthma to the extent that *a mother eating yogurt while pregnant can increase her newborns likeliness of developing asthma at birth by sixty percent.* This was determined from researching 61,912 women in Denmark, who were a part of the *Danish National Birth Cohort Study.* The information was presented at the *European Respiratory Society's Annual Congress* in September of 2011.

Animal fats contain an inflammatory carcinogen known as arachidonic acid. This acid worsens the symptoms of asthma and is found in all high-fat animal products. When animal proteins are metabolized, they also form uric acid. A report in the April 2011 *Immunity Journal* declared that *uric acid is released in the airways of allergen-challenged asthmatic patients.* The researchers found that *uric acid is an essential initiator and amplifier of allergic inflammation.* To alleviate asthmatic conditions, it is important to avoid all meat and animal products, including eggs. Many people successfully reverse asthma by resorting to the low-fat raw vegan diet rich in fruits and vegetables – and they find it to be much easier to do cardiovascular exercise.

Asthma indicates that your body has increased production of histamine. The histamine regulates the bronchial muscle contraction and when you have excess amounts, the result is less water evaporation (due to the bronchial restriction) during breathing.

When asthmatic attacks or issues occur, mucus is secreted to protect the lung tissues. This narrows the airways. Therefore it is important to eat mucus dissolving foods. Good mucus-dissolving foods include, black radishes/radishes, figs, olives, raisins and spinach. Raw organic apple cider vinegar can also be helpful.

Clinical Immunology published a study in 2009 concluding that a compound in cruciferous vegetables prevents respiratory inflammation. The compound is a protective antioxidant enzyme known as sulforaphane. These enzymes are found in broccoli, cabbage, kale, cauliflower, collards, and other cruciferous vegetables. They help to reduce the risk of respiratory inflammation that leads to chronic diseases, such as asthma and COPD. *Researchers found that participants who were given the highest dose of sulforaphane had as much as three times as many antioxidant enzymes in their upper airway cells compared to baseline.*

Goji berries, being rich in beta carotene, are considered helpful in the reduction of asthma attacks. Kiwis may also be beneficial because they contain highly absorbable Vitamin C. Organic virgin unrefined coconut oil may also be beneficial because of one of the medium chain fatty acids, monolaurin, which has highly antibacterial, antihistamine, antiviral, and antifungal properties. Making tea with comfrey or even drinking comfrey juice can also help.

It was recently reported that a group of researchers from the United Kingdom developed a method of studying asthma by growing lung cells from asthma patients in a laboratory. They now can study the tissues to see how they differ from tissues of a non-asthmatic person and test potential therapies for them. This new method will reduce the unethical experimentation on animals for asthma studies that have been conducted in the past. This information was presented by Kristie Sullivan, M.P.H. from the *Research Ethics Department of the Physician's Committee for Responsible Medicine.*

FROM MS TO NORMAL

Multiple Sclerosis (MS) is one of the most common neurological diseases in the United States. Nearly five-hundred thousand Americans suffer from MS, while it is believed that nearly 2.5 million worldwide do. Those who suffer from MS experience recurrent attacks on their nervous system, which alters their senses and various bodily functions. The good news is that many people are improving from multiple sclerosis by cleaning up their diet.

It is important to understand that MS is an autoimmune disease, so an autoimmune reaction is disrupting the electrical signals carrying messages to and from the brain and spinal cord, which are the two components of the central nervous system. There is a sheath of myelin, which is a fatty substance that covers each of your nerves. This sheath helps transmit these messages between the brain and other parts of the body. The messages then control movements and motor skills. The autoimmune reaction destroys this myelin sheath.

Dr. Roy swank is considered to be the first to link diet to MS. In the 1940's he began conducting a study on 144 patients with the disease. His idea was that there was a link between animal-based foods high in saturated fats and this autoimmune disease. In *The China Study,* Dr. Campbell writes about Swank and how, *"He divided patients up into two groups, one group eating a diet low in saturated fats, and the other eating more than twenty grams a day of saturated fats. After keeping records on them for thirty-four years, he concluded that, of those following the low saturated fat diet, about ninety-five percent remained only mildly disabled and only five percent of them died. Of the group following a high fat diet, eighty percent of them died from MS."*

In a 2005 issue of *Multiple Sclerosis Journal,* an article was published on nutrition and its link to MS. It reported that, *"Several investigations noted a higher prevalence of MS in correlation with greater intakes of fat and protein, specifically, higher intake of saturated fats found in foods of animal origin. These foods included meat, milk, butter, and eggs."*

Dr. John McDougall treats his MS patients with a whole food vegan diet free from added oils. In an article published in the *Vegetarian Times* journal, titled *Treating Multiple Sclerosis with Diet – Fact or Fraud?,* he states that, *"To arrest MS, the diet must be as low in saturated fat as possible, approximately six percent of total calories. This translates into a low-fat vegan diet."* In this same article, he suggests that, *"MS attacks could be caused by a decreased supply of blood to the brain tissues. Dietary fat has this effect by entering the bloodstream and coating the blood cells. As a result, the cells stick together, forming clumps that slow the flow of blood to vital tissues."*

In addition to animal products, drinking soda also contributes to the onset of this disease. While aspartame has been linked multiple times to developing MS, the phosphoric acid found in the chemical concoctions known as sodas, also do damage to the myelin sheath. Researchers from the *Department of Neurology at the University Hospital* in the Netherlands conducted a study on thirty-nine patients with MS and fifteen healthy subjects. They found that, "*The MS spectra had increased levels of creatine phosphates. This increase was correlated with the severity of the handicap and was greater in patients with a progressive course of the disease.*"This study was published in the *Archives of Neurology* in 1992. Uric acid from meats, and arachidonic acid from animal fats, do similar damage to the sheath.

By drinking sodas, ingesting chemical sweeteners, eating meats, eggs, and dairy products, and through exposure to mercury (amalgam fillings, fish, and other animal foods), the myelin sheath erodes. This is the cause of MS. The acidity from the soda and other foods eats away at the sheath. When the sheath is no longer present, or is damaged, the electrical signals from the brain and spinal cord no longer work efficiently.

If you suffer from MS, be sure to nourish yourself with an adequate amount of B vitamins and magnesium. Because most B vitamins are created by friendly bacteria, probiotics are very helpful with overcoming MS. Vitamin B1, magnesium, B6, and B12 are also needed from food sources. The best foods for these nutrients are, sea vegetables, leafy green vegetables, and raw fruits. These foods will create an alkaline state in the body, which could speed up the recovery process. Along with eliminating all sodas, meat, eggs, dairy, artificial sweeteners, MSG, excitotoxins, and mercury from the diet, you should incorporate these nutrient-rich foods. Remember that we are exposed to mercury from eating fish and other animal foods. It also bioaccumulates in the environment from industrial pollutants, such as coal plants, cement kilns, and fossil fuels. Be sure to avoid mercury.

If I were diagnosed with MS, I would take an organic greens superfood supplement, such as *Infinity Greens, Vitamineral Green, Green Vibrance,* or *Field of Greens,* twice daily for the enzymes, probiotics, and alkalizing nutrients. Enzymes are best derived from raw fruits and veggies, not from packaged products, so I would be sure to eat plenty of raw fruits and vegetables as well. I would also eat sulfur-rich foods, such as kale, broccoli sprouts, arugula, wild greens, dandelion, brussels sprouts, cabbage, kelp, onions, garlic, broccoli, and radishes, to go along with organic spirulina, pure phycocyanin, and AFA super blue green algae daily. The sulfur acts as an opposite to mercury, so by eating sulfur-rich foods, it is possible to eliminate mercury from the body.

FIBER AND DIVERTICULA

"As food moves through the small intestine, the nutrients (proteins, fats, carbohydrates, vitamins, and minerals) are absorbed through the intestinal wall and into the bloodstream. Left behind are non-digestible matter (dietary fiber), colon bacteria, and many dead cells that will soon become the stool. This material passes into the right side of the large intestine and is then moved to the left side by rythmic contractions known as peristalsis. According to the well-known law of physics, the Law of Laplace, contractions at small diameters cause high pressures. If there is minimal fiber in the diet, and therefore very little stool mass, these contractions occur at high pressures. Years of elevated pressures produce ruptures in the walls of the intestine (balloon-like bulges) known as diverticula. Half of people who have followed the Western diet (meat, dairy, eggs, sugars, gluten grains) for more than fifty years have diverticular disease." – **Dr. John McDougall, Digestive Tune-Up**

The *National Digestive Diseases Information Clearinghouse* reports that half of people between the ages of sixty and eighty have diverticular disease and nearly all people over eighty have some level of it. The reason for the occurrence is a lack of fiber in the diet and a lack of healthy bacteria in the system. This lack of fiber is a result of eating animal products, bleached foods, and cooked oils. All meat, eggs, and dairy products are void of fiber. The intestinal flora become damaged as a result of a combination of poor quality foods and diverticula accumulate in the bowels.

The addition of fiber to the diet is important for reversing diverticular disease. Therefore, it is important to know the difference between soluble and insoluble fibers. *Soluble fiber* dissolves in water and converts to a gel-like substance in the small intestine, slowing digestion, and delaying the absorption of nutrients. Beta-glucans, gums, and pectins are soluble fibers. These can be found in apples, beans, citrus fruits, ground flaxseeds, lentils, mushrooms, oats, pears, peas, prunes, and psyllium. *Insoluble fiber* does not dissolve in water and increases the bulk of the stool, thus relieving constipation, and helping to alleviate symptoms of this disease. This fiber can be found in fruits, such as apples, avocados, cherries, melon, and pineapple, and vegetables such as cabbage, cauliflower, celery, chard, cucumber, kale, leafy greens, parsnips, spinach, and turnips. These fibers can also be found in beans and lentils. All fruits, veggies, nuts, and seeds contain fiber, but people with diverticulitis may have difficulty with ungerminated and unsprouted seeds, and seeds that have been heated.

The *American Dietetic Association* recommends eating twenty to thirty-five grams of fiber rich food every day to prevent the disease. Fiber is the indigestible part of plant foods. Plants contain cellulose fibers and when we chew them up, they release cellulase enzymes, which aid in their digestion.

In July 2011, *BMJ Journal* reported a study that examined the associations of a vegetarian diet and dietary fiber intake with risk of diverticular disease. The study was conducted by the *Nuffield Department of Clinical Medicine* at Oxford University. They studied 47,033 men and women living in Scotland and England. 15,459 of them reported consuming a vegetarian diet. All subjects were measured for dietary fiber intake. After a mean follow-up time of 11.6 years, they determined that, "*Vegetarians had a thirty-one percent lower risk of developing diverticular disease than meat eaters. After mutual adjustment, both a vegetarian diet and a higher intake of fiber were significantly associated with a lower risk of diverticular disease.*"

The researchers concluded that, "*Consuming a vegetarian diet and a high intake of dietary fiber were both associated with a lower risk of admission to hospital or death from diverticular disease.*"

The best way to go about reversing diverticulitis is to cleanse internally, and to eliminate all processed foods, animal products, and foods that contain bleached flours and bottled oils, while incorporating raw fruits and vegetables into your diet. These foods are rich in fibers and may be beneficial.

THE THYROID SOLUTION

The *National Thyroid Institute* declares that millions of Americans suffer from hyperthyroidism and hypothyroidism. The cause of the two conditions is said to be unknown and there is no known cure, only treatment with synthetic thyroid chemicals. What many are not aware of is the direct link between fluoride and the altering of thyroid function. The *National Research Council of the National Academies* released a report in 2006, stating that, "*Fluoride is an endocrine disruptor in the broad sense of altering normal endocrine function.*" Thyroid dysfunction is considered the most prevalent of all endocrine diseases in the U.S. The thyroid gland maintains the body's overall metabolic rate. When its function is altered, metabolism is disrupted. Because fluoride disrupts the function of the thyroid gland, if you are having thyroid issues, it is important to avoid tap water, certain teas, non-organic or conventional grapes (including wine), coffee (even decaf), and dental procedures that require the use of fluoride.

An article in *Food and Toxicology*, published in 2003, clarifies that *tea plants accumulate fluoride in their leaves. In general, the oldest tea leaves contain the most fluoride.* According to the *Organic Consumer's Association*, California grape growers use cryolite to control two insects that can devastate vineyards. Cryolite is a naturally occurring inorganic substance; however, it contains an aminofluoride ion. Researchers from *California State University* in Fresno conducted a 5 year study from 1990-1994 on vineyards throughout the San Joaquin Valley. They found that, "*Multiple applications of cryolite during the growing season significantly increased fluoride levels in wines.*" Coffee is also known to contain high amounts of fluoride because of the pesticides used on the leaves. This helps to explain the rise in thyroid issues.

The main contributor to poor thyroid function, however, may not be fluoride; it could be a chemical that is used to treat flour during processing known as bromide. Because of this, whenever you are dealing with any type of issue involving the endocrine (glandular) system, it is important to give up all foods that contain flours, especially bleached flours. A report published in the *Journal of Clinical Pathology* in 1993 suggests that, *"An increase in bromine potentiates an increase in thyroid stimulating hormone, thus affecting thyroid function."* When this hormone is over-stimulated, the function of the thyroid is disrupted.

An analogy I will use to help explain why bromide has an effect on the thyroid gland carries us over to the problem with cigarette smoking and why people get addicted. Chemically, the nicotine in cigarettes is almost identical to nicotinic acid, niacin, and niacinamide. These four compounds form a subgroup which is related to vitamin B3 (niacin). When a person smokes, they ingest that nicotine and the nicotine occupies the vitamin B3 receptor site. Because of this, they may become deficient in vitamin B3. As a result, they may crave B3 while believing they are retrieving B3 from cigarettes because of the false occupancy of the receptor site from nicotine.

The thyroid gland relies on iodine to function healthfully. It is the primary fuel for the gland, just like glucose is the primary fuel for the brain. Iodine is an essential compound for the thyroid to function at its optimal level.

Iodine happens to be nearly identical, chemically, to another compound known as "bromide." Just like the body uses nicotine as B3 because of its occupation of the B3 receptor site, the body is also tricked into using bromide as iodine when it is ingested into the body because it falsely occupies the iodine receptor site in the thyroid. When these receptor sites in the thyroid are pre-occupied by bromide, an adequate amount of iodine will not be absorbed.

Many flour products contain bromide, which is added during the treatment process. After it is added, the flours are used to make bread and dough. Pizza is one of the worst foods to eat when one has a thyroid condition because of the doughy bread. If you want to improve your thyroid condition, you must eliminate all foods that contain flour.

This does not mean you can never eat bread again. You can make your own sprouted bread using a dehydrator or purchase oil-free sprouted grain breads in the refrigerated section of your natural foods store. Avoid sprouted breads containing wheat gluten. Be sure to check for gluten grains in the ingredients label and avoid those products.

Maca is an endocrine boosting food, and adding it to your smoothies could be helpful for treating a thyroid condition. Try taking one daily teaspoon of organic maca powder, accompanied by eating two to four tablespoons of organic virgin raw coconut oil, whether as a dressing or in a smoothie. Add a handful or two of goji berries, some watercress, and kelp for the iodine boost. A couple of tablespoons of raw organic hemp seeds, or freshly ground flaxseed meal can be beneficial for the omega-3 content. The body uses the omega-3s to create DHA, which can also improve thyroid conditions.

I am not a medical doctor, but if I were told that I had a thyroid condition, those are the steps I would take.

YOUR LIVER IS NOT YOUR ENEMY

"The liver is the master controller of all the bodily functions. It depends on the other glands, organs of elimination and circulation to carry out its vital roles. Because the liver is the major organ of detoxification, it determines the health of the organs and the blood. The foods of the modern diet, especially meats, fried foods, refined oils, and foods with chemical additives weaken the liver." – Ann Wigmore, The Hippocrates Diet

When you have an overload of toxicity in your liver from excess alcohol, chemicals, and pharmaceutical drugs, fasting on distilled water, or fresh, raw organic juices can be beneficial and restorative. A lot of people suggest milk thistle. Go for raw, organic whole thistle seeds over a synthetic packaged option. It is far better to eat raw, organic whole milk thistle seeds after soaking them.

To learn more about fasting, I suggest you read Patricia Bragg's *Miracle of Fasting.* Juice and raw food cleanses can be found in Penni Shelton's, *Raw Food Cleanse*, and Natasha Kyssa's, *The Simply Raw Living Foods Detox Manual,* and more in John McCabe's, *Sunfood Diet Infusion.*

Because the liver produces bile, which is stored in the gallbladder, a gallbladder flush can be of great benefit to anyone. Many people have gallstones that have accumulated in their gallbladder. If you would like to find a liver/gallbladder flush that works for you, simply visit the website *curezone.com/cleanse/liver/default.asp.*

If you want to reach a level of optimal health, you must take good care of your liver. Avoiding alcohol, animal proteins, bleached grains, fried oils, gluten, illicit drugs, and synthetic food chemicals is a great way to maintain liver health.

BE GOOD TO YOUR COLON

According to Dr. Bernard Jensen, *"The intestines of newborn children lack many organisms, yet the adult colon is a complex ecosystem of around five-hundred species of microorganisms."* As we progress with age, some of us are regressing in health. As we continue to poison our bodies with drugs, alcohol, animal products, chemical food additives, pesticide residues, foods deficient in nutrients, foods that are physically and chemically changed by food processing, farming chemicals, and soil contaminants and components, we accumulate more microorganisms in our colon.

Many diseases can be directly linked to toxic residues in the system. Toxins in the colon are one reason disease develops and premature aging occurs. By keeping our colon and bowels clean, we increase longevity, preserve our youth, prevent disease, and feel more healthful. These poisons pollute the bloodstream and deteriorate every tissue, gland, and organ of the body over time.

Meat, eggs, dairy, synthetic food additives, heat-generated chemicals, and chemical drugs present a toxic mix to the bowel. When our colon becomes over-intoxicated, it stagnates and assimilates these toxins into the blood. This leads to many degenerative diseases. The lymph, heart, lungs, immune system, and digestive organs also become tainted. As a result, we are left with feeling bloated, having unhealthy skin, having foul breath, and prematurely aging with arthritic conditions and low levels of energy.

Some of the symptoms of toxemia are: irritable bowel syndrome, depression, anxiety, headaches, insomnia, dull or pallid skin, eczema, sores, acne, psoriasis, arthritis, cysts, tumors, and the list goes on.

A great way to start your journey back to good health would be by avoiding all animal products, only eating organic, eating raw, and most importantly, going in for seasonal colon hydrotherapy sessions to keep the colon clean.

GIVE YOUR KIDNEYS A CHANCE

Kidneys filter blood and are partially responsible for eliminating drugs, pollutants, and bacterial waste from the body. Because of the thousands of additives and drugs in our food and water, these organs are being overly taxed, and may function poorly. Sometimes, one or both of the kidneys can become so compromised that they may fail.

The first step to kidney cleansing is to avoid all refined and processed foods, salt, refined sugars, meat, eggs, dairy, cooked oils, coffee, tea, cola, caffeinated "energy" drinks, "sports" drinks, alcohol, tobacco, and plastic tainted bottled water. A diet rich in animal protein, gluten grains, acrylamides, glycotoxins, heterocyclic amines, polycyclic aromatic hydrocarbons, nitrates, and synthetic chemicals is rough on the kidneys, as all of those substances, or the digested residues and components of them, must be filtered out of the blood, and that process taxes and can damage the kidneys – even to the point of causing kidney stones, cancer, and failure. Each day we pump up to four thousand quarts of blood through our kidneys in order to cleanse them of all of the waste that we put into our bodies, as well as the waste our cells create.

The January 2012 edition of the *American Journal of Clinical Nutrition* published a study revealing a link between eating red meat and grilled and fried foods, with increased risk of kidney cancer. *Researchers followed the diets of nearly 500,000 men and women in the NIH-AARP Diet and Health Study and found that those who ate the most meat, around 4.5 ounces per day (the size of a hamburger), had a higher risk of kidney cancer.*

In December 2011, the *Clinical Journal of the American Society of Nephrology* published a study equipping us with the knowledge that vegetarian diets are healthier for kidney patients, compared with animal-based diets. They found that *patients following vegetarian diets had lower serum phosphorus levels, compared with those who consumed meat.* The article then explains how, *"Maintaining normal phosphorus levels is critical for patients with chronic kidney disease and is controlled by restricting intake of meat."*

Dr. Michael Greger states that, *"Kidney failure can be treated with a plant based diet because the kidneys are highly vascular organs which filter our entire bloodstream. The Standard American Diet is toxic to the blood vessels."* He then mentions how Harvard researchers found three risk factors for declining kidney function. These risk factors are: animal protein, animal fat, and cholesterol.

We should always be good to our kidneys. This means we should not poison them with meat, dairy, eggs, food additives, chemical drugs, or alcohol. Be sure to drink plenty of water and incorporate fresh organic green juices in your diet. This will help rejuvenate your kidneys.

BLOOD PURIFYING

Keeping our blood free of dietary cholesterol, animal fats, gluten, cooked oils, chemical food additives, and chemical drugs, will help free us from sickness and disease. By eliminating acidic foods and toxic beverages, we can maintain an alkaline pH, thereby avoiding acidosis. Cooked oils, meats, eggs, and dairy, and heat-generated food chemicals slow the blood, trigger an immune reaction, and interfere with the function of the endothelial cells lining the cardiovascular system. Avoiding these impurities will help keep our blood pure, and assure better health. A clean blood supply is a key to reversing diseases.

Fasting with wheatgrass juice and incorporating wheatgrass enema implants can help build a clean blood supply. A wheatgrass juice fast can be done by drinking a four to six-ounce glass of wheatgrass juice four times a day and only drinking the juice of watermelon in between drinks of wheatgrass. This should be fresh juice that has not been pasteurized or heated.

IT IS NEVER TOO LATE

No matter what your condition or how advanced your disease may be, it is always important to remember that it is never too late. Common degenerative and chronic diseases can be greatly reduced and avoided with a lifestyle change and the incorporation of raw organic foods. Do not be discouraged. Do not let a doctor or anyone else convince you that it is too late to turn your health around. Always believe that your health can improve. Envision yourself being healthy again, and take actions to make it happen.

The detoxification process may take longer, depending on how advanced your condition is, and the job will become more difficult for me or whoever your health coach or naturopathic doctor may be, but we will always find ways to make you healthy again. Do not give up and do not succumb to the allopathic medical theory that your condition is incurable, that a clean diet will not make a difference, or that chemical drugs and surgery are your only choices.

Choose raw, organic fruits and vegetables, sprouts and berries, and daily exercise. Choose health.

After analyzing the diseases I mentioned in chapter ten, you most likely noticed a common trend occurring with each one. Many of these diseases are linked in some way to eating animal products. There are vast numbers of studies concluding that eating meat, dairy, eggs, excess fats, synthetic chemical additives, and clarified sugars will speed up the process of developing degenerative and chronic diseases.

If you are sick, the best option you have is to change your diet and lifestyle. We cannot rely on chemical drugs to save us. Many living by the philosophy that prescription drugs will save us from common disease have found a sure way to a low-quality life and an earlier grave.

By converting to a low-fat, raw vegan diet, you will notice that your health improves steadily. You will gain more energy and begin to adapt a more active lifestyle. When you live this way, you no longer have room for sickness or disease in your life. Now is our time to change. Together we can make the world a better place.

THE FINAL LESSON:

WE CAN CHANGE

HEALING THE POISONS

"Throughout time, as human beings, we have poisoned our hearts with bitterness. We have poisoned our thoughts with jealousy and greed. We have poisoned our bodies with unhealthy foods and artificial substances. We have poisoned our spirits with our lack of gratitude. In this sickened state, the human race has lost sight of what this crooked trail has done to the world around us.

We have dumped chemicals into the waters, buried the toxins in the soil, poisoning the Earth, the creatures, and the plant people. Many humans feel helpless to stop the ravaging that is taking place on the Earth Mother. To find the solutions, we must begin at home by being conscious of how we can contribute to the answers and the clean up. We are being asked to recycle, to reuse, and to be conscious of our consumption.

On a personal level, we are being asked to clean up and heal our thoughts, our emotions, our intentions, our old pain, our denials, our physical health, and our actions. When we become personally responsible for the healing of every thought, action, intention and deed in our lives, the rest of the world will heal along with us."

— *Jamie Sams, Excerpt from her book, Earth Medicine*

Chapter 11: WHAT CAN WE DO?

"'How does one become a butterfly?' she asked. 'You must want to fly so much that you are willing to give up being a caterpillar.'" – *Hope for the Flowers*

In order to change the world, we first need to correct ourselves. We should prepare ourselves for the next level of achievement that waits. This means it is necessary that we change the way we eat and adjust our lifestyles to make healthier choices. This can be done by breaking away from tradition and creating new traditions. The ways of the past have not worked for us. To reach an optimal level of health, the best decision we can make is to transition to a vegan lifestyle. Removing all animal products from our diet will free us from much of the sickness and disease with which we are afflicted, and it will help heal the world and protect wildlife.

"Correcting oneself is correcting the whole world. The sun is simply bright. It does not correct anyone. Because it shines, the whole world is full of light. Transforming yourself is a means of giving light to the whole world." – *Ramana Maharshi*

Each action we take should be influenced by love and respect for everyone else around us. Our strengths lie in our refusal to give in to what makes less out of us. We become stronger by detoxifying our spirits, rejuvenating our souls, cleansing our internal organs, and exercising our intellect by keeping our minds active and engaged in positive things. Being active and incorporating physical exercise into our lives will help us gain this strength, while preserving our beauty and extending longevity.

As we shift away from being spectators watching the world erode from our homes, glued to our television sets, suggesting to ourselves that perhaps one day we will change our ways, and we begin to take action and make things happen for ourselves, we will contribute to making the world a better place. The time to act is now. There is no better time and no better way to create positive change.

"History will have to record that the greatest tragedy of this period of social transition was not the strident clamor of the bad people, but the appalling silence of the good people." – *Dr. Martin Luther King, Jr.*

The best way to show self-dignity, self-pride, and self-love is to make it official, and make a commitment to yourself right now, that you will never again eat food products that have been contaminated with chemicals. Make a pact with yourself that you will refrain from eating food sold at commercial fast food restaurant chains and that you will free yourself from eating animal products. Choose raw fruits, vegetables, nuts, seeds, sprouts, and seaweeds.

"When health is absent, wisdom cannot reveal itself, art cannot manifest, strength cannot fight, wealth becomes useless, and intelligence cannot be applied." – *Herophilos*

Other than a clean diet rich in raw, edible plant matter, there are absolutely no combatants for poor nutrition and poor lifestyle choices. No matter how fast you run, how hard or how often, if you are eating cooked oils, refined sugars, meat, dairy, eggs, and processed foods, and additionally drinking alcohol and smoking cigarettes, chances are, you will still develop sickness, disease, and ailments. You will never win this way.

If you ignore your health... It will go away

We are all in this together. We are a team. Many of us have thought the same thoughts, we have faced the same struggles, and we have dreamed the same dreams. We simply take on a different appearance. We use our energy in different ways. This does not mean we should distance ourselves from a common ground. We should help each other as much as possible.

"As humans we experience our selves, thoughts, and feelings as something separated from the rest of the universe. This delusion is a kind of prison for us, restricting us to our personal desires and to affection for a few persons nearest to us. Our task must be to free ourselves from this prison by widening our circle of compassion to embrace all living creatures & the whole of nature in its beauty." – Albert Einstein

We will not erase sickness or disease until we banish the slaughtering of animals and refrain from eating all animal products. Additionally, we need to grow our own organic culinary gardens, and support organic polycropping to help put an end to conventional monocropping farming methods. We are destroying our health and the health of the environment by eating chemical-laden crops and the flesh of dead and diseased animals.

We can change the world. It is going to take a lot of work. We are going to have to correct a lot of the problems we create for ourselves; however, it can be done. Each day we have to commit to being better and we have to know that we will prevail. We could start by changing some of the laws that are out there today. But, the first way we can change the world is through our food choices. The most healthful foods are derived from organically-grown plants.

"If you think we can't change the world, it simply means you are not one of those who will." – Jacque Fresco

GOING VEGAN

"There is absolutely no nutrient, no protein, no vitamin, no mineral that we know of that cannot be obtained from plant-based food." – Michael Klaper, MD

Animals are not food, they are life. We have no business eating them. We have no business enslaving them or torturing them. When we do, we become stricken with disease and premature death. While vegans have a longer average lifespan than meat-eaters, we are also less likely to develop common chronic and degenerative diseases. Meat-eaters not only live shorter lives, but they are much more likely to spend a majority of their years fighting off disease and sickness. Many die from complications due to obesity, or from cardiovascular disease, cancer, osteoporosis, diabetes, Alzheimer's, MS, kidney disease, or some other easily avoidable condition.

In *The China Study*, Dr. T. Colin Campbell lists *Eight Principles of Food and Health*. Principle number three is, *"There are virtually no nutrients in animal-based foods that are not better provided by plants."* Dr. Campbell provides a chart that shows us plant-based foods have a significantly greater amount of antioxidants, fiber, and minerals than animal foods. The chart shows us that animal foods only contain higher amounts of cholesterol, fat, and poor quality proteins, which all cause common human diseases.

I believe going vegan is the most important first step to be taken to improve your quality of life. If you want to prevent disease, reverse disease, save the environment, protect wildlife, and save our civilization, it is a wise choice to permanently refrain from eating and drinking animal products. By following a diet rich in raw fruits and vegetables, you will find that there are much better food options available to you than just eating meat, cheese, eggs, and other dairy products. You will also find that your energy improves, your weight balances, your vibe increases, and your desire to get things done, and to use your talent, skills, and intellect increase.

CHART 11.2: NUTRIENT COMPOSITION OF PLANT AND ANIMAL-BASED FOODS (PER 500 CALORIES OF ENERGY)

Nutrient	Plant-Based Foods*	Animal-Based Foods**
Cholesterol (mg)	—	137
Fat (g)	4	36
Protein (g)	33	34
Beta-carotene (mcg)	29,919	17
Dietary Fiber (g)	31	—
Vitamin C (mg)	293	4
Folate (mcg)	1168	19
Vitamin E (mg_ATE)	11	0.5
Iron (mg)	20	2
Magnesium (mg)	548	51
Calcium (mg)	545	252

* Equal parts of tomatoes, spinach, lima beans, peas, potatoes

** Equal parts of beef, pork, chicken, whole milk

"To be a vegetarian is to disagree, to disagree with the course of things today. Things like starvation, world hunger, cruelty, waste and wars. We must make a statement against these things. Vegetarianism is my statement. And I think it is a strong one." – Isaac Bashevis Singer

Making the decision to follow a vegan diet is something I strongly advise for anyone who would like to preserve their youth, beautiful features, and beautiful mind. As you make the transition to a vegan lifestyle, and shop for only fresh organic foods, as well as eliminate refined sugars and synthetic chemicals from your diet, while concurrently avoiding meat and dairy products, your body begins to balance itself out and properly adapt to its new, more wholesome, and vital environment.

The *American Dietetic Association* has also promoted this philosophy for quite some time. In 1988 they released a statement about the positive relation between a vegetarian diet and lifestyle and the decrease of several conditions, including hypertension, heart disease, and obesity. I'm sure many of us have never had the chance to read this, which is not surprising, since the meat, dairy, and egg industries pay millions of dollars to cover up these statements and saturate the media with misleading articles that quickly revert our minds back to the lies that lured us into believing that eating meat and consuming dairy is somehow good for our bones, makes us stronger, and provides us with energy and health.

"Nothing will benefit health and increase the chances for survival of life on Earth as the evolution to a vegetarian diet." – Albert Einstein

Meat, milk, and eggs nourish us with nothing that we cannot obtain from plant-based foods. There is no reason to be consuming any of them. All they have provided for us over the years is sickness, disease, and fatigue. Meat, milk, and eggs slow us down, age our skin, drain the life from our complexion, and rob us of our youth and vitality.

Meat, dairy, and egg products provide us with no nutrients we cannot obtain from plant-based foods. They inhibit our ability to absorb, assimilate, and utilize other nutrients, especially calcium, leading to many nutrient deficiencies, while increasing the incidence of osteoporosis, arthritis, cardiovascular disease, kidney disease, diabetes, asthma, cancer, macular degeneration, erectile dysfunction, and obesity.

"I would rather eat cardboard than go back to eating animals." – Ellen Degeneres

You are responsible for implementing the changes you need to make today in order to better yourself. You make the choice as to whether or not you want healthy skin, healthy organs, a fit body, and a life free from disease. To improve your quality of life, you can start by eliminating animal products, and increasing consumption of leafy greens, and raw fruits and vegetables.

"We collectively raise, feed, water, kill, and eat over sixty-five billion animals each year for food. This is ten times as many people as we have on the entire earth. We have developed a complex system of producing more and more animals that use more and more of our resources, while leaving a massive amount of waste, pollution, and adverse climate change in their wake. This system is heavily intertwined with our culture, politics, economics, and the suppression of the reality of its effect on our planet." – Dr. Richard Oppenlander, Comfortably Unaware

THE GROUND IS DISEASED

"The ground is wrongly cultivated when it is fertilized too much and too uniformly with chemical manure. We may run the risk that the ground becomes just as diseased as man. Over-acidified, undernourished, and yields sick plants not fit for human food." – Dr. Kirstine Nolfi

Today, the ground has become diseased. Not only from the pesticides and chemicals we use in fertilizer, but from growing millions of acres of monocropped grains and grasses to feed the livestock industry. By planting genetically modified seeds and using toxic farming chemicals that are not natural to Earth, we are laying the foundation for disaster. Our ground is diseased from the trillions of cigarette remnants that are being littered around the world. The ground is diseased, sickened, corrupted, tainted, and poisoned from the fossil fuels industries, toxic farming chemical industries, and by raising the billions of animals being slaughtered annually in the Animal Holocaust. What we do to the Earth and other living creatures always comes back to us. For as long as the ground is diseased, we will be diseased.

Just like the human body, we cannot rely on medicine for the ground to get well. We cannot feed the ground more chemicals and expect it to get better. We must discontinue the use of chemicals. We must polycrop organically rather than monocrop chemically. Once we do this, the ground, just like the human body, will heal.

PLANT YOUR WAY TO HAPPINESS

"Your food choices not only impact your health, they impact the health of the environment and wildlife. Whatever you put into your body ends up in the environment, and in wildlife. All of the substances used to grow, ship, process, package, market, and prepare your foods end up in you, in the environment, and in wildlife. If any of those substances can make you sick, they can also degrade the health of the environment and wildlife. Therefore, it is important to follow a clean diet. One way to do that is to plant and maintain an organic garden that utilizes compost made from your organic food scraps." – John McCabe, author of *Sunfood Diet Infusion*

Now is a better time than any to plant your own garden. While you restore nature in doing so, you also could save yourself from depression. An article written by Robyn Francis and published on the website for *Permaculture College Australia* reports that, *"Getting our fingers dirty and harvesting our own food can trigger our natural production of "happy chemicals" that suppress depression."* The article cites research that contact with soil, and a specific soil bacteria known as *mycobacterium vaccae*, triggers the release of serotonin in our brain. Serotonin is a neurotransmitter that acts as an anti-depressant and strengthens the immune system. A lack of this chemical has shown to be linked to depression.

In this same article, research is cited showing a release of dopamine from the brain when we harvest crops from the garden. Dopamine is another neurotransmitter that triggers a state of bliss or mild euphoria, inhibiting the onset of depression. The author, Robyn Francis, also links chemicals sprayed on crops that are referred to as *glyphosates*, to a depletion of serotonin and dopamine levels. A commonly used chemical product known as *Round-Up* contains many of these glyphosates. She informs us that, *"A recent study in 2008 discovered that glyphosate, the active ingredient of Round-Up, depletes serotonin and dopamine levels in mammals. Contrary to Monsanto claims, glyphosate and other Round-Up ingredients do perpetuate in the environment, in soil, water, plants and in the cells and organs of animals. One study found glyphosate residues in cotton fabric made from Round-Up ready GM cotton can absorb into the skin and into our nervous and circulatory systems."*

By planting our own gardens, we can guarantee that our food does not contain these chemicals that deplete our neurotransmitters that we need for our happiness. We also raise levels of serotonin and dopamine. These two "happy chemicals" can free us from depression. In addition to creating vivacity, gardening rebuilds our top soil and contributes to a healthy environment. I urge you to make an attempt to get your own garden started. I also recommend placing house plants in each room of your home. This way you are adding life to materialism; you are providing living energy. You may discover that you are an overall much happier person by doing so.

BREAKING AWAY FROM TRADITION

"The definition of insanity is doing the same thing over and over again and expecting the results to be different." – Albert Einstein

All of the bad habits we have attached to traditional events have caused traditions to regress into contributors of sickness and ill health. The Christmas dinners that are centered on ham, or another piece of dead flesh, are contributing to degenerative disease. The turkey and processed foods on Thanksgiving are doing the same. On holidays such as Valentine's Day and

Halloween, we give out candy that contains mixtures of harmful chemicals and is lacking healthful ingredients. We bake cookies full of clarified sugars, cooked oils, and refined gluten grain flours for the holidays. In the summer, we enjoy frozen popsicles and ice cream that consists of preservatives, dairy, and refined sugars, leading to common illnesses. In winter, we delight ourselves with hot chocolate that is also a mixture of harmful chemicals.

Major food companies have used marketing tactics to turn the common foods we eat on holidays into chemical-laden, processed food look-a-like substances that rob us of our health and induce sickness. Candy is not food and is not safe for human consumption. It is poison in a package. Do you ever notice why so many people get sick around the holidays? It is not "seasonal," it is because we load up on the worst foods during these holidays.

Late October, going into November, is when the most cases of influenza and the common cold are documented in public schools across the country. Why do you think this is? The reason is that kids are given permission to eat gobs of candy and this is literally poisoning them.

"Halloween is just two weeks away, and most parents are worried about the frightening amount of sugar children consume. That's understandable. But Halloween is just one day. What really scares me are the meat and dairy products lurking in children's diets every day and everywhere – from fast food to school lunches. Unfortunately, some parents don't share this fear. Some parents may not yet realize how healthful a plant-based diet can be for their children.

Meat and dairy products are loaded with fat and cholesterol that lead to childhood obesity, diabetes, cancer, and heart disease. A new study in the British Medical Journal found that obese children as young as five years old were already showing signs of heart disease that could seriously increase their risk of heart attacks and stroke as they get older. Now that gives me nightmares." – Dr. Neal Barnard

In school, candy is passed out as a treat. Some teachers order pizza for kids as a reward for good behavior. This means they are being poisoned as a reward. Then you get the people who say, "Oh let them live, they are just kids." Well, that is exactly what I want them to do. I want them to live. Unfortunately, the school lunches, pizza days, and candy being handed out play a role in cutting their lives short. Children do not enjoy being sick. If we would simply explain to them that sickness does not come from germs, and instead, we inform them of the truth: that the candy, meat, eggs, dairy, sugar, and fried foods they are being served in school, and are often eating at home, are making them sick, then chances are they would be less likely to indulge in them. There is no reason to be scared of telling your child the truth about bad foods. If you want your child to "live a little," as so many say, then you should allow them to live with good health and give them real food while educating them on the dangers of the poison they are being served in school.

Another common time for sickness to develop is around Christmas. From the end of October all the way up until mid January, we see the most sickness. This is not because of cold weather, it is because so many eat candy on Halloween, overload on animal protein and processed foods on Thanksgiving, and eat too many cookies and other sweets around Christmas. Then, to top it off, they wash them down with the pus and secretions (cow's milk) of a six-hundred pound animal that has been enslaved since birth, and fed an unnatural diet that gets them so sick they are treated with drugs.

Another common tradition is hunting. Hunting is not only cruel, but completely unnecessary. The animal farming industry and ranching has killed off the predator animals, which has created an overpopulation of certain other animals, creating an imbalance of both prey and plant life.

"Thanksgiving dinner's sad and thankless,
Christmas dinner's dark and blue,
when you stop and try to see it
from the turkey's point of view.
Sunday dinner isn't sunny,
Easter feasts are just bad luck,
when you see it from the viewpoint
of a chicken or a duck.
Oh how I once loved tuna salad,
Pork and lobsters, lamb chops too.
'Til I stopped and looked at dinner,
from the dinner's point of view."

– Shel Silverstein

Massive road construction, urban sprawl, drainage of wetlands, damming of rivers, and loss of topsoil from intensive industrial monocropping of millions upon millions of acres of land to grow food for billions of farm animals, all points to one thing that is destroying Earth, as well as our civilization – meat eating. I had a friend who responded to a message I had made public about eradicating hunting. This was his response:

"Eradicate hunting? Are you out of your mind? What's next; hand all of our guns over to the government? Sorry Jesse, but I'm going to have to dislike this one. Being healthy and eating healthy is one thing, but hunting is and will always be an American tradition."

My friend had a good point, hunting is an American tradition and it is an unnecessary one. You kill an animal, steal its life, and then eat its dead, decayed flesh, develop disease, and after suffering the last few years of your life with cancer or some other degenerative disease linked to meat-eating, you die prematurely.

Everyone is entitled to their opinion and I am glad he responded the way he did. I don't look at him as any less of a person. All I did was try my best to educate him on why the hobby is unnecessary.

It has also become American tradition to be obese, develop cancer, develop heart disease, and cut our life expectancy in half. It has become American tradition to drink our lives away with alcohol and smoke our lungs away with cigarettes, while trashing our body systems with garbage foods. It is American tradition to support the fast food industry and other corporations that are major contributors to the destruction of the rainforests, and are largely responsible for the crisis of global warming. It is traditional to eat GMO foods that cause cancer, and then vote no for the laws that would force these GMO companies to label the food products they sell so we are aware of what we are eating.

"Vegetarian food leaves a deep impression on our nature. If the whole world adopts vegetarianism, it can change the destiny of humankind." – Albert Einstein

The point I am making is that American tradition is leading to American suffering. We have to break away from tradition, cleanse ourselves, change our diets, stop considering animals as food, and build our new traditions based on love, good health, prosperity, and protecting wildlife and the environment if we want to see our health progress. This is how we will eradicate sickness.

I dream big dreams. I know that we are on the verge of positive change. We are getting closer every day to putting an end to this cycle of sickness, disease, and death that we have created through greed, ignorance, and miseducation.

Wouldn't it would be great if we could create laws — the same way lawmakers teamed up with industry leaders to preserve pharmaceutical industry profits, and those of the huge corporations that have been poisoning us — but rather to enact laws which preserve our health and longevity, and that of nature?

We shouldn't have to wait for these laws to be created until we begin to do what is right. We cannot rely on politicians to tell us how to live. This is giving up our power, and perpetuating ignorance and laziness. While we are waiting around, the ground, waterways, and our food supply continue to be poisoned as wildlife suffers. Disease continues to spread. It is up to us to implement the change we need.

If you don't understand it by now, you can participate in The Raw Cure by eliminating unhealthful foods from your life, supporting organic farmers, growing at least some of your foods using organic methods, and composting your organic food scraps into soil. You can participate in The Raw Cure by following a diet rich in raw organic fruits and vegetables, and by eliminating all meat, milk, and egg products from your diet. By doing these things, you will be healthier, and so will the environment and wildlife.

EVERY ACT MUST COME FROM LOVE

"My elders have taught me that anything we do, speak, think or make is our creation. When we make something with our own hands, whether it is a meal, a drawing, a sculpture, a plan, a written story, a fence, a toy, or a song, the attitude we have at that time we create those things will show forever.

A song may sound happy, but if it is written while the person is too busy, it won't flow for the listener. If a meal is thrown together, the love isn't there and the food will not be as nourishing. If people are angry or resentful when they build a fence, the job may be filled with problems and the fence may hinder friendships with neighbors. Every attitude is invested into our creations. If one fears that the things they have made to sell will not be appreciated, that fear will keep the clients away.

If we change our attitudes and create everything from joy, the happiness allows our creations to touch the lives of others. The missions of our creations are then unhindered, bringing bounty, beauty and good feelings to all connected."

— *Jamie Sams, Excerpt from her book,* **Earth Medicine**

Chapter 12: PURITY WITHIN

Living a sedentary life without exercise, eating processed foods, drinking alcohol, smoking cigarettes, and indulging in meat, eggs, clarified sugars, oil extracts, and dairy are all practices increasing the risks of experiencing degenerative disease. When we make that big step towards bettering our lives, we face quite a journey. On this journey we will experience the greatest moments of our lives, however, things will get tough at certain points. During these rough patches it is required that you never give up.

The best way to break old habits is to develop new habits. To help break your lazy habits you can start by exercising. To help break your chemical addictions, you can incorporate healthy, organic raw foods into your diet. In order for you to break these habits faster, it is also important to cleanse your system using some sort of internal cleansing procedure. Be sure to educate yourself on anything you decide to do prior to doing it.

I watched a documentary titled, *May I Be Frank*. It features a man named Frank Ferrante. Frank was more than a hundred pounds overweight; he was taking several medications, positive for hepatitis C, depressed, and lacked a love life. His life changed one day while eating at a raw vegan restaurant in San Francisco, called *Café Gratitude*. Frank was embraced by the health coaches in the establishment and embarked on a forty-two day journey that would forever change the way he approaches life. In the film you see the great impact that converting to a vegan lifestyle, exercising, and implementing internal cleansing services can have on your health. Frank loses over a hundred pounds, frees himself from all medications, cures his hepatitis C and depression, and revives his libido. The documentary is heart-warming and is a must-watch for anyone, especially men serious about restoring their health.

EXERCISE

Exercise does not have to be physically exhausting. Brisk walking, taking a bike ride, or even being involved in a recreational sport all account for exercise. The most important thing is that you start moving. When you exercise, you expand your lung capacity. You move your lymph fluid around and this helps to eliminate some of the toxins that are hiding within that lymph. Additionally, you provide oxygen to your cells, gain more energy throughout the day, feel better, look better, and live better.

"Our bloodstream carries nutrients, extracted from the food we eat, to every cell in our body. Exercise helps this journey of these nutrients while generating enormous amounts of oxygen in the bloodstream." – Dr. Brian Clement, LifeForce

For nearly ten years, I have been working with clients to assist them with weight loss, nutrition, and proper exercise techniques. I can honestly say that each of the hundreds of clients I have worked with have all improved in all aspects of life from changing their lifestyles to incorporating more of the ideas I have shared with you. If you are looking for a great book that will teach you how to exercise and eat properly, check out Jeff Sekerak's the *Super Fit Vegan* (*thesuperfitvegan.com*). Of all of the exercise modalities, my absolute favorite is yoga.

YOGA

Real men do yoga. Yoga is a chance to connect with intention, spiritual love, and inner peace. It is a chance to unite with nature and find harmony. Practicing yoga helps to cleanse of all deadening foods, slothful energy, and negative thoughts. Yoga simply works in tune with following a clean vegan diet rich in raw fruits and vegetables. It helps to align with nature and the vibe of your spirit, which can improve through a clean diet.

I had a yoga instructor walk into the room before class on one occasion, and before class began he spoke about how he had a great burger for lunch. First of all, there is no such thing as a great burger; unless of course it is some kind of raw sun burger or garden burger. I immediately had a bad impression and decided I would not attend the class again. I could feel the dead energy swarming the room and did all I could to put up a shield and reflect it away.

Practicing yoga helps to be aware of levels of energy and to clear the mind of negativity. If you are not yet aware of who you are, and if you still have not gained a relationship with nature, yoga is a perfect starting point.

Incorporating yoga into your life is an intelligent way to bring balance between your mind, body, and spirit. There is always a place somewhere within each community where yoga is practiced. Get online and type yoga, along with your zipcode or county, into a search engine and you will most likely find a yoga class or community nearby. If not, you can always get yoga DVD's or even do yoga from a live webstream in the comfort of your own home.

There is a website, *physiiq.com*, which offers live yoga classes online. On the site, look for *Pele Chen* and try one of her classes.

REVERSING OBESITY

According to the *World Health Organization*, there are an estimated 1.6 billion overweight adults and almost five-hundred million who are obese. I can guarantee that a high percentage of them eat a high intake of dairy products. If not now, then they most likely did during childhood or adolescence. Dairy is among the worst foods for your health.

"Fat tissue is the body's largest endocrine organ and its volume is impressive, even in people who are 'physically fit.' The main function of the fat cells is to store excess calories. In someone who is obese, the fat cells swell to three times their usual size. As people gain more weight, they create more fat cells, which store even more calories. As the cycle continues, the cumulative excess becomes deadly. All fat cells emit weight-increasing chemicals that assault every organ of the body. These cells store chemical, synthetic toxins as well that are absorbed from food, medicines and consumer products." – Dr. Brian Clement, LifeForce

By adding more alkaline foods to your diet and shifting your pH to an alkaline level, fat absorption from the intestine has a greater impact, making us feel fuller. By eating more phosphorus rich fruits and vegetables, the appetite will be depressed and weight loss will occur.

The *American Journal of Clinical Nutrition* published an article in March of 2010, titled, *Vegetarian Diets and Childhood Obesity Prevention*, in which *epidemiologic studies indicated that, "Vegetarian diets are associated with a lower body mass index (BMI) and a lower prevalence of obesity in adults and children. A meta-analysis of adult vegetarian diet studies estimated a reduced weight difference of 7.6 kg for men and 3.3 kg for women, which resulted in a 2-point lower BMI (in kg/m^2). Similarly, compared with non-vegetarians, vegetarian children are leaner, and their BMI difference becomes greater during adolescence. Studies exploring the risk of overweight and food groups and dietary patterns indicate that a plant-based diet seems to be a sensible approach for the prevention of obesity in children. Plant-based diets are low in energy density and high in complex carbohydrate, fiber, and water, which may increase satiety and resting energy expenditure. Plant-based dietary patterns should be encouraged for optimal health and environmental benefits."*

In a 2012 article titled *Meat Consumption and Prospective Weight Change in Participants of the EPIC-PANACEA Study*, the *American Journal of Clinical Nutrition* shares the results of a study conducted on a total of 103,455 men and 270,348 women between the ages of twenty-five to seventy. They were followed to assess the association between consumption of total meat, red meat, poultry, processed meat, and weight gain after a five year follow up. *Total meat consumption was positively associated with weight gain in men and women, in normal weight and overweight subjects.* This was established even after controlling for calories, meaning that the intake of 250g of meat daily resulted in annual weight gain higher than the weight gain experienced from an isocaloric diet with lower meat content (same amount of calories, less meat). The conclusion of the study was that *a decrease in meat consumption can improve weight management.*

The very best way to tackle your obesity problem is to remove all animal products from your diet. This means no meat, eggs, or dairy of any kind. The fatty tissue in obese people is deficient in lipase, which is the enzyme that breaks down fats into simpler substances. When we do not provide our bodies with any fats, our lipogenic enzymes are activated, and these are our fat-storing enzymes. They protect us from running out of fat. When we do not provide our bodies with any fat whatsoever, we activate these enzymes, and as a result, we store the fat we already have.

When we eat foods with plant-based fats, while cutting out animal fats and cooked fats, we activate our lipolytic enzymes and these are more like fat-burning enzymes. They help us to rid our bodies of unwanted fat deposits. Many people struggle with losing weight because they get lost in these "fad" diets that have them limit caloric intake. In doing so, these diets also limit their nutrient intake. So while some may lose weight, they are far from becoming healthy. All of the chemicals they are given permission to eat on these diets continue to accumulate in their bodies and increase the risk of common degenerative and chronic diseases. Dr. Robert Atkins was the man who created the low carbohydrate, high protein, Atkins diet. Atkins himself died from heart disease by following this diet. Additionally, the thirteen billion dollar a year weight loss supplement industry caters to the struggles by continuing to promote diet pills that are of no benefit.

"Did you know that our bodies protect us from toxins by storing them in our fat cells, and in order to allow our body to lose weight, we must reduce the intake of toxins (such as pesticides, chemicals, drugs, artificial sweeteners, high fructose corn syrup, partially hydrogenated oil and substances found in processed food). These toxic chemicals are also affecting our hormones and liver functions in charge of metabolism. So instead of reducing calories, reduce toxins to lose weight, regain health and youth, and enjoy life." – The Detox Advisor

In November 2010, Helena Gibson-Moore published an article in the *Nutrition Bulletin* titled, *Do Slimming Supplements Work?* In the article, she includes research from two studies that were presented at the *11th International Congress on Obesity* in Stockholm, Sweden in July 2010. The two studies tested the results of common slimming supplements versus placebo pills consisting of clarified sugars. After completion of the studies, the conclusion was made that there is no difference between the supplements and placebo pills, and their impact on test subjects. In a separate study, the *Weight Management Center* at *Johns Hopkins University* made a similar conclusion about diet pills. Researchers concluded that, *"It is fitting to highlight that perhaps the most general and safest 'alternative' approach to weight control is to substitute low-energy density foods in place of high-energy density, and processed foods, thereby reducing total energy intake. By taking advantage of the low-energy density and health-promoting effects of plant-based foods, one may be able to achieve weight loss, or at least assist weight maintenance without cutting down on the volume of food consumed or compromising its nutrient value."*

If you want to lose weight, stop worrying so much about calories. Shift your attention to eating organic living foods that are full of vitamins, minerals, enzymes, biophotons, essential fatty acids, amino acids, antioxidants, and fiber. As I stated, the first step that you must take for gaining true health is transitioning to a vegan diet. If you want to lose weight and become healthy while doing it, you have to start by eliminating all animal products from your diet. Calories are not everything. Eat raw, organic fruits, sprouts, and vegetables, and some raw nuts and seeds. Drink plenty of water and be sure to do internal cleansing. Avoid the nine worst food groups, which are, meat, dairy, eggs, clarified sugars, flours, cooked oils, gluten, foods containing synthetic chemicals, and processed salts. By following this advice, you can expect to experience a reduction in weight.

"Calories are far less important than the quality of the food you are ingesting. Your body absorbs the vitamins and minerals from raw, natural foods far more effectively than the Standard American Diet foods. The helpful fats in nature actually help your body burn fat. Stop counting calories and feed your body nutrient rich foods that sustain and regenerate it." – Karyn Calabrese, Soak Your Nuts

INTERNAL CLEANSING

I believe cleansing your colon is one of the more effective ways to start the detoxification process. This procedure alone can help lose weight. The health and vitality of the immune system can be dependent on the cleanliness of the colon. After cleansing your colon, the most efficient way to keep the weight off and stay healthy is to eat clean, raw, low-fat vegan, and organic.

The average American walks around each day with plaque hardened to their bowels. This is one reason why many people wake up with bad breath. This is also a source of where body odor comes from. This is where sickness may start to develop. If you have any sort of sickness, condition, or disease, it is helpful to do internal cleansing regularly. When your internal organs are clean, you reduce the chance of having bad breath, are less likely to have body odor, and your skin will begin looking healthier. You also assist with the prevention and reversal of disease.

One major problem that negatively impacts many people is the calcification of the pineal gland. When we drink water contaminated with chemicals, especially fluoride, and eat combinations of pharmaceutical drugs, along with farming chemical residues, and chemical food additives, we calcify this gland. When the pineal gland is blocked, we no longer generate sufficient amounts of melatonin. This hormone keeps us happy and elevates our harmony. A lack of melatonin can dull our senses, lower our intellect, make us feel sluggish, and drain our desire to achieve more in life. To avoid this it is important to avoid chemical contamination. There are many *YouTube* videos explaining the guidelines for decalcifying the pineal gland. You may want to access these.

There are several books on detoxification and cleansing that I recommend. *Soak Your Nuts*, written by Karyn Calabrese provides a twenty-eight day cleansing program. *Raw Food Cleanse*, by Penni Shelton, is about restoring health and losing weight by eating raw foods. Natasha Kyssa wrote a detox manual, titled, *The Simply Raw Living Foods Detox Manual*.

One procedure for cleansing internally is colon hydrotherapy. This is a simple procedure where a tube is inserted rectally and water is pumped into your colon to loosen up the hardened fecal matter for expulsion. It may not sound like something we would jump for joy about having done, but I assure you it will improve your health.

Another method for cleansing the colon is using an enema bucket. This can be much more cost efficient and can also be done in the privacy of your home without assistance. You can purchase an enema bag and kit online for less than ten dollars and search on any online search engine for instructions guiding you through the process. If you go this route, be sure to use distilled water rather than the saline solution provided.

WHAT IS A COFFEE ENEMA?

The *Gerson Hospital and Healing Centre, CHIPSA*, uses coffee enemas for detoxifying the liver, removing toxic bile, and destroying free radicals due to an increase in the antioxidant enzyme, Glutathione S-transferase.

I am, however, more sold on the chlorophyll implant over coffee, because coffee contains free radicals and acrylamides. Chlorophyll can be implanted in enemas and has a better detoxifying power. Most places offering colon hydrotherapy will provide a chlorophyll implant if you ask. Caffeine is a stimulant, so it is always best to avoid. You cannot opt for decaf either because the purpose behind the coffee enema is for the stimulant to detoxify the liver.

According to Charlotte Gerson, in her book *The Gerson Therapy*, "*When you do a coffee enema you should retain the coffee inside for up to fifteen minutes before expelling. During the time the coffee is inside, all of the body's blood is said to pass through the liver every three minutes.*"The reason why I recommend chlorophyll over coffee, then, is that chlorophyll is almost identical to hemoglobin in structure, but is centered on the magnesium atom rather than the iron atom, which hemoglobin centers around. A magnesium deficiency may trigger the health problems that would call for a coffee enema.

If you wish to do a coffee enema, which many prefer, I have provided the guidelines for you.

The guidelines for doing a self-administered coffee enema from the Gerson Institute are as follows:

    1.) Use 3 rounded tablespoons of organic drip-grind coffee (not instant) and add them to a quart of boiling water (use distilled).

    2.) Let it boil for 3 minutes uncovered and then simmer for about 15 minutes while covered

    3.) Strain the solution in a very good, fine strainer to catch all of the coffee grounds. Then after straining, add hot distilled water back until you have 1 quart again.

    4.) Let the solution cool to body temperature and then fill the enema bag and get to work.

LYMPHATIC DRAINAGE

"The cell is immortal. It is merely the fluid in which it floats that degenerates. Renew this fluid at regular intervals, give the cells what they require for nutrition, and as far as we know, the pulsation of life can go on forever." – Dr. Alexis Carrell – Nobel Prize winner

    Because the lymph fluid filters our cells, it is important to keep our lymph moving and clean from toxins. Many people who have been sedentary for years have tainted lymph fluid, and while exercise helps to move the toxins, there is also an internal cleansing service that will speed up the process for you.

    Most holistic health centers provide the lymphatic drainage. This is a cost efficient and non-invasive procedure that moves mucus out of the lymph, making it easier to breathe, and revitalizing your energy. Anyone who has trouble with congestion or lung disorders would benefit by undergoing this procedure. By simply typing "lymphatic drainage" along with your zipcode into an online search engine, you will find a place that offers this service. If you live on an island, or in a random place that does not offer this service, try jumping on a mini trampoline daily. This is known as "rebounding," and also helps to move the lymph. Running uphill can also be helpful.

OXYGEN BATH

    The oxygen bath is an internal cleansing service that submerges your body in ozone and draws toxins and heavy metals out of your blood. Many people who do this service see the evidence of heavy metal toxins being expelled from their skin immediately after the procedure. When they dry off after each session, the white towels they use become discolored from the toxins being released.

Most internal cleansing services are non-invasive and rather simple procedures. After utilizing these services you feel terrific. They rev up your energy levels and provide a positive boost. By typing "oxygen bath" into an online search engine, you should find a place nearby that offers this service. Living in the Chicago area, I personally send my clients to ***Karyn's Raw Café and Inner Beauty Center*** (karynraw.com), where they offer each of these internal cleansing services at affordable prices. If you cannot find this service in your area, research skin brushing, and try it out.

As I stated, the key to implementing change is to start by bettering ourselves. Once we do this we are ready to unite as one. Now that you have learned how to change your diet, cleanse your body, and live more harmoniously with nature, we are ready to move forward into a peaceful, loving world where the slaughtering of billions of farm animals does not exist.

I urge you to share what you have learned about eating a clean diet to revitalize health and vigor with everyone you know so we can elevate our level of consciousness, away from the usual, routine way of living, to a higher and more enlightening way of not only living, but enjoying each breath we take.

It is now time for us all to come together and unite as one. It is time to combine our ideas, build on them, and create a world full of good health, happiness, smiles, and laughter.

Chapter 13: UNITING AS ONE

Learning in depth about nutrition taught me to appreciate all of nature equally. Everything is connected. From the microorganisms to the plants, from the roots to the soil to the trees, from the fruits to the winds, from the grains to the rain, from the sun to the animals on land, from the birds on the mountains to the fish in the distant seas; everything is connected with nature. Once we find that connection, we are ready to connect with each other and unite.

"Many people, especially ignorant people, want to punish you for speaking the truth, for being correct, for being you. Never apologize for being correct, or for being years ahead of your time. If you are right and you know it, speak your mind. Even if you are a minority of one, the truth is still the truth." – Mahatma Gandhi

We need leaders in this revolution. The power of voice goes a long way. I am dedicated to doing all I can to end our dependence on chemical drugs, and to spread awareness about the dangers of eating meat, dairy, eggs, fried oils, gluten, food additives, farming chemical residues, and clarified sugars. I am willing to do whatever it takes to end the corruption and greed that contributes to millions of unnecessary deaths each year. How close are you to saying these words? How close are you to feeling this way?

What we really need is for those people who already have power and influence to shift their ways of thinking and join our movement. We need to inform the wealthy, in addition to the less fortunate, of what is taking place and engage them in this quest for change.

THE LEADERS OF THE REVOLUTION

I cannot bash the intelligence of Bill Gates; however, I do question his sphere of influence and why he would choose to accept in his life the people who feed lies into his head. There are many intelligent people with vast amounts of more accurate, helpful, and truthful information and that would be more beneficial to his apparent desire to improve world conditions.

His speech on the topic of genetically modified crops, in addition to his speech about health care and vaccinations, where he admits healthcare will decrease our population if executed "properly," demonstrate how important it is to analyze the people you learn from before absorbing the information they present to you. While favoring the production and distribution of cancer-causing GMO crops, Gates declared in a speech, *"I think the right way to think about GMO's is the same way we think about drugs. Whenever someone creates a new drug, you have to have very smart people looking at lots of trial-based data to make sure the benefits far outweigh any of the dangers."* Well, this trial based data has been released, and I included these studies in Chapter One, justifying my labeling of GMO's as cancer-causing. If you have not seen the speeches he presented, search for them on YouTube by typing in his name with GMO, and separately with population control. In his speech on population control, he announced that, *"The world today has over 6.8 billion people, and we are headed to nine billion. If we do a really great job on new vaccines, healthcare, and reproductive health services, we could lower our population by about fifteen to twenty percent."*

Gates needs to realize that many of the problems that exist today are due to the spreading of genetically modified crops, and these suicide seeds. Wildlife is being sickened by the plants, the chemicals used on them, and the alteration of plant DNA – nature's creation throughout millions of years. These GMO companies are putting animal genes in plants, and are putting farmers under strict contracts. Thousands of farmers are committing suicide because of their circumstances, and we don't really know, and cannot know, what these GMO plants will form into over thousands of years, nor the extent of what they can do to nature.

While the U.S. unloads huge amounts of GMO foods in Third World countries, this only helps to collapse their farming industries, leading to more starvation. Rather than considering what we really are doing, we continue to produce GMO corn, soy, and wheat crops, which are not necessary for health or well-being, and ship them out. Then, we continue to develop more toxic drugs to treat conditions that are the result of bad diet, and get more people believing in the false cure these harmful drugs are said to provide.

Through our ignorance, we are getting sick and people in these drought stricken countries are dying. We need more people of influence to step up and become a part of the real solution, in tune with nature. Gates should be using his money to change the agricultural industry so we shift to organic polycropping growing methods. This will not only save us from extinction, but will prevent us from getting sick. The sad thing is that Gates has already admitted that he supports the GMO, medical, and healthcare industries because it, "Helps keep our population under control." But it helps corporate profits most of all.

KINDNESS TRUST

Philip Wollen started the *Kindness Trust* fund (kindnesstrust.com). He funds projects and organizations that bring kindness to our world. At the age of thirty-four, Philip became the Vice President of *Citibank*. By the age of forty, after visiting a factory farm where animals are slaughtered, he resigned, and put his money, and energy, towards ending the factory farming industry, and enriching us with kindness. He believes we must remove animal products from the menu. He is well known for a speech he delivered at the *St. James Ethics Debate*, where he argued for the removal of animal products from our menus.

It is among the greatest speeches of our era. Following is an excerpt of his speech:

"Victor Hugo said, 'Nothing is more powerful than an idea whose time has come.' Well, animal rights today is now the greatest social justice issue since the abolition of slavery. Do you know there are over 600 million vegetarians in this world? And that is bigger than the United States, England, France, Germany, Spain, Italy, Canada, Australia, New Zealand – all put together. And despite this massive demographic footprint, we are still drowned out by the huntin,' shootin,' killin' cartels who believe that violence is the answer when it should not even be a question.

We are facing the perfect storm. If any nation had developed weapons that could wreak such havoc on the planet – as the livestock industry does – we would launch a preemptive military strike and bomb it back into the Bronze Age. But it is not a rogue state, it is an industry. The good news is we don't have to bomb it; we can just stop buying it. So George Bush was wrong. The Axis of Evil does not run through Iraq, Iran or North Korea, it runs through our dining tables. Weapons of Mass Destruction are our knives and forks.

Animals are not just other species, they are other nations. And we murder them at our peril. The Peace Map is drawn on a menu. Peace is not just the absence of war; it is the presence of justice. Justice must be blind to race, color, religion or species; if she's not blind, she will be a weapon of terror. And tonight there is unimaginable terror in those ghastly Guantanamo's we call factory farms or slaughterhouses. Believe me, if slaughterhouses had glass walls, we would not be having this debate tonight. You see, I believe another world is possible. Let's get animals off the menu and out of these torture chambers. Please vote tonight for those who have no voice." – Philip Wollen, founder of **The Kindness Trust.**

We need more leaders like Philip, who are kind, loving, and passionate, and willing to devote their energy to good causes. Please check out his website, and watch the video clips of his speeches on YouTube. You will learn a lot from him.

CELEBRITY INFLUENCE

"There's cleanliness to how I eat now. I'm much more in tune with my body. I am now so in tune based on having become a vegan, that I can tell what foods affect energy levels. I can tell when I've been eating particularly high nutrient foods or I can tell when my glycemic levels are all over the place. The detox and veganism really allowed me to tune into the subtleties of how food affects my body. This has really helped for my training especially. Kale is my best friend. I eat kale salad. I put kale in my smoothies, kale in my soup. Kale, kale, kale! I feel like Popeye. I love it!" – Alanis Morissette, talented musician.

After a health scare, the amazing American tennis star, Serena Williams, announced she had made the transition to a raw vegan diet. Soon after, she took home the gold medal for her country, and most recently, she won the US open title.

Ellen DeGeneres, TV personality, is an advocate, and follower of a vegan diet. The actors, Russell Brand and Ben Stiller, both announced in 2012 they have transitioned to a vegan diet. Jared Leto, Joaquin Phoenix, Russell Brand, Tobey Maguire, and Woody Harrelson follow vegan diets. Actresses, Alyssa Milano, Jenny McCarthy, and Michelle Pfeiffer, abide by a vegan diet. The well-known musician, Alanis Morissette, also announced her transition to a vegan diet and claims to be feeling better than ever. How ironic is that?

The singers, Carrie Underwood, Erykah Badu, Fiona Apple, Jason Mraz, Michael Franti, follow vegan diets. Musicians, Moby, and Ozzy Ozbourne do not include animal products in their diets. Mike Tyson converted to veganism and claims to feel better than he ever has. The NFL running back Arian Foster successfully adopted a plant-based lifestyle and is having an impressive season. Andre 3000, musician of OutKast, eats vegan. Def Jam founder, Russell Simmons, abides by a vegan diet as well and he is a shining example of good health.

With more celebrities and influential people stepping up and making the transition to veganism, we are beginning to see a rise in the trend. Not one of us is capable of transforming our society on our own; this only becomes possible by uniting as one. We need you, your family, and your friends to join us as well.

Chapter 14: PRESCRIPTION DRUGS DO NOT EXIST

"Your pain, misery and illness result from your own dietary mistakes and drugs. You are suffering because you are filled with toxic wastes caused by your diet of poorly selected food filled with artificial flavorings, preservatives, synthetics, over-processed ingredients – too much stimulating food, too few natural vitamins from vegetables and fruits. Even if you selected wholesome, natural foods, they were probably improperly prepared, boiled to death or overheated in oil, then covered with harmful condiments. The normal chemistry of your digestion is upset not only by these toxic wastes but also by harmful drugs, unhealthy living habits that include lack of exercise. So, highly poisonous materials – toxins – which have stagnated in your blood, impair the filters and eliminative organs, chief of which are the kidneys, liver, bowels and skin." – **Dr. Henry Bieler,** *Food Is Your Best Medicine*

The best way to avoid a dependence on chemical drugs is to simply believe in your mind that these drugs are not an option, and do not exist. In doing so, you will begin to look for alternatives. You will find that the best solution to sickness is a change in diet and lifestyle.

"The necessity of teaching mankind not to take drugs and medicines is a duty incumbent upon all who know their uncertainty and injurious effects; and the time is not far distant when the drug system will be abandoned." – *Charles Armbruster, M.D.*

I envision a world where chemical drugs do not exist. I see a future where hospitals will not be necessary, other than for emergency medicine, rehab, defects, and very few "conditions." Good health will be contagious and spread all around, rather than sickness and disease. This vision of mine is not too far from becoming reality. When we finally shift from chemical drugs to organic polycropped foods as our main source of medicine, we will reach a new paradigm where we are more than likely to know good health and happiness.

"Drugs never cure disease. They merely hush the voice of nature's protest, and pull down the danger signals she erects along the pathway of transgression. Any poison taken into the system has to be reckoned with later on, even though it palliates present symptoms. Pain may disappear, but the patient is left in a worse condition, though unconscious of it at the time." – *Daniel. H. Kress, M.D.*

OUR ECONOMY AT ITS STRONGEST

My ultimate goal in life would be to influence the end of poverty and sickness through optimal, plant-based, organic nutrition, awareness, and education.

We can completely rebuild our economy through the growth, production, and sale of organic produce and superfoods, by utilizing optimal nutrition to cure and treat sickness and disease, and by switching to sustainable materials and energy, such as industrial hemp, and truly Earth-friendly energy sources. By opening raw organic vegan restaurants all over the world, we can not only build our economy stronger, but also build true health. In this situation, we would not have to continue to rely on medicine to keep our economy going, we can quit fooling people into believing chemical drugs are an elixir for sickness and we can end the profits from the sickness campaign that is the pharmaceutical industry, GMO monocropping, and the animal farming, and fast food and junk foods industries that induce illness.

We can combat sickness with raw, organic foods. We can end disease by properly nourishing our bodies. We can end our dependency on drugs.

The way this can and will be done is through educating our society on the dangers of eating animal products and downing mass quantities of pharmaceutical drugs, by exposing the marketing schemes of the pharmaceutical industry, and by providing organic fruits, vegetables, herbs, seeds, and superfoods all over the world.

The solution can be simple if we each work together as a team. The answers have been right in front of our eyes the entire time.

LONGEVITY RETREATS

We can strengthen our economy by replacing hospitals with longevity retreats that will only grow and serve organic foods. I am ready to open these retreats. If you would like to join me and help get this started, please reach out to me. I have a business plan ready. The patients will not receive any drugs, only internal cleansing and real organic food and juices. They will see sunlight daily. They will be provided with yoga, exercise, massage, and intellectual stimulation.

These new retreats will be so diverse with treatments that they will create millions of new jobs. As we become healthier and happier as a society, we will also gain our health.

Our economy will be stronger than it has been in all of history. We will no longer worry about wars, power, or resources. We will have the greatest resources of all: true health, happiness, and love.

Chapter 15: IS THIS CHANGE REALLY POSSIBLE?

"The end of the human race will be that it will eventually die of civilization." –
Ralph Waldo Emerson

The most beneficial way to solve the problems of this world is to shift the power and profit from corporations, deleterious foods, and chemical drugs, to good health. By providing everyone with optimal nutrition, we can change attitudes, we can heal sickness, we can reverse imbalances stealing life from the mentally challenged, and we can reduce frustration, anxiety, and desperation that play out in social ills and crimes.

At the *Victor Valley Medium Community Correctional Facility* in Adelanto, California, new inmates attended an orientation where they received two clear choices. They could live on one side of the prison which operated using the standard *California Department of Corrections (CDC)* guidelines and food menus; or, they could live on the side of the prison operated under the *"NEWSTART"* program which included a vegan diet, job training, and anger management. Initially, the *State of California* was very supportive of the *NEWSTART* concept; however, they did not believe that any of the five-hundred inmates would accept this kind of a diet. They announced that inmates would most likely, *"Burn the place down before they became vegetarians."* Surprisingly to them, once the program was in progress, the opposite became true.

On average, eighty-five percent of the inmates chose the **NEWSTART** side, while only fifteen percent chose the **CDC** program. Throughout the **NEWSTART** program, the improvements in their attitudes and behavioral changes were astonishing, and could even be seen outside in the prison yard. Prison officials declared that not one of the inmates on the program "owned," or controlled the yard. Typical lines that were drawn between Blacks, Whites, Hispanics, gang members, and other groups were non-existent. Those on the *NEWSTART* program were instead seen playing basketball together, developing fellowship, and finding purpose in life. Those living with CDC regulations, eating typical prison diets most likely prepared from the Basic Four food groups, experienced the typical racial divisions seen at any other prison.

In testimonials, the inmates shared that they were surprised by how good the food tasted, felt much better after eating it, noticed improved energy levels, increased their stamina, gained mental clarity, and reduced problems with acne. This study is scientific proof that a vegan diet can be effective with rehabilitation, and can change the thinking patterns of criminals. When **Victor Valley** nutrition services coordinator **Julianne Aranda** explained the effectiveness of the program, she stated, *"What we eat not only affects us physically, but it affects our mental attitude, our aggressiveness, and our*

307

ability to make good decisions." This study was published in the January 2011 issue of *Vegetarian Spotlight* magazine (*vegetarianspotlight.com*).

If we were to eliminate the factory farms, banish dairy farms, and put an end to growing unnecessary crops for the purpose of fattening the livestock; we could ultimately change the world.

We can save the rainforests. We can save thousands of species from extinction. We can be a nation that thrives on good health, intelligence, and happiness rather than one saturated with greed, crime, sickness, and premature death. We can do all of this by simply changing our approach to eating, and avoiding all animal products.

When outsiders consider the "land of the free," they may not see a land full of freedom. They might see a country run by cannibals, terrorizing animals, killing them for profit and feeding the dead flesh to millions of sick and diseased citizens. They may see a country ruled by corporate terrorists intentionally poisoning their own people with chemicals in the food and water supply, and then deceiving them with more poison in the form of prescription drugs and fossil fuels.

How is this referred to as the land of the free? We do not have the freedom to choose how we want to be treated for our health conditions. If we discover a cure for cancer, or a cure for any disease, we face criminal charges for releasing it. When we video record what is happening in the factory farms and slaughterhouses, where billions of animals are being stripped of their lives in the Animal Holocaust, or if we protest the crimes of the animal farming industry, the government and corporations refer to the act of recording these atrocities and protesting as "acts of terrorism." If we discover the truth we seem to be reprimanded for refusing to conceal it.

"You can never change things by fighting the existing reality. To change something, build a new model that makes the existing model obsolete." – Richard Buckminster Fuller

Why is it that we cannot unite and restructure the way our country is being manipulated by the criminals in charge? Many of the criminal acts in the world are being committed by those who are in charge of determining who is or is not the criminal.

So I wonder, is it possible to change? I think we most definitely can – and must. A good way to begin is by educating ourselves on what is really happening. We have to stop feeding into the lies and stop supporting the chemical companies, GMO industry, and pharmaceutical industry. We must eat only organic and refuse to eat processed foods. If we do not purchase these chemicals in the form of food, then eventually the companies will have to quit making them.

To continue your studies on these issues, please read John Robbins' book, *The Food Revolution*; Vandan Shiva's book, *Making Peace With The Earth*; Dr. T. Colin Campbell's book, *The China Study*; John McCabe's books, *Sunfood Diet Infusion* and *Extinction*; and Sergei Boutenko's book, *Wild Edibles*, to be published in 2013.

HOW WILL THE GOVERNMENT RESPOND?

"We need to have a fat and cholesterol tax, a protein and phosphorus tax, and a sucrose and caffeine tax, to cover the true costs of food abuse." – Sapoty Brook

I'm beginning to think government leaders and politicians may not realize how much stronger our economy would grow to be if we were to find more natural ways to end sickness, and to quit relying on chemicals and chemical drugs. The marketing schemes of the huge corporations may be conning them into believing the economy will collapse without chemicals, sickness, and prescription drugs. When we look at it from a neutral perspective, our economy has already collapsed. When life ends, the economy will no longer matter. We choose if we want to preserve life, or continue to let our "leaders" lead us astray.

"If people let the government decide what foods they eat and what medicines they take, their bodies will soon be in as sorry a state as the souls who live under tyranny." – Thomas Jefferson

It is up to us whether or not we will choose to permit the government to do as Thomas Jefferson said in that famous quotation. We must be ready to stand for what we believe in. We cannot continue to be subjects in this big experiment we will never win, where sickness never goes away, and we accept misery as a part of life. Do you like being weak? Do you enjoy giving your paychecks to the government so they can poison you in return? If you are one of those who does not enjoy this at all, it is time for you to stand up and make some changes in your life, starting with your health.

By eliminating all meats, dairy, processed foods, fast foods, dependency on prescription drugs and synthetic chemicals, gluten, flours, sugars, alcohol, and cigarettes from your life, you no longer support the profits of corporations feeding on misfortunes they created. One of the most powerful things you can do is plant and maintain your own organic food garden enriched with compost from your own organic food scraps.

CRIMINAL CHARGES

"The Earth is alive. Like our own bodies, she has organs, blood and intelligence. Since the functions of our being are synchronized with the planet, we must adhere to the law that created and maintains the Earth. Only in this way will true ecology and world peace be secured. Any misuse of any part of the Earth can disturb life's stability. Today, 'super powers' compete for leadership, but none of them can ever establish their 'one world order' with laws other than the law that maintains true world order. In the attempt to attain exclusive planetary authority with man-made laws, the opposite is accomplished. No one can compete with the power that authorized us to exist on planet Earth. Only ignorance can make one persist on following the dead-end path that ignorance produces." – **Martin Gashweseoma**

The Wall Street protests were the first sign of action many of us living today have seen take place. This was a great first step. We saw how the government responded. They filed criminal charges. They pepper sprayed elderly folks faces. They did everything they could to protect the corporations over the people. This truly criminal "bullying" needs to stop, and as long as we continue to go forth with non-violence we will eventually break away from the axis of evil that looms over our home land and spreads into poorer countries.

"The right to search for truth implies also a duty; one must not conceal any part of what one has recognized to be true." – **Albert Einstein**

How many criminal charges can there be for revealing the truth? How many criminal charges can exist for expressing individuality? How many times can they continue to arrest us and beat us down for demonstrating peace and revealing corporate and government crimes and corruption?

We can change this world. We can live better lives. We can spread the truth. We shall start by improving our health individually, by being wiser with what we consume, and by becoming more self-sufficient.

CHECKMATE

"When the power of love overcomes the love of power, this is when the world will know peace." – **Jimi Hendrix, Legendary guitarist**

We are all acting as pawns and the pharmaceutical reps are playing the chess board. We are getting used like puppets and the miseducated medical doctors are our ventriloquists. We are being brainwashed, abused, mishandled, and mistreated. These huge corporations and industries do not care about us. They care about their profits.

We have been welcomed to play them in a big game of chess, on their board, where they make the rules, and they make the first move. They have blinded us so we play at the novice level while they are chess masters. When we go in blind like we do, we have no chance.

310

This is why I urge you to educate yourself further on what is really going on. Get involved in nutrition. Plant your own gardens and grow your own food. Break away from the traditions that are holding you back. Take back your health. It is 2013, this does not mean the *Armageddon* is going to come and end the world, this means we are going to shift to a higher level of consciousness and transform the world into a better place.

I hope I have equipped you to lead your own revolution towards taking back your health. I hope I have inspired you to pull yourself out of the trap of sickness and despair. I hope I have motivated you to eat right.

I encourage you to spread the word to everyone you know, everyone you care about, and each person you love. Once we help ourselves and we discover the paradise that awaits us in the world of organic, raw vegan foods, the best thing we can do is share the experience with those around us.

The raw vegan (term coined by John McCabe) community is building globally with places like *Living Light Culinary Institute* in California, and *Samudra* in Australia; websites and bloggers on every continent, such as Angie Curtis in Africa, and FreeLee Frugivore and Harley "DurianRider" Johnstone in Australia; raw food books in many languages, such as Eduardo Corassa in Brazil with his raw food books, and the Boutenko family publishing their raw food books in many languages. There are raw food companies in many countries, such as Andrei Andi in Romania, where he makes raw vegan cakes. There are raw vegan cafes in many diverse countries, such as in Bali, Germany, Switzerland, New Zealand, Thailand, and Turkey. For more on the international raw vegan industry, join the Facebook group page, *Raw Vegan Restaurants, Chefs, Retreats, and Produce*. Also, see the book *Sunfood Traveler*, by John McCabe.

Let's create our own *Armageddon*, where we put an end to the world of sickness, disease, processed foods, chemicals, drugs, and greed. Together we can unite in a place where peace, laughter, smiles, and happiness are abundant; and we dance to the sounds of music, with the energy from raw foods.

ANYWAY

People are often unreasonable, illogical and self centered;
forgive them anyway.

If you are kind, people may accuse you of selfish, ulterior motives;
be kind anyway.

If you are successful, you will win some false friends and some true enemies;
succeed anyway.

If you are honest and frank, people may cheat you;
be honest and frank anyway.

What you spend years building, someone could destroy overnight;
Build anyway.

If you find serenity and happiness, they may be jealous;
be happy anyway.

The good you do today, people will often forget tomorrow;
do good anyway.

Give the world the best you have, and it may never be enough;
Give the world the best you've got anyway.

You see, in the final analysis, it is between you and your journey;
It was never between you and them anyway.

—   *Mother Teresa*

JUST WALKED AWAY

Earth is crumbling. The soil is poisoned.

We eat what does not come from nature and call it food; we plant seeds that are genetically altered, it is no wonder we lose.

The bark on the trees is starting to decay; the roots are drying. Ancient Sequoia's collapse, while arrogant hunters end the lives of beautiful animals, shooting them dead in their tracks.

It all stacks up and soon the sun will be under attack.

The Iceberg's are already melting away, while radioactive elements taint marine life and stain what it once was.

Imaginations no longer exist because our nutrients were robbed by pasteurization and refinement.

These processed foods steal the magic from children's minds and lower our intelligence quotient, so we go from being radiant and always shining to sedentary and without motion, while lacking our true emotions.

Where is the potion, the elixir? Is there still hope? Can we save the last plant before its life force withers with famine? Can we change the planet before thousands more species vanish?

Rather, humans disrupt the life cycle trying to manage factory farms.

These fellow humans are not even real, they are money controlled savages, poisoned by corporations and marketing tactics.

The pharmaceuticals have murdered generation after generation and we all drowned in the devastation, praying for some type of "cure" with looks and feelings of desperation. We seek doctor after doctor for consultations that only lead to more deadly combinations of chemicals and false obligations. What happened to this entire nation?

We fail to look around and actually see, too familiar with sitting in front of the TV that misleads us into living in distorted realities and guides us into buying fast foods, new cars, and chemical pills. These practices eventually induce disease.

We mask our hunger malnourishing ourselves day after day by eating garbage, to give us temporary feelings of success, driven from ego and to "treat" the ailments that have developed from our ignorance.

It's no wonder why so many resort to crime, their heads are so polluted with medical lies. Prozac for kids and other drugs for all of the so-called "mental illnesses" to compliment their frozen dinners at home, because devalued time is too valuable to prepare fresh, nurturing meals, so there goes another winner.

No more home sweet home, now it's full of sickness and misery and poverty eats up the ones we look past on our quest to prove all others wrong, so we can shine in our own spotlight that is really only greed. Or is it really a lack of knowledge? Or is it the only way to feel free when ninety percent of us are locked up behind alcoholism, animal products, drug abuse, nicotine, overeating, caffeine, synthetic foods, obesity, and disease?

Rainy days are no longer spent relaxing in bed, but instead, we labor through them to pay mortgages so we don't lose our homes and life savings to the feds that work for big banks that would rather see us dead than lower their profits for some to get a chance to live before their time comes; something they have never once did.

America's traditions have moved from turkeys on Thanksgiving to celebrate the overtaking of cultures they decimated, to pig dinners at Christmas turned into a corporate fiasco, to alcohol with every meal, every break, every moment, to smoking for "relief" of stress, to chemicals in the food and water supply, to poisons everywhere, to premature aging, to cancer at any age, to diseases we never before heard of, to a life expectancy of just over sixty; But we cannot change tradition, right? How could we ever let this be?

All of those steak dinners just made another widow; cardiovascular disease never warns it just hits you. We all might as well let our dreams escape through that open window.

We've been "dumbed down" so much that we've become numb to the things that are important; like love, like loyalty, like trust, like family, like promises never broken.

We have lost our capacity to feel pain with each cooked animal vein, each synthetic drug coating our brains, each drink the bartender makes, each dollar the corporate companies take.

This audacity of hope, well, it just walked away.

— **Jesse J. Jacoby**

MY VISION FOR THE FUTURE

In a society full of sickness, disease, misfortunes, dishonesty, deceit, greed and unnecessary deaths, I always search for the positive. Through all of these negative characteristics, I have found love, prosperity, warmth, generosity, truth, passion, and life. For every up there is a down, for every wrong there is a right, and from all of my research, I have discovered that for most every disease there is a cure.

As a society, together, we have cried enough tears to build waterways grieving over the millions of loved ones we have lost due to unnecessary deaths from being misdiagnosed and given chemical drugs that were not helpful in any way. We have suffered through unimaginable pains and we have swallowed death sentences handed out by doctors who have never been educated on proper ways to cure the ailments with which they are being presented. We have been lied to, kicked while we are down, and forced to go through radiation and chemotherapy treatments that are never necessary to begin with. We have been poisoned through our food supply and our water supply for years with added chemicals approved of by the administration that was established with the sole purpose of keeping us safe (FDA), and with dissolved solvents which we have never been warned about, that linger in water sources we use for drinking, for food, and for bathing.

We have allowed ourselves to be pawns. We have permitted huge corporations and pharmaceutical empires to turn us into these puppets which they control. Our ventriloquists are the doctors who lie in our faces to hit their quota each month so they will receive bonuses that will allow them to take their tropical vacations each season, or to pay for their homes that are often so large they do not know what to do with the extra rooms, all at the expense of our health. The outcome of our lives, the lives of our loved ones, and all of our misfortunes have been placed at the fingertips of these men and women who, in most cases, believe what they are doing is right, because they are following concepts they were taught in the medical schools they attended – which are greatly influenced by pharma and medical technology companies.

Each written prescription may result in a death, either suddenly, or in the future. Each false diagnosis results in more sickness, and unnecessary surgery. Each penny spent continues to add up and contributes to the profits of the richest, greediest, most lousy, most inhumane, and most unethical businesses.

We have reached an era in society. An era where we can no longer lay back and tell our children that mommy is no longer here because she was "meant to evolve" into a sick individual, and develop a disease which "somehow" has no cure. We are in an era where our children should no longer have to grow up without a father because "daddy had heart disease." An era where we should never again have to watch our newborn children, or our young children, go through painful, life-destructing medical treatments using toxic drugs, radiation, and chemotherapy, when we all know there are natural cures.

We are at a critical time and a critical juncture in life. We are at the crossroads of life and death and the only thing standing in our way, the only barricade blocking us from life, and the only obstacle we face, is whether or not we choose to believe that we were not meant to evolve this way and stand up and demand the truth, or whether we shall accept the doctor's orders and lay on our death beds, allowing the hospitals and banks to take over our lives and our properties.

Amongst these reckoning grounds, we still can cling to this hope. We have access to knowledge we have never before unveiled. We have access to foods from every region of the world providing us with the nutrients our food supply once lacked. We now know what real superfoods are, and what the plants and fruits of the earth can and will do for us when we ingest them in their wild, natural, and organic state. We have an army of bright, intelligent young men and women, who demand the truth, and dedicate and devote their lives to spreading the word, while reclaiming our evolution and civilization.

We must act now.

RECOMMENDED RESOURCES

My Top Ten Recommended Books:
1.) Becoming Raw, by Vesanto Melina and Brenda Davis
2.) Sunfood Diet Infusion, 2nd Edition 2012 by John McCabe
3.) The China Study, by Dr. T. Colin Campbell
4.) Preventing & Reversing Heart Disease, by Dr. Caldwell Esselstyn
5.) The Food Revolution, by John Robbins
6.) Raw Food For Dummies, by Cherie Soria & Dan Ladermann
7.) Comfortably Unaware, by Dr. Richard Oppenlander
8.) The World Peace Diet, by Will Tuttle
9.) Conscious Eating, by Dr. Gabriel Cousens
10.) The 80/10/10 Diet, by Dr. Douglas Graham

Other Excellent Reads:
1.) Green For Life, by Victoria Boutenko
2.) Sunfood Traveler, by John McCabe
3.) Eco-Eating, by Sapoty Brook
4.) Rawsome!, by Brigitte Mars
5.) The Country Almanac of Home Remedies, by Brigitte Mars
6.) Making Peace With the Earth, by Vandana Shiva
7.) The Gerson Therapy, by Charlotte Gerson
8.) 21-Day Weight Loss Kickstart, by Dr. Neal Barnard
9.) The Starch Solution, by Dr. John McDougall
10.) LifeForce, by Dr. Brian Clement
11.) Hooked On Raw, by Rhio
12.) The Spectrum, by Dr. Dean Ornish
13.) The Simply Raw Living Foods Detox Manual, by Natasha Kyssa
14.) Health and Nutrition Secrets, by Dr. Russell Blaylock
15.) Wild Edibles, by Sergei Boutenko
16.) Overdosed America, by Dr. John Abramson
17.) Igniting Your Life, by John McCabe
18.) Fats That Heal, Fats That Kill, by Dr. Udo Erasmus
19.) Soak Your Nuts, by Karyn Calabrese
20.) Creating Healthy Children, by Karen Ranzi
21.) There Is A Cure for Diabetes, by Dr. Gabriel Cousens
22.) Raw Food Cleanse, by Penni Shelton
23.) Green For Life, by Victoria Boutenko
24.) Thrive Foods, by Brendan Brazier
25.) The Detox Miracle Sourcebook, by Dr. Robert Morse
26.) The Raw Food Revolution Diet, by Cherie Soria
27.) The Super Fit Vegan, by Jeff Sekerak
28.) Eating Animals, by Jonathan Safran Foer
29.) Nourished, by Silvie and Maryl Celiz
30.) Waist Away: How to Joyfully Lose Weight, by Dr. Michael Greger
31.) The Pleasure Trap, by Dr. Doug Lisle

Raw Recipe Books:
    1.) I am Grateful, by Terces Engelhart
    2.) The Raw Truth, by Jeremy Safron
    3.) Hooked On Raw, by Rhio
    4.) Ani's Raw Food Kitchen, by Ani Phyo
    5.) Live Raw, by Mimi Kirk
    6.) Viva La Raw, by Eric Rivkin
    7.) Rainbow Green Live-Food Cuisine, by Dr. Gabriel Cousens
    8.) Raw Food Real World, by Matthew Kenney
    9.) Easy To Be Raw, by Megan Elizabeth
    10.) Rawlicious Recipes, by Andrea Cox
    11.) Living Raw Food, by Sarma Melngailis
    12.) Rawlicious, by Peter Daniel
    13.) 101 Frickin' Raw Recipes, by Chris Kendall
    14.) Simple Vegan Classics, by Jason Wrobel

Recommended DVD's:
    1.) Forks Over Knives
    2.) May I Be Frank
    3.) The Big Fix
    4.) Earthlings
    5.) Fresh
    6.) Fat, Sick, and Nearly Dead
    7.) Food Matters
    8.) The Gerson Miracle
    9.) The Beautiful Truth
    10.) Food, INC
    11.) The Future of Food
    12.) Simply Raw: Reversing Diabetes in 30 Days
    13.) Farmageddon
    14.) Acid Test by NRDC
    15.) The World According to Monsanto
    16.) Dying To Have Known
    17.) King Corn
    18.) Ingredients
    19.) Vegucated
    20.) Folks, This Ain't Normal
    21.) A Delicate Balance
    22.) Cancer Is Curable Now

Recommended Websites:
    1.) Therawcure.com
    2.) Nutritionfacts.org
    3.) Kindnesstrust.com
    4.) Ignitingyourlife.com
    5.) Fullyraw.com

6.) Plantpoweredliving.com
7.) Rawfullytempting.com
8.) Rawfoodinfo.com
9.) Rawpowerkids.com
10.) Superhealthychildren.com
11.) Rawfoodexplained.com
12.) Almondblossomlive.com
13.) Welikeitraw.com
14.) Livingfoodsinstitute.com
15.) Ecopeaceful.com
16.) Therawadvantage.com
17.) Pcrm.org
18.) 30bananasaday.com
19.) Healthyhaven.net
20.) Rawfoodrehab.ning.com
21.) VegWorldMagazine.com

Organizations, Movements, Activism:
1.) Kindness Trust
2.) Foodnotlawns.com
3.) Kitchengardens.com
4.) Urban Homesteaders
5.) Food Routes
6.) Organic Consumers Association
7.) Food Not Bombs
8.) Sea Shepherd
9.) Earth Island Institute
10.) Physician's Committee for Responsible Medicine
11.) Natural Resources Defense Council
12.) Earth Echo
13.) Earth First
14.) Fracking
15.) Mountain Top Removal
16.) Stop Tar Sands
17.) Votehemp.com
18.) Rainforest Action Network
19.) Farm Sanctuary
20.) School Gardens

Seed and Gardening Websites:
1.) Edibleforestgardens.com
2.) SeedAlliance.org
3.) Theorganicgardener.net
4.) Permaculture.net
5.) Rareseeds.com
6.) SavingOurSeed.org

ABOUT THE AUTHOR

Jesse Jacoby is a dedicated raw foodist who has devoted his life to the movement. He abides by a raw, organic vegan diet, lives a natural lifestyle, and encourages compassion towards all animals.

Jesse is a longevity expert, nutritionist, certified raw organic nutritionist, certified lifestyle and weight management consultant, certified personal trainer, and holistic health coach. He truly believes he can help anyone greatly improve their quality of health no matter what age or how severe their issues may be, without having to rely on chemical drugs.

You can reach Jesse by e-mail at:
Jesse@therawcure.com, or find him on Facebook.
Join his facebook group: The Raw Cure

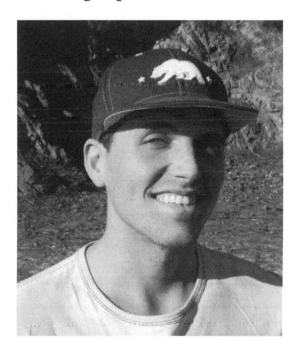

BIBLIOGRAPHY

Intro:

-Campbell, T.Colin. *The China Study*. Ben Bella Books, 1ˢᵗ Edition, 2006.

-"AERS Patient Outcomes by Year," Food and Drug Administration (Washington, DC: U.S. Department of Health and Human Services, March 31, 2010).

-Howlader N, Noone AM, Krapcho M, Neyman N, Aminou R, Waldron W, Altekruse SF, Kosary CL, Ruhl J, Tatalovich Z, Cho H, Mariotto A, Eisner MP, Lewis DR, Chen HS, Feuer EJ, Cronin KA, Edwards BK (eds). *SEER Cancer Statistics Review, 1975-2008*, National Cancer Institute. Bethesda, MD, http://seer.cancer.gov/csr/1975_2008/, based on November 2010 SEER data submission, posted to the SEER web site, 2011.

-Substance Abuse and Mental Health Services Administration. Results from the 2010 National Survey on Drug Use and Health: volume 1: summary of national findings. Rockville, MD: Substance Abuse and Mental Health Services Administration, Office of Applied Studies; 2011.

-Preston-Martin, S. et al. "N-nitroso compounds and childhood *brain tumors*: A case-control study." Cancer Res. 1982; 42:5240-5.

-Adams, Kelly M. MPH, RD; Kohlmeier, Martin MD; Zeisel, Steven H. MD, PhD. Nutrition Education in U.S. Medical Schools: Latest Update of a National Survey. Academic Medicine: September 2010 - Volume 85 - Issue 9 - pp 1537-1542

Chapter 1:

-"New Evidence Confirms the Nutritional Superiority of Plant-Based Organic Foods," State of Science Review, March 2008

-Shelton, Herbert. *Food Combining Made Easy*. Ontario: Willow Publishing, 1982.

-Wigmore, Ann. *The Hippocrates Diet and Health Program*. NJ: Avery Penguin Putnam, 1984.

-McCabe, John. *The Sunfood Traveler*. Carmania Books, 2011

-Carrington, Hereward. *Vitality, Fasting and Nutrition*. General Books LLC, 2009.

-McKenna, Terrence. *Food of the Gods*. Bantam, 1993.

-Clement, Brian. *Hippocrates LifeForce*. Healthy Living Publications, 1ˢᵗ Edition, 2007.

-Rothkranz, Markus. *Heal Yourself 101*. Rothkranz Publishing, 1ˢᵗ Edition, 2011.

- Vallejo, F., Tomás-Barberán, F. and García-Viguera, C. (2003), Phenolic compound contents in edible parts of broccoli inflorescences after domestic cooking. J. Sci. Food Agric., 83: 1511–1516. doi: 10.1002/jsfa.1585

-Howell, Edward. *Enzyme Nutrition*. Avery Publishing Group, 1ˢᵗ Edition, 1995.

-Holbrook, M.L. *Eating For Strength*. Nabu Press, 2010.

-Melngailis, Sarma. *Raw Food Real World*. William Morrow Cookbooks, 1ˢᵗ Edition, 2005.

Chapter 2:

-Blaylock, Russell. *Health and Nutrition Secrets*. Health Press NA Inc, Revised Edition, 2006.

-Bragg, Paul and Patricia. *The Miracle of Fasting*. Health Science, 3ʳᵈ Edition, 1999.

-Kulvinskas, Viktoras. *Survival into the 21ˢᵗ Century*. IA: 21ˢᵗ Century Publications, 1975.

-*Food Matters*. Documentary, 2009.

-Price, Weston A. *Nutrition and Physical Degeneration*. Price Pottenger Nutrition, 8ᵗʰ Edition, 2008.

- Pan A, Sun Q, Bernstein AM; et al. Red meat consumption and mortality: results from 2 prospective cohort studies [published online March 12, 2012]. *Arch Intern Med.* doi:10.1001/archinternmed.2011.2287

-Robbins, John. *Diet for a New America*. HJ Kramer, 2ⁿᵈ Edition, 1998.

322

-Harris, Robert S. *Nutritional Evaluation of Food Processing.* AVI Publishing Company, 1973.

-Ers.usda.gov(USDA Economics research Service)

-Graham, Douglas. *The 80/10/10 Diet.* Foodnsport Press, 2006.

-Primack, Jeff. *Conquering Any Disease.* Press On QI Productions, 2011

-Lappe, Frances Moore. *Diet for a Small Planet.* Ballantine Books, 20th Anv Edition, 1991.

-Erasmus, Udo. *Fats That Heal, Fats That Kill.* Alive Books, Revised Edition, 1993.

- Potera, Carol. "The artificial food dye blues." Environmental Health Perspectives 118.10 (Oct 2010) A428(1).

- Kanigel, Rachele. "It Raises Diabetes Risk And Robs Bone. It's Wrecking Our Teeth. And It's Making Us Fat. The Culprit? SODA." *Prevention* 58.10 (2006): 160-207. *Academic Search Premier.* Web. 21 Mar. 2012.

-Campbell, T.Colin. *The China Study.* BenBella Books, 1st Edition, 2006.

-Denise Grady Scientists See Higher Use Of Antibiotics on Farms, New York Times, January 2001

-McCabe, John. *The Sunfood Traveler.* Carmania Books, 2011

-McCabe, John. *Sunfood Living.* North Atlantic Books, 2007

-DeGeneres, Ellen. *My Point and I do Have One.* Bantam, 2007.

-Barnard, Neal. *Breaking the Food Seduction.* St. Martin's Griffin, 2004.

-Langley, Gill. *Vegan Nutrition.* Vegan Society Ltd, 1988.

-Cohen, Robert. *www.notmilk.com*

- Ziegler, Ekhard E. "Consumption Of Cow's Milk As A Cause Of Iron Deficiency In Infants And Toddlers." *Nutrition Reviews* 69.(2011): S37-S42.

- Sonneville KR, Gordon CM, Kocher MS, Pierce LM, Ramappa A, Field AE. Vitamin D, Calcium, and Dairy Intakes and Stress Fractures Among Female Adolescents. *Arch Pediatr Adolesc Med.* March 5, 2012.

-McCabe, John. *Sunfood Diet Infusion.* Carmania Books, 2011

- Steen Stender, et al. "Nutrition Transition And Its Relationship To The Development Of Obesity And Related Chronic Diseases." *Obesity Reviews* 9.(2008): 48-52.

-Dietary Sugars Intake and Cardiovascular Health: A Scientific Statement From the American Heart Association *Circulation. 2009;120:1011-1020*

- Erin L. Richman, Stacey A. Kenfield, Meir J. Stampfer, Edward L. Giovannucci, June M. Chan. ***"Egg, red meat, and poultry intake and risk of lethal prostate cancer in the prostate specific antigen-era: incidence and survival"*** *Cancer Prev Res* Published Online First 19 September 2011; DOI:10.1158/1940-6207.CAPR-11-0354

- Seafood Choices: Balancing Risks and Benefits. *Institute of Medicine:* Washington, D.C., 2007.

-Journal of the American College of Cardiology, 2006; 48: 1666

- Hurrell, R.F., 2003. Influence of vegetable protein sources on trace element and mineral bioavailability. J. Nutr., 133: 2973S-2977S.

-Batmanghelidj, Fereydoon. *Your Body's Many Cries for Water.* Global Health Solutions, Inc, 3rd Edition, 2008.

Chapter 3:

Klaper, Michael. *Vegan Nutrition.* HI: Gentle World INC, 4th edition, 1998.

Real Food Pyramid. *www.vegan-raw-diet.com.*

Food guide pyramid. *www.usda.gov.*

Kulvinskas, Viktoras. *Survival into the 21st Century.* IA: 21st Century Publications, 1975.

- Lairon D. Nutritional quality and safety of organic food. A review. *Agron Sustain Dev* 2009.

Rothkranz, Markus. *Heal Yourself 101*. Rothkranz Publishing, 1st Edition, 2011.
- Recker, R., "The Effect of Milk Supplements on Calcium Metabolism, Bone Metabolism, and Calcium Balance," American Journal of Clinical Nutrition, 41:254, 1985.
- Smith SR. A look at the low-carbohydrate diet. *N Engl J Med*. 2009;361(23):2286-2288
Kervran, C.L. *Biological Transmutations*. Happiness Press, 1989.
Graham, Douglas. *The 80/10/10 Diet*. Foodnsport Press, 2006.
Price, Weston A. *Nutrition and Physical Degeneration*. Price Pottenger Nutrition, 8th Edition, 2008.
Brook, Sapoty. *Eco-Eating*. Lothian Pub Co, 1997
Shelton, Herbert. *Food Combining Made Easy*. Ontario: Willow Publishing, 1982.
Harris, Robert S. *Nutritional Evaluation of Food Processing*. AVI Publishing Company, 1973.
- Asuman SUNGUROĞLU, et al. "Antiproliferative, Apoptotic And Antioxidant Activities Of Wheatgrass (Triticum Aestivum L.) Extract On CML (K562) Cell Line." *Turkish Journal Of Medical Sciences* 41.4 (2011): 657-663.
- Bilsborough S, Mann N. A review of issues of dietary protein intake in humans. Int J Sport Nutr Exerc Metab. 2006;16(2):129–152.   -Edmunds JW, Jayapalan S, DiMarco NM, Saboorian MH, Aukema HM. Creatine supplementation increases renal disease progression in Han:SPRD-cy rats. Am J Kidney Dis. 2001 Jan;37(1):73-78.
-Cousens, Gabriel. *Conscious Eating*. North Atlantic Books, 2nd Edition, 2000.
- Bolland MK, Grey A, Avenell A, Gamble GD, Reid IR. Calcium supplements with or without vitamin D and risk of cardiovascular events: reanalysis of the Women's Health Initiative limited access dataset and meta-analysis. *BMJ*. Published ahead of print April 19, 2011.

Chapter 4:
Price, Weston A. *Nutrition and Physical Degeneration*. Price Pottenger Nutrition, 8th Edition, 2008.
Graham, Douglas. *The 80/10/10 Diet*. Foodnsport Press, 2006.
Tuttle, Will. *The World Peace Diet*. Lantern Books, 2005.
Gandhi, Mahatma. *The Health Guide*. Crossing Press, 2004.
Robbins, John. *Diet for a New America*. HJ Kramer, 2nd Edition, 1998.
Horne, Ross. *Cancerproof Your Body*. Angus and Robertson, 1996.
Chopra, Deepak. *Perfect Weight*. Crown Publishing, 1996.
Cousens, Gabriel. *Conscious Eating*. North Atlantic Books, 2nd Edition, 2000.

Chapter 5:
Primack, Jeff. *Conquering Any Disease*. Press On QI Productions, 2011
Osho. *Being In Love*. Harmony, 2008.
McCabe, John. *Igniting Your Life*. Carmania Books, 2011
Horne, Ross. *Cancerproof Your Body*. Angus and Robertson, 1996.

- Tatsuya Kunisue, Zhen Chen, Germaine Buck Louis, Rajeshwari Sundaram, Mary Hediger, Liping Sun, and Kurunthachalam Kannan. Urinary Concentrations of Benzophenone-type UV Filters in US Women and Their Association with Endometriosis. Environmental Science & Technology

- Moan J, Porojnicu AC, Dahlback A, Setlow RB. Addressing the health benefits and risks, involving vitamin D or skin cancer, of increased sun exposure. Proc Natl Acad Sci USA. 2008;105:668–673.

Chapter 6:
Morse, Robert. *The Detox Miracle Sourcebook*. AZ: Kalindi Press, 2004.

Carrington, Hereward. *Vitality, Fasting and Nutrition*. General Books LLC, 2009.

Tilden, John. *Toxemia: The Basic Cause of Disease*. FL: Nat'l Health Assoc, 1974.

- Breslow NE, Enstrom JE. Geographic correlations between cancer mortality rates and alcohol-tobacco consumption in the United States. *J Natl Cancer Inst*. 1974;53:631-639.

- James Morris, George Stone. **Children and Psychotropic Medication: A Cautionary Note**. *Journal of Marital and Family Therapy*, 2009; DOI:

Chapter 7:

-Trall, R.T. *Water Cure for the Millions*. Russell Thacher Trall, 1860.

-Batmanghelidj, Fereydoon. *Your Body's Many Cries for Water*. Global Health Solutions, Inc, 3rd Edition, 2008.

-Mercola, Joseph. *Sweet Deception*. Nelson Books, 2006

-Blaylock, Russell. *Health and Nutrition Secrets*. Health Press NA Inc, Revised Edition, 2006.

-Jacka FN, Kremer PJ, Berk M, de Silva-Sanigorski AM, Moodie M, et al. (2011) A Prospective Study of Diet Quality and Mental Health in Adolescents. PLoS ONE 6(9): e24805.

-Lakhan SE, Vieira KF. Nutritional therapies for mental health disorders. Nutr J. 2008;7:2.

-Fournier JC, DeRubeis RJ, Hollon SD, Dimidjian S, Amsterdam JD, Shelton RC, et al. *Antidepressant drug effects and depression severity: a patient-level meta-analysis*. *JAMA 2010; 303: 47–53*.

-Robbins, John. *Diet for a New America*. HJ Kramer, 2nd Edition, 1998.

-Shutto Y, Shimada M, Kitajima M, Yamabe H, Razzaque MS. Lack of awareness among future medical professionals about the risk of consuming hidden phosphate-containing processed food and drinks. PLoS One. 2011;6(12):e29105.

-Oliveira A, Rodríguez-Artalejo F, Gaio R, Santos AC, Ramos E, Lopes C. Major habitual dietary patterns are associated with acute myocardial infarction and cardiovascular risk markers in a southern European population. J Am Diet Assoc. 2011 Feb;111(2):241-50.

- Charles S. Lieber, M.D., M.A.C.P. Relationships Between Nutrition, Alcohol Use, and Liver Disease. National Institute on Alcohol Abuse and Alcoholism

- Barr, L., Metaxas, G., Harbach, C. A. J., Savoy, L. A. and Darbre, P. D. (2012), Measurement of paraben concentrations in human breast tissue at serial locations across the breast from axilla to sternum. J. Appl. Toxicol., 32: 219–232.

-Gerson, Charlotte. *The Gerson Therapy*. Kensington Books, 2001.

- Lin SW, Wheeler DC, Park Y, Cahoon EK, Hollenbeck AR, Michal Freedman D, Abnet CC. Prospective study of ultraviolet radiation exposure and risk of cancer in the U.S. Int J Cancer. 2012 Apr 26. doi: 10.1002/ijc.27619.

Chapter 8:

Clement, Brian. *Hippocrates LifeForce*. Healthy Living Publications, 1st Edition, 2007.

- Ford ES, Bergmann MM, Kröger J, Schienkiewitz A, Weikert C, Boeing H. Healthy living is the best revenge: findings from the European Prospective Investigation Into Cancer and Nutrition-Potsdam study. Arch Intern Med. 2009;169(15):1355-1362.

Garner, Ron. *Conscious Health*. Beaufort Books, 2006.

Chapter 9:

-Price, Weston A. Nutrition and Physical Degeneration. Price Pottenger Nutrition, 8th Edition, 2008.

- Jiang R, Camargo CA Jr, Varraso R, Paik DC, Willett WC, Barr RG. Consumption of cured meats and prospective risk of chronic obstructive pulmonary disease in women. Am J Clin Nutr. 2008 Apr;87(4):1002-8.

- Varraso R, Jiang R, Barr RG, Willett WC, Camargo CA Jr. Prospective study of cured meats consumption and risk of chronic obstructive pulmonary disease in men. Am J Epidemiol. 2007 Dec 15;166(12):1438-45. Epub 2007 Sep 4.
- Jiang R, Paik DC, Hankinson JL, Barr RG. Cured meat consumption, lung function, and chronic obstructive pulmonary disease among United States adults. Am J Respir Crit Care Med. 2007 Apr 15;175(8):798-804. Epub 2007 Jan 25.
- Wahju Aniwidyaningsih, Raphaëlle Varraso, Noel Cano, and Christophe Pison. Impact of nutritional status on body functioning in chronic obstructive pulmonary disease and how to intervene. Curr Opin Clin Nutr Metab Care. 2008 July; 11(4): 435–442.
- Varraso R, Fung TT, Barr RG, et al. Prospective study of dietary patterns and chronic obstructive pulmonary disease among US women. Am J Clin Nutr. 2007;86:488–495.
- David J. Margolis, MD, PhD; Matthew Fanelli, MD; Eli Kupperman, BA; Maryte Papadopoulos, BA; Joshua P. Metlay, MD, PhD; Sharon Xiangwen Xie, PhD; Joseph DiRienzo, PhD; Paul H. Edelstein, MD. **Association of Pharyngitis With Oral Antibiotic Use for the Treatment of Acne.** *Arch Dermatol.* 2012;148(3):326-332.
- Adebamowo CA, Spiegelman D et al. High school dietary dairy intake and teenage acne. J Am Acad Dermatol. 2005 Feb;52(2):207-14.
- J.McFadden, J Collins,B Beaman, M Arthur, G Gitnick. Mycobacteria in Crohn's disease: DNA probes identify the wood pigeon strain of Mycobacterium avium and Mycobacterium paratuberculosis from human tissue. **Journal of Clinical Microbiology 1992;30(12):3070-3073**
- R W Sweeney, R H Whitlock, A E Rosenberger. Mycobacterium paratuberculosis cultured from milk and supramammary lymph nodes of infected asymptomatic cows. **Journal of Clinical Microbiology 1992;30(1):166-171**
- Nackmoon Sung and Michael T. Collins. Effect of Three Factors in Cheese Production (pH, Salt, and Heat) on *Mycobacterium avium* subsp. *paratuberculosis* Viability. Appl Environ Microbiol. 2000 April; 66(4): 1334–1339.
- D. Mishina, P. Katsel, S.T. Brown, E.C.A.M. Gilberts, R.J. Greenstein. On the Etiology of Crohn disease. Proceedings National Academy of Sciences USA, Vol 93, pp 9816-9820, September 1996.
- Romano C, Cucchiara S, Barabino A, Annese V, Sferlazzas C. Usefulness of omega-3 fatty acid supplementation in addition to mesalazine in maintaining remission in pediatric Crohn's disease: a double-blind, randomized, placebo-controlled study. World J Gastroenterol. 2005 Dec 7;11(45):7118-21.
- Malin M, Suomalainen H, Saxelin M, Isolauri E. Promotion of IgA immune response in patients with Crohn's disease by oral bacteriotherapy with Lactobacillus GG. Ann Nutr Metab. 1996;40(3):137-45.
- Ling PR, Boyce P, Bistrian BR. Role of arachidonic acid in the regulation of the inflammatory response in TNF-alpha-treated rats. JPEN J Parenter Enteral Nutr 1998;22:268–75.

Chapter 10:
Horne, Ross. *Cancerproof Your Body.* Angus and Robertson, 1996.
Clement, Brian. *Living Foods for Optimum Health.* Three rivers Press, 1998.
Rath, Matthias. *Why Animals Don't Get Heart Attacks, But People Do.* MR Publishing, 4th Edition, 2003.
Blaylock, Russell. *Health and Nutrition Secrets.* Health Press NA Inc, Revised Edition, 2006.

- Kanigel, Rachele. "It Raises Diabetes Risk And Robs Bone. It's Wrecking Our Teeth. And It's Making Us Fat. The Culprit? SODA." *Prevention* 58.10 (2006): 160-207. *Academic Search Premier*. Web. 21 Mar. 2012.

Robbins, John. *Diet for a New America*. HJ Kramer, 2nd Edition, 1998.

Brook, Sapoty. *Eco-Eating*. Lothian Pub Co, 1997

- Liu W, Huang XF, Qi Q, Dai QS, Yang L, Nie FF, Lu N, et al. Asparanin A induces G(2)/M cell cycle arrest and apoptosis in human hepatocellular carcinoma HepG2 cells. Biochem Biophys Res Commun. 2009 Apr 17;381(4):700-5.

- Asuman SUNGUROĞLU, et al. "Antiproliferative, Apoptotic And Antioxidant Activities Of Wheatgrass (Triticum Aestivum L.) Extract On CML (K562) Cell Line." *Turkish Journal Of Medical Sciences* 41.4 (2011): 657-663.

- Bachran C, Bachran S, Sutherland M, Bachran D, Fuchs H. Saponins in tumor therapy. Mini Rev Med Chem. 2008 Jun;8(6):575-84.

- Carroll KK, Braden LM, Bell JA, et al. "Fat and cancer." Cancer 58 (1986): 1818-1825.

-Dong JY, He K, Wang P, et al. Dietary fiber intake and risk of breast cancer: a meta-analysis of prospective cohort studies. Am J Clin Nutr 2011.

-Zhang M, Huang J, Xie X, et al. Dietary intakes of mushrooms and green tea combine to reduce the risk of breast cancer in Chinese women. Int J Cancer 2009;124:1404-1408.

-Thompson LU, Chen JM, Li T, et al. Dietary flaxseed alters tumor biological markers in postmenopausal breast cancer. Clin Cancer Res 2005;11:3828-3835.

- Bonkhoff H, Fixemer T, Hunsicker I, Remberger K. Progesterone receptor expression in human prostate cancer: correlation with tumor progression. Prostate. 2001 Sep 15;48(4):285-91.

- Fradet Y, Meyer F, Bairati I, Shadmani R. Dietary fat and prostate cancer progression and survival. Eur Urol. 1999;388:391.

- Chan JM, Stampfer MJ, Ma J, Ajani U, Gaziano JM, Giovannucci E. Dairy products, calcium, and prostate cancer risk in the Physicians' Health Study. Presentation, American Association for Cancer Research, San Francisco, April 2000.

-Enos WF, Holmes RH, Beyer J. Coronary disease among United States soldiers killed in action in Korea: preliminary report. *J Am Med Assoc* 1953;152:1090–3.

- Yang SY, Zhang HJ, Sun SY, et al. Relationship of carotid intima-media thickness and duration of vegetarian diet in Chinese male vegetarians. Nutr Metab. 2011;8:63.

-Jean A. Welsh, MPH, RN, Andrea Sharma, PhD, MPH, Jerome L. Abramson, PhD, Viola Vaccarino, MD, PhD, Cathleen Gillespie, MS, Miriam B. Vos, MD, MSPH. Caloric Sweetener Consumption and Dyslipidemia Among US Adults. *JAMA*. 2010;303(15):1490-1497

- Breslau NA, Brinkley L, Hill KD, Pak CYC. Relationship of animal protein-rich diet to kidney stone formation and calcium metabolism. *J Clin Endocrinol*. 1988;66:140-146.

- Remer T, Manz F. Estimation of the renal net acid excretion by adults consuming diets containing variable amounts of protein. *Am J Clin Nutr*. 1994;59:1356-1361.

- Feskanich D, Willett WC, Stampfer MJ, Colditz GA. Milk, dietary calcium, and bone fractures in women: a 12-year prospective study. American Journal of Public Health. 1997

- Case-Control Study of Risk Factors for Hip Fractures in the Elderly. American Journal of Epidemiology. Vol. 139, No. 5, 1994

- S. Soriano et al. Rapid insulinotropic action of low doses of bisphenol-A on mouse and human islets of Langerhans: Role of estrogen receptor ß. PLoS ONE, Vol. 7, February 8, 2012, p. e31109.

- Thomas L Halton, Walter C Willett, Simin Liu, JoAnn E Manson, Meir J Stampfer, and Frank B Hu· Potato and french fry consumption and risk of type 2 diabetes in women. American Journal of Clinical Nutrition, Vol. 83, No. 2, 284-290, February 2000

-Tuomilehto J, Lindstrom J, Eriksson JG, Valle TT,Hämäläinen H, Ilanne-Parikka P, Keinänen-Kiukaanniemi S,Laakso M, Louheranta A, Rastas M, Salminen V, Uusitupa M,Finnish Diabetes Prevention Study Group. Prevention of type 2diabetes mellitus by changes in lifestyle among subjects withimpaired glucose tolerance. *N Engl J Med* 2001; **344**: 1343–1350.

- Knowler WC, Barrett-Connor E, Fowler SE, Hamman RF,Lachin JM,Walker EA, Nathan DM, Diabetes Prevention ProgramResearch Group. Reduction in the incidence of type 2 diabeteswith lifestyle intervention or metformin. *N Engl J Med* 2002; **346**: 393–403.

- Fretts AM, Howard BV, McKnight B, et al. Associations of processed meat and unprocessed red meat intake with incident diabetes: the Strong Heart Family Study. *Am J Clin Nutr.* Published ahead of print Jan 25, 2012.

- Barnard RJ, Lattimore L, Holly RG, Cherny S, Pritikin N. Response of non-insulindependent diabetic patients to an intensive program of diet and exercise. *Diabetes Care.* 1982;5(4):370-374.

- Tonstad S, Steward K, Oda K, Batech M, Herring RP, Fraser GE. Vegetarian diets and incidence of diabetes in the Adventist Health Study-2 among individuals following therapeutic diets for type 2 diabetes. J Nutr. 2011;141:1469-1474.

- Siepmann T, Roofeh J, Kiefer FW, Edelson DG. Hypogonadism and erectile dysfunction associated with soy product consumption. Nutrition. 2011 Jul-Aug;27(7-8):859-62.

-Dong JY, Zhang YH, Qin LQ. Erectile dysfunction and risk of cardiovascular disease: meta-analysis of prospective cohort studies. J Am Coll Cardiol. 2011 Sep 20;58(13):1378-85.

-Beezhold BL, Johnston CS, Daigle DR. Vegetarian diets are associated with healthy mood states: a cross-sectional study in Seventh Day Adventist adults. *Nutr J.* 2010;9:26.

- Shaheen E Lakhan, Karen F Vieira. Nutritional and herbal supplements for anxiety and anxiety-related disorders: systematic review. Nutr J. 2010; 9: 42.

- Bourne,E.J.,(1995) 'The Anxiety and Phobia Workbook, p.333 -337 passim.

- Shi Z, Hu X, He K, Yuan B, Garg M. Joint association of magnesium and iron intake with anemia among Chinese adults. Nutrition. 2008 Oct;24(10):977-84

- Soma Mukhopadhyay, Phd, Ashis Mukhopadhyay, MD, Pinaki Ranjan Gupta, MBBS, Manoj Kar, Phd, and Arpita Ghosh, MS. The Role of Iron Chelation Activity of Wheat Grass Juice in Blood Transfusion Requirement of Intermediate Thalassaemia. Blood (ASH Annual Meeting Abstracts) 2007 110: Abstract 3829

- Morris MC, Evans DA, Bienias JL et al. Dietary fats and the risk of incident Alzheimer disease. *Arch Neurol.* 2003;60:194-200.

- Giem P, Beeson WL, Fraser GE. The incidence of dementia and intake of animal products: preliminary findings from the adventist health study. *Neuroepidemiology.* 1993;12:28-36.

- Dawson R, Simpkins JW, Wallace DR. Age and dose-dependent effects of neonatal monosodium glutamate (MSG) administration to female rats. Neurotox Teratol 1989;11:331-337.

- Dawson R. Acute and long lasting neurochemical effects of monosodium glutamate administration to mice. Neuropharmacology 1983;22:1417-1419

328

- Mattson MP, Cheng B, Davis D, Bryant K, Lieberburg I, Rydel RE. *β-Amyloid peptides destabilize calcium homeostasis and render human cortical neurons vulnerable to excitoxicity.* J Neurosci 12: 376–389, 1992.
- The 9th International Conference on Alzheimer's Disease and Related Disorders in Philadelphia, July 17-22, 2004. Jae Kang P2-283. Fruit and Vegetable Consumption and Cognitive Decline in Women (Mon., 7/19, 12:30 p.m.)
- Elaine W.-T. Chong, MD, PhD, MEpi; Luibov D. Robman, PhD; Julie A. Simpson, PhD; Allison M. Hodge, PhD; Khin Zaw Aung, MD; Theresa K. Dolphin, BAppSci, Dallas R. English, PhD; Graham G. Giles, PhD; Robyn H. Guymer, MD, PhD. Fat Consumption and Its Association With Age-Related Macular Degeneration. Arch Ophthalmol. 2009;127(5):674-680
- "Journal of Agricultural and Food Chemistry": Phytosterol Composition of Nuts and Seeds Commonly Consumed in the U.S.
- *Elaine W.-T. Chong, Julie A. Simpson, Luibov D. Robman, Allison M. Hodge, Khin Zaw Aung, Dallas R. English, Graham G. Giles, Robyn H. Guymer. Red Meat and Chicken Consumption and Its Association With Age-related Macular Degeneration.* Am. J. Epidemiol. *(2009) 169 (7): 867-876.*
- Appleby PN, Allen NK, Key TJ. Diet, vegetarianism, and cataract risk. *Am J Clin Nutr.* Published ahead of print March 23, 2011.
- Kahn A, Mozin MJ, Rebuffat E, Sottiaux M, Muller MF. Milk intolerance in children with persistent sleeplessness: a prospective double-blind crossover evaluation. Pediatrics. 1989 Oct;84(4):595-603.
- Haensch, Carl-Albrecht. Cerebrospinal Fluid Magnesium Level in Different Neurological Disorders. Neuroscience & Medicine, 2010, 1, 60-63
- Food Matters. Documentary, 2009
- Cousens, Gabriel. *Conscious Eating.* North Atlantic Books, 2nd Edition, 2000.
- Bieler, Henry. *Food Is your Best Medicine.* Ballantine Books, 1987.
- Walker, Norman A. *Become Younger.* AZ: Norwalk Press, 2nd Edition, 1995.
- Robert F. Grimble. The Effects of Sulfur Amino Acid Intake on Immune Function in Humans. *J. Nutr.* June 1, 2006 vol. 136 no. 6 1660S-1665S
- Schaeffer DJ, Krylov VS. Anti-HIV activity of extracts and compounds from algae and cyanobacteria. Ecotoxicol Environ Saf. 2000 Mar;45(3):208-27.
- Coulter, Harris. *AIDS, Syphilis and the Hidden Link.* North Atlantic Books, 1996.
- Batmanghelidj, Fereydoon. *Your Body's Many Cries for Water.* Global Health Solutions, Inc, 3rd Edition, 2008.
- Ellison, Bryan. *Why We Will Never Win the War on AIDS.* Inside Story Communications.
- Barefoot, Robert, *Death by Diet.* Deonna Enterprises, 2002.
- Ehret, Arnold. *Mucusless Diet Healing System.* Benedict Lust Publications, Inc., 2001.
- Josling P. Preventing the common cold with a garlic supplement: a double-blind, placebo-controlled survey. Adv Ther. 2001 Jul-Aug;18(4):189-93.
- CHUTER, ROBYN. "Early Stage Prostate Cancer." *Natural Health & Vegetarian Life* (2010): 48-50.
- Berger, Stuart. *The Immune Power Diet.* Dutton Adult, 1st Edition, 1985.
- Jensen, Bernard. *Guide to Diet and Detoxification.* McGraw-Hill, 2000.
- Price, Weston A. *Nutrition and Physical Degeneration.* Price Pottenger Nutrition, 8th Edition, 2008.
- Wigmore, Ann. *The Hippocrates Diet and Health Program.* NJ: Avery Penguin Putnam, 1984.

- Tunev SS, Hastey CJ, Hodzic E, Feng S, Barthold SW, et al. (2011) Lymphoadenopathy during Lyme Borreliosis Is Caused by Spirochete Migration-Induced Specific B Cell Activation. PLoS Pathog 7(5): e1002066.
- Primack, Jeff. *Conquering Any Disease.* Press On QI Productions, 2011
- Kulvinskas, Viktoras. *Survival into the 21st Century.* IA: 21st Century Publications, 1975.
- Wolters M. Diet and psoriasis: experimental data and clinical evidence. Br J Dermatol. 2005 Oct;153(4):706-14.
- Abrar A. Qureshi, MD, MPH; Patrick L. Dominguez, MD; Hyon K. Choi, MD, DrPH; Jiali Han, PhD; Gary Curhan, MD, ScD. Alcohol Intake and Risk of Incident Psoriasis in US Women. *Arch Dermatol.* 2010;146(12):1364-1369.
- British Journal of Dermatology, Volume 142, Number 1, January 2000, pp. 44-51(8)
- Zackheim HS, Farber EM. Low-protein diet and psoriasis. A hospital study. Arch Dermatol. 1969 May;99(5):580–586.
- Businco L, Businco E, Cantani A, Galli E, Infussi R, Benincori N. Results of a milk and/or egg free diet in children with atopic dermatitis. Allergol Immunopathol (Madr). 1982 Jul-Aug;10(4):283-8.
- Taussig SJ, Batkin S. Bromelain, the enzyme complex of pineapple (Ananas comosus) and its clinical application. An update. J Ethnopharmacol. 1988 Feb-Mar;22(2):191-203.
- Abrar A. Qureshi, M.D., assistant professor of dermatology, Harvard Medical School, Boston; Joel M. Gelfand, M.D., medical director, department of dermatology clinical studies unit, University of Pennsylvania, Philadelphia; January 2012, American Journal of Epidemiology
- Arthritis Care Res 2007;57:1439-1445 [Data Source: 2001–2004 National Ambulatory Medical Care Survey and 2001–2004 National Hospital Ambulatory Medical Care Survey]
- Arthritis & Rheumatism 2006;54(1):226-229 [Data Source: 2003 NHIS]
- McDougall J, Bruce B, Spiller G, Westerdahl J, McDougall M. Effects of a very low-fat, vegan diet in subjects with rheumatoid arthritis. *J Altern Complement Med.* 2002;8(1):71-75.
- Hanninen, Kaartinen K, Rauma AL, Nenonen M, Torronen R, Hakkinen AS, Adlercreutz H, Laakso J. Antioxidants in vegan diet and rheumatic disorders. *Toxicology.* 2000;155(1-3):45-53.
- Riedl MA, Saxon A, Diaz-Sanchez D. Oral sulforaphane increases Phase II antioxidant enzymes in the human upper airway. Clin Immunol. 2009;130:244-251.
- Mirjam Kool, Monique A.M. Willart, Menno van Nimwegen, Ingrid Bergen, Philippe Pouliot, J. Christian Virchow, Neil Rogers, Fabiola Osorio, Caetano Reis e Sousa, Hamida Hammad, Bart N. Lambrecht . An Unexpected Role for Uric Acid as an Inducer of T Helper 2 Cell Immunity to Inhaled Antigens and Inflammatory Mediator of Allergic Asthma. Immunity. 22 April 2011; Vol. 34, Issue 4, pp. 527-540.
- Maslova E, Halldorsson TI, Stom M, Olsen SF. Low-fat yoghurt intake in pregnancy associated with increased child asthma and allergic rhinitis risk: a prospective cohort study. Poster presented as part of the European Respiratory Society's Annual Congress, Amsterdam, Netherlands, 25 September 2011.
- Crowe FL, Appleby PN, Allen NE, Key TJ. Diet and risk of diverticular disease in Oxford cohort of European Prospective Investigation into Cancer and Nutrition (EPIC): prospective study of British vegetarians and non-vegetarians. BMJ. 2011 Jul 19;343:d4131.

- Cao J, Zhao Y, Liu J, et al. Brick tea fluoride as a main source of adult fluorosis. Food Chem Toxicol. 2003;41(4):535-542.
- Cao J, Luo SF, Liu JW, Li YH. Safety evaluation on fluoride content in black tea. Food Chemistry. 2004;88(2):233-236.
- Ostrom GS. Cryolite on grapes/Fluoride in wines - A guide for growers and vintners to determine optimum cryolite applications on grapevines. CATI Publication #960601.
- National Research Council. 2006. *Fluoride in Drinking Water: A Scientific Review of EPA's Standards*. National Academies Press: Washington, DC. 507 pp.
- P Allain, S Berre, N Krari, P Laine, N Barbot, V Rohmer, and J C Bigorgne. Bromine and thyroid hormone activity. J Clin Pathol. 1993 May; 46(5): 456–458.
- Schwarz S, Leweling H. Multiple sclerosis and nutrition. *Mult Scler*. 2005;11:24–32.
- Minderhoud JM, Mooyaart EL, Kamman RL, Teelken AW, Hoogstraten MC, Vencken LM, Gravenmade EJ, van den Burg W. In vivo phosphorus magnetic resonance spectroscopy in multiple sclerosis. Arch Neurol. 1992 Feb;49(2):161-5.
- McDougall, John, M.D. Treating Multiple Sclerosis with Diet: Fact or Fraud?. Vegetarian Times.
- Moe SM, Zidehsarai MP, Chambers MA, et al. Vegetarian compared with meat dietary protein source and phosphorus homeostasis in chronic kidney disease. *Clin J Am Soc Nephrol*. 2011;6:257-264.
- Daniel CR, Cross AJ, Graubard BI, et al. Large prospective investigation of meat intake, related mutagens, and risk of renal cell carcinoma. *Am J Clin Nutr*. 2012;1:155-162.

Chapter 11:
Price, Weston A. *Nutrition and Physical Degeneration*. Price Pottenger Nutrition, 8th Edition, 2008.
Schweiss, Alexander. *Diet, Crime and Delinquency*. Life Sciences PR, 1981

Chapter 12:
Klaper, Michael. *Vegan Nutrition*. HI: Gentle World INC, 4th edition, 1998.

Chapter 13:
Clement, Brian. *Hippocrates LifeForce*. Healthy Living Publications, 1st Edition, 2007.
-Vegetarian diets and childhood obesity prevention *Am J Clin Nutr 2010 91: 1525S-1529S*
- de Gonzalez AB, Hartge P, Cerhan JR, et al. Body mass index and mortality among 1.46 million white adults. *N Engl J Med*. 2010;363:2211-2219.
Calabrese, Karyn. *Soak Your Nuts*. Healthy Living Publications, 2011
Gerson, Charlotte. *The Gerson Therapy*. Kensington Books, 2001.

Chapter 15:
Bieler, Henry. *Food Is your Best Medicine*. Ballantine Books, 1987.

331

INDEX

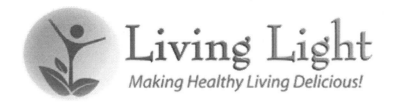

Living Light
Making Healthy Living Delicious!

LIVING LIGHT CULINARY INSTITUTE is the world's leading gourmet raw vegan chef school. Located on the beautiful Mendocino coast of northern California, it was founded in 1997 by Cherie Soria, who is known as "The mother of gourmet raw vegan cuisine." Her graduates are a virtual who's who in the world of raw foods.

People from over 50 countries have attended the Institute to study raw vegan culinary arts and the science of raw food nutrition to become certified chefs, nutritional consultants, instructors, and recipe book authors. Many of the raw restaurants around the world are owned by graduates of Living Light.

To subscribe to the Living Light newsletter, access their site, RawFoodChef.com. Scroll down and enter your email address in the "subscribe" box.

Besides Living Light Culinary Arts Institute, Cherie and her husband, Dan Laderman, own and operate several other eco-friendly, raw vegan businesses.

The Living Light Café and Living Light Marketplace share the same building as the Institute. The Marketplace also has an online store providing gifts for chefs and products for healthful living. (Access: RawFoodChef.com/store/marketplace). The historic Living Light Inn is located nearby in a restored mansion.

Cherie and Dan have received numerous awards and accolades for Living Light International, which is recognized as one of the leading raw food businesses in the world.

ARISE

Some people are their own life architects. Others are their own demolition crew. Which one are you?

Each person is a power source and tool. Each body is generating energy that is manifested in its thoughts, actions, words, relationships, and results.

By plugging into your potential, using your talents and skills, guiding your thought processes, and actively choosing what to do with your energy and time, you can fuel a life that you want to lead. Or, like many people, you can do none of it, and end up in a life that you may not care to have as you are surrounded by the disaster you helped to create while you point blame at other people.

"Some men see things as they are and say, 'Why?' I dream of things that never were, and say, 'Why not?'" – George Bernard Shaw

Don't settle into being an excuse-maker who continually dismisses any possibility of getting out of the life they are leading, and negates those around them who are driven to make a difference. You know you are in that mind space if, whenever you are presented with opportunities, you easily and even habitually spew excuses and drone on about why things cannot be a more satisfying possibility - when you would be better off formulating solutions and working toward them as an active, driven participant in creating a better life for yourself and those around you.

Lead your way into the solution. Believe in your self. Use your talents, skills, intellect, power, time, and resources to formulate the answers and situations you wish to see.

There are dreamers who make their dreams come true and remain engaged in creating the life they want. And there are the dwellers of the dull and mundane, those who do not rise up, who get stuck in the rut of repetitive conformity to a deadened society of manufactured thoughts and manufactured foods and manufactured lifestyles that replicate commercial imagery produced by greed-driven corporations dictating an unsustainable, chemically-saturated way of living based on purchasing products by those corporations.

Are you among those who gave up on their talents and skills, who gave up on ever leading the life you wish to have, who feed on deadened, chemically-saturated foods manufactured by greed-driven corporations while continually filling your mind with commercial imagery and what is broadcast out of the tell-a-vision?

One clue as to how much you are ingrained in commercialized society, or are working to stay out of it, is on your plate. How much of it is processed corporate food, and how much of it is organic, non-GMO, locally grown fruits and vegetables? Do you grow some of your own food and support regional organic farmers? Or, like most people these days, are you totally reliant on stores and restaurants for your food?

It is always time to latch onto your own vision, to fuel yourself with plant foods free of corporate chemicals and processing, to get daily exercise, and to set and work toward specific goals.

If you had a sad or unsatisfactory past, and want a happy future, choose not to dwell in the past. Decide for yourself that you will not be a walking wound. Look forward, not backward. Be constantly involved in creating a better future.

If Leonardo Da Vinci had never envisioned and painted his amazing works, they would not exist. If you do not envision and work toward the amazing life you wish to have, it will never exist.

It is up to you.

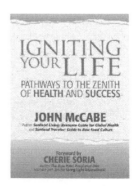

Arise.

– John McCabe, Igniting Your Life

MEET ANDREA COX

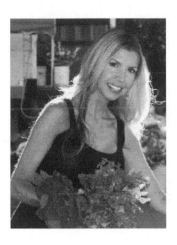

"After almost losing my life, and more importantly my zest for life, on a high protein diet as a pin-up girl and fitness model, I knew I needed a change. By incorporating juice fasting, water fasting, sweating, and raw living foods in my life, I found that change I desired. I cannot tell you how many times I see it over and over again, women and men just want to be able to get back to their 'happy place' and maintain a stable weight. With the simple practices I teach through my daily You tube videos, Digital Detox program, and cleansing retreats, people can and do achieve these goals. More importantly, they get to that 'happy place!'"

"Jesse J. Jacoby's book, 'The Raw Cure,' uses the same principles and practices that I use at my cleansing retreats. This book is filled with a plethora of factual knowledge that anyone can use. Get ready folks, and let the peeling of the onion begin. Your beauty will come shining through as each layer is peeled away.

Bravo to you, Jesse J. Jacoby, for shining your light!"

Learn more about Andrea by accessing these sites:

www.alkalizewithandrea.com
www.healthyhaven.net
www.youtube.com/user/TheHealthyHavennet1?feature=mhee

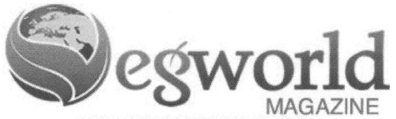

MAGAZINE
THE EVOLUTION OF VEGGIE LIVING

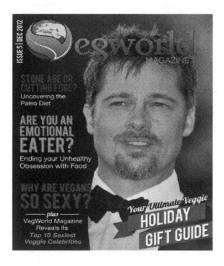

VegWorld Magazine is the world's first digital vegetarian magazine to connect you to the leaders, authors, and luminaries in veggie living.

Each issue is packed with mouthwatering recipe videos, entertaining audio interviews with guest celebrities, and vital information on natural health from the world's top medical doctors.

Visit *vegworldmag.com* to subscribe and access the digital publication that has been voted the number one health app in the *Itunes* store.

Printed in Great Britain
by Amazon

32978611R00199